Gluteal Augmentation

Editors

ROBERT F. CENTENO
CONSTANTINO G. MENDIETA

CLINICS IN PLASTIC SURGERY

www.plasticsurgery.theclinics.com

April 2018 • Volume 45 • Number 2

ELSEVIER

1600 John F. Kennedy Boulevard • Suite 1800 • Philadelphia, Pennsylvania, 19103-2899

http://www.theclinics.com

CLINICS IN PLASTIC SURGERY Volume 45, Number 2
April 2018 ISSN 0094-1298, ISBN-13: 978-0-323-58322-0

Editor: Jessica McCool
Developmental Editor: Meredith Madeira

Clinics in Plastic Surgery (ISSN 0094-1298) is published quarterly by Elsevier Inc., 360 Park Avenue South, New York, NY 10010-1710. Months of issue are January, April, July, and October. Business and Editorial Offices: 1600 John F. Kennedy Blvd., Suite 1800, Philadelphia, PA 19103-2899. Periodicals postage paid at New York, NY and additional mailing offices. Subscription prices are $525.00 per year for US individuals, $882.00 per year for US institutions, $100.00 per year for US students and residents, $595.00 per year for Canadian individuals, $1050.00 per year for Canadian institutions, $636.00 per year for international individuals, $1050.00 per year for international institutions, and $305.00 per year for Canadian and international students/residents. To receive student/resident rate, orders must be accompanied by name of affiliated institution, date of term, and the *signature* of program/residency coordinator on institution letterhead. Orders will be billed at individual rate until proof of status is received. Foreign air speed delivery is included in all *Clinics* subscription prices. All prices are subject to change without notice. **POSTMASTER:** Send address changes to *Clinics in Plastic Surgery*, Elsevier Health Sciences Division, Subscription Customer Service, 3251 Riverport Lane, Maryland Heights, MO 63043. **Customer Service: 1-800-654-2452 (US and Canada). From outside of the United States and Canada, call 314-447-8871. Fax: 314-447-8029. E-mail: JournalsCustomerService-usa@elsevier.com (for print support); JournalsOnlineSupport-usa@elsevier.com (for online support).**

Reprints. For copies of 100 or more of articles in this publication, please contact the Commercial Reprints Department, Elsevier Inc., 360 Park Avenue South, New York, New York 10010-1710. Tel.: +1-212-633-3874; Fax: +1-212-633-3820; E-mail: reprints@elsevier.com.

Clinics in Plastic Surgery is covered in *Current Contents, EMBASE/Excerpta Medica, Science Citation Index, MEDLINE/PubMed (Index Medicus), ASCA, and ISI/BIOMED.*

Contributors

EDITORS

ROBERT F. CENTENO, MD, MBA, FACS
Diplomate, American Board of Plastic Surgery, Adjunct Assistant Clinical Professor, Department of Plastic Surgery, The Ohio State University, Private Practice, Columbus Institute of Plastic Surgery, Columbus, Ohio, USA

CONSTANTINO G. MENDIETA, MD, FACS, FICS
Diplomate, American Board of Plastic Surgery, Private Practice, Miami, Florida, USA

AUTHORS

GUILLERMO ERNESTO ALVARENGA, MD
Aesthetic Surgery Fellow, Plastic Surgery Institute, Hospital Ángeles Lomas, Mexico City, Mexico

LÁZARO CÁRDENAS-CAMARENA, MD
Plastic Surgeon, International Society of Aesthetic Plastic Surgery (ISAPS), Iberolatinoamerican Plastic Surgery Federation (FILACP), Mexican Association of Plastic Esthetic and Reconstructive Surgery (AMCPER), American Society of Plastic Surgeons (ASPS)

ROBERT F. CENTENO, MD, MBA, FACS
Diplomate, American Board of Plastic Surgery, Adjunct Assistant Clinical Professor, Department of Plastic Surgery, The Ohio State University, Private Practice, Columbus Institute of Plastic Surgery, Columbus, Ohio, USA

JOHN C. CRANTFORD, MD
Fellow, Hunstad Kortesis Bharti Plastic Surgery & MedSpa, Huntersville, North Carolina, USA

MARK A. DANIELS, MD
Fellow, Hunstad Kortesis Bharti Plastic Surgery & MedSpa, Huntersville, North Carolina, USA

JOSE ABEL DE LA PEÑA SALCEDO, MD, FACS
Director, Plastic Surgery Institute, Hospital Ángeles Lomas, Mexico City, Mexico

HÉCTOR DURÁN, MD
Plastic Surgeon, International Society of Aesthetic Plastic Surgery (ISAPS), Iberolatinoamerican Plastic Surgery Federation (FILACP), Mexican Association of Plastic Esthetic and Reconstructive Surgery (AMCPER), American Society of Plastic Surgeons (ASPS)

OSMAN ERHAN ERYILMAZ, MD
Estetik Istanbul, Istanbul, Turkey

GUILLERMO J. GALLARDO, MD
Plastic Surgeon, Plastic Surgery Institute, Hospital Ángeles Lomas, Mexico City, Mexico

ASHKAN GHAVAMI, MD
Assistant Clinical Professor, Department of Surgery, Division of Plastic and Reconstructive Surgery, David Geffen School of Medicine at UCLA, Los Angeles, California, USA; Private Practice, Ghavami Plastic Surgery, Beverly Hills, California, USA

PAULO MIRANDA GODOY, MD
Hospital Moriah, São Paulo, São Paulo, Brazil

RAUL GONZALEZ, MD
Assistant Professor of UNAERP Medicine School, Head, Clinica Raul Gonzalez, Ribeirao Preto, São Paulo, Brazil

RICARDO GONZALEZ, MD
Clinica Raul Gonzalez, Ribeirao Preto, São Paulo, Brazil

JORGE E. HIDALGO, MD
Faculty of Medicine, Post Graduate Professor, University San Martin de Porres, Lima, Peru

JOSEPH P. HUNSTAD, MD, FACS
Founder, Plastic Surgeon, Hunstad Kortesis Bharti Plastic Surgery & MedSpa, Huntersville, North Carolina, USA

CONSTANTINO G. MENDIETA, MD, FACS, FICS
Diplomate, American Board of Plastic Surgery, Private Practice, Miami, Florida, USA

ALEXANDRE MENDONÇA MUNHOZ, MD, PhD
Hospital Moriah, Hospital Sírio-Libanês, Cancer Institute of São Paulo, University of São Paulo, Plastic Surgery Division, University of São Paulo School of Medicine, São Paulo, São Paulo, Brazil

DOUGLAS M. SENDEROFF, MD, FACS
Mount Sinai Beth Israel Medical Center, New York, New York, USA

BIVIK SHAH, MD
Private Practice, Columbus Institute of Plastic Surgery, Assistant Clinical Professor, The Ohio State University, Columbus, Ohio, USA

ADITYA SOOD, MD, MBA
Aesthetic Surgery Fellow, Columbus Institute of Plastic Surgery, Department of Plastic Surgery, The Ohio State University Wexner Medical Center, Columbus, Ohio, USA

SADRI OZAN SOZER, MD
El Paso Cosmetic Surgery, El Paso, Texas, USA

NATHANIEL L. VILLANUEVA, MD
Department of Plastic Surgery, The University of Texas Southwestern Medical Center, Dallas, Texas, USA

VERNON LEROY YOUNG, MD
Director, Mercy Clinic Research Institute, Washington, Missouri, USA

Contents

Improvement of the Gluteal Contour: Modern Concepts with Systematized Lipoinjection **237**

Lázaro Cárdenas-Camarena and Héctor Durán

Buttock enlargement with lipoinjection is a procedure that has had a very high demand in the last 5 years. Changes in aesthetics have made more patients request greater volume in their buttocks and hips. The procedure requires not only liposuction, in which the fat is obtained, but also a systematization of the fat injection process in the buttock to obtain the appropriate aesthetic results according to the characteristics of each patient. The procedure achieves very satisfactory results because it can transform the patient's physical appearance significantly.

Gluteal Augmentation and Contouring with Autologous Fat Transfer: Part I **249**

Ashkan Ghavami and Nathaniel L. Villanueva

Video content accompanies this article at http://www.plasticsurgery.theclinics.com/.

Gluteal augmentation with autologous fat transfer is an increasingly popular procedure that has the ability to transform a patient's entire body silhouette and gluteal appearance. Proper patient selection, preoperative evaluation, and planning are critical to the success of the procedure. Using the preoperative planning, surgical technique, and postoperative care described, the procedure can be performed safely with powerful and consistent results and avoidance of complications associated with gluteal fat transfer.

Autologous Flap Gluteal Augmentation: Purse-String Technique **261**

Joseph P. Hunstad, Mark A. Daniels, and John C. Crantford

The ideal patient for purse-string gluteoplasty has buttock deflation and ptosis and wishes to improve projection. Key elements of the procedure are buttock lifting combined with autoaugmentation, no undermining of autoaugmentation tissue, and use of a purse-string suture to enhance projection of autoaugmentation tissue. Purse-string gluteoplasty is a safe and effective technique to correct buttock ptosis and atrophy.

Autologous Flap Gluteal Augmentation: Split Gluteal Flap Technique **269**

Sadri Ozan Sozer and Osman Erhan Eryilmaz

Video content accompanies this article at http://www.plasticsurgery.theclinics.com/.

Postbariatric, cosmetic, and circumferential body lift patients seek to avoid a flattened buttock contour. Gluteal implants have been described with various rates of complications and difficulties. Lipografting moderately increases buttock volume; neither procedure directly addresses ptosis. The procedure described in this article addresses the volume deficit and ptosis. Most adipocutaneous flaps originate within the superior gluteal region and maintain volume in the top half of the buttocks, lacking the ability to reach the midportion of the buttocks. The ideal flap should be versatile, result in a superior gluteal concavity, and give the maximum projection at the midlevel of the buttocks.

Autologous Gluteal Augmentation with the Moustache Transposition Flap Technique **277**

Robert F. Centeno

Video content accompanies this article at http://www.plasticsurgery.theclinics.com/.

Patients with massive weight loss and aesthetic patients can present with significant gluteal contour abnormalities. Gluteal ptosis, skeletal deformities, severe platypgia, and a paucity of donor fat for autologous transfer are common problems. Excisional procedures are used to treat massive-weight-loss contour abnormalities. These procedures present an opportunity to address severe gluteal deformities using autologous tissue augmentation. With a working knowledge of the relevant anatomy, sound surgical technique, and meticulous postoperative care, autologous gluteal autoaugmentation with circumferential body lift/excisional buttock lift using the "Moustache" flap technique will enhance massive weight loss body contouring outcomes and improve patient satisfaction.

CLINICS IN PLASTIC SURGERY

FORTHCOMING ISSUES

July 2018
Gender Confirmation Surgery
Loren Schechter and Bauback Safa, *Editors*

October 2018
Lower Facial Rejuvenation: A Multispecialty Approach
Shai Rozen and Lisa Ishii, *Editors*

January 2019
Plastic Surgery After Weight Loss
Jeffrey A. Gusenoff, *Editor*

RECENT ISSUES

January 2018
Contemporary Indications in Breast Reconstruction
Jian Farhadi, Stefan O.P. Hofer, and Jaume Masia, *Editors*

October 2017
Burn Care: Rehabilitation, Reconstruction, and Recovery
Charles Scott Hultman and Michael W. Neumeister, *Editors*

July 2017
Burn Care: Rescue, Resuscitation, and Resurfacing
Charles Scott Hultman and Michael W. Neumeister, *Editors*

ISSUE OF RELATED INTEREST

Dermatologic Clinics, Volume 36, Issue 1 (January 2018)
Cosmetic Dermatology for Men
Neil S. Sadick, *Editor*

Preface

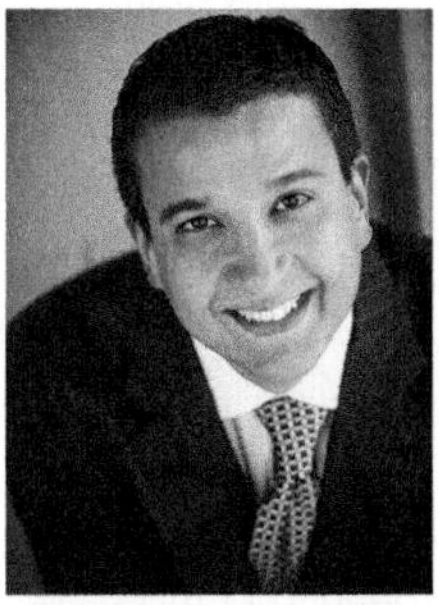
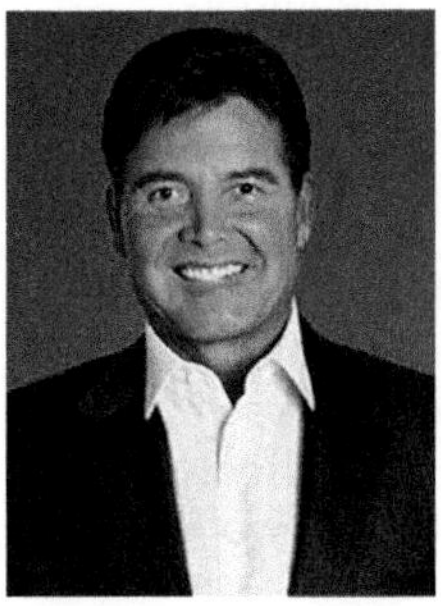

Robert F. Centeno, MD, MBA, FACS Constantino G. Mendieta, MD, FACS, FICS
Editors

A decade ago, the publication of the *Clinics in Plastic Surgery* "Gluteal Augmentation" issue, edited by V. Leroy Young, MD and Thomas Roberts, MD, helped to usher in a new era for this heretofore uncommonly performed procedure. The publication and US-based teaching courses helped gluteal augmentation to become part of the mainstream of plastic surgery procedures in the United States and solidified its place abroad. Our esteemed colleagues in Central and South America as well as US-based plastic surgeons valiantly took up the charge to not only improve upon the work of early pioneers but also bring a more rigorous approach to delivering consistent and safe outcomes to our patients.

During the ensuing time, the aesthetic surgery patients' demand for gluteal augmentation procedures here in the United States has eclipsed anything that we could have predicted. In 2017, gluteal augmentation was the fastest growing procedure in aesthetic surgery. By necessity, this procedure has become part of the armamentarium of virtually all plastic surgeons today. Demographic changes, media awareness, and "pop" culture influencers will likely ensure that gluteal augmentation remains a regularly requested procedure in the future.

While significant progress has been made, due to anatomical and device associated limitations, gluteal augmentation remains a technically demanding procedure. A thorough knowledge of all the available techniques, clinical anatomy, and management strategies is critical to successful outcomes and high patient satisfaction. Recently published mortality data associated with the popular autologous fat transfer procedure have given us pause regarding the widespread adoption of this procedure. As with any aesthetic surgery procedure, in untrained hands, gluteal augmentation of any kind can be potentially harmful to the patients entrusted to our care.

This *Clinics in Plastic Surgery* Gluteal Augmentation issue is certain to become a valuable addition to the aesthetic surgery literature and help to further improve the outcomes associated with aesthetic gluteal-contouring procedures. Toward that end, this issue includes access to procedural videos to supplement the articles. We have also included multiple articles for the most popular procedures so that the reader can glean the commonly accepted principles and identify the nuances that may lead to safer and more refined outcomes. While you are perusing the articles, there are a few emerging themes that should be noted. As our gluteal-contouring practices have all matured, the authors uniformly emphasize prioritizing improving gluteal shape or contour over size. Large, poorly shaped buttocks rarely meet anyone's aesthetic ideals. Furthermore, irrespective of technique used, increasing buttock size or patient body mass index seems to be associated with increasing complications. Notably in this issue, most authors openly

Clin Plastic Surg 45 (2018) xi–xii
https://doi.org/10.1016/j.cps.2018.01.001
0094-1298/18/© 2018 Published by Elsevier Inc.

discuss combining different techniques to further refine outcomes and to address shortcomings inherent to their preferred technique. The importance of meticulous technique and patient management in aesthetic gluteal contouring cannot be overstated.

We would like to thank each of the authors for their commitment to furthering this body of work as well as their generosity in sharing it with their colleagues. Finally, we would like to thank our families, spouses, partners, and editors for their forbearance in bringing this work to fruition.

Robert F. Centeno, MD, MBA, FACS
Department of Plastic Surgery
The Ohio State University
Columbus Institute of Plastic Surgery
6499 East Broad Street, Suite 130
Columbus, OH 43213, USA

Constantino G. Mendieta, MD, FACS, FICS
Private Practice, 2310 South Dixie Highway
Miami, FL 33133, USA

E-mail addresses:
drcenteno@instituteplasticsurgery.com (R.F. Centeno)
DrMendieta@4beauty.net (C.G. Mendieta)

Clinical Anatomy in Aesthetic Gluteal Contouring

Robert F. Centeno, MD, MBA[a,b,*], Aditya Sood, MD, MBA[a,b], Vernon Leroy Young, MD[c]

KEYWORDS

- Gluteal anatomy • Gluteal augmentation • Body contouring • Buttock lift • Circumferential body lift
- Autologous fat transfer • Brazilian butt lift • Gluteal implants

KEY POINTS

- A robust knowledge of gluteal anatomy is critical to the safe execution of gluteal contouring procedures.
- Favorable aesthetic outcomes with the various techniques also require precise anatomic mastery.

TOPICAL ANATOMIC LANDMARKS

Fig. 1 illustrates several superficial anatomic landmarks that have clinical relevance to gluteal augmentation with either alloplastic implants or autologous tissue.[1–8] Not only do these landmarks provide a road map for the procedure, but they have significant implications for the postoperative appearance of specific gluteal features (**Fig. 2**) judged to be appealing in society.[9]

The iliac crest, which forms the superior border of the buttocks, is a palpable and often visible landmark for guiding incision placement in a posterior buttock lift or circumferential body lift (CBL) with autologous gluteal augmentation (AGA) (please see Robert F. Centeno article, "Autologous Gluteal Augmentation with The Moustache Transposition Flap Technique," in this issue). The incision placement is varied superiorly or inferiorly with respect to the iliac crest to achieve a more aesthetically pleasing postoperative result.

The posterior superior iliac spines (PSIS) form two distinct depressions in the sacral region that result from the confluence of the PSIS, the multifidus muscles, the lumbosacral aponeurosis, and the insertion of the gluteus maximus. These anatomic depressions are characteristics of attractive buttocks and attempts should be made to preserve, define, or unmask this anatomic structure to improve surgical outcomes.[9]

These depressions serve as the superior corners of the sacral triangle, which is defined by the two PSIS and the coccyx as the inferior border of the triangle.[1] This triangle is aesthetically pleasing and its borders should be enhanced during surgery if possible. Liposuction and inverted triangle modification of the posterior CBL incision (**Fig. 3**) are surgical maneuvers aimed at enhancing the sacral triangle.[10,11] The original publication on gluteal aesthetic units, which are illustrated in **Fig. 4**, describes how to enhance the sacral triangle and other gluteal units during

Disclosure Statement: The authors have nothing to disclose.
This article originally appeared in *Clinics in Plastic Surgery*, Volume 33, Issue 3, July 2006.
[a] Department of Plastic Surgery, The Ohio State University, 915 Olentangy River Road, Suite 2100, Columbus, OH 43212, USA; [b] Private Practice, The Columbus Institute of Plastic Surgery, 6499 East Broad Street, Suite 130, Columbus, OH 43213, USA; [c] Mercy Clinic Research Institute, 901 Patients First Drive, Washington, MO 63090, USA
* Corresponding author. The Columbus Institute of Plastic Surgery, 6499 East Broad Street, Suite 130, Columbus, OH 43213.
E-mail address: drcenteno@instituteplasticsurgery.com

Clin Plastic Surg 45 (2018) 145–157
https://doi.org/10.1016/j.cps.2017.12.010

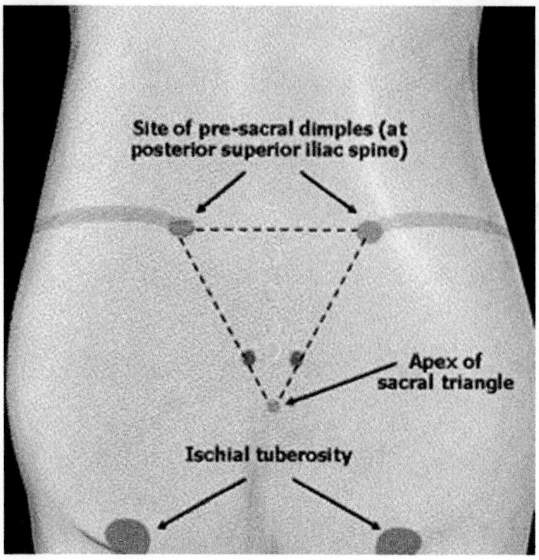

Fig. 1. Superficial anatomic landmarks: iliac crest, posterior-superior iliac spine, sacrum, coccyx, and ischial tuberosity.

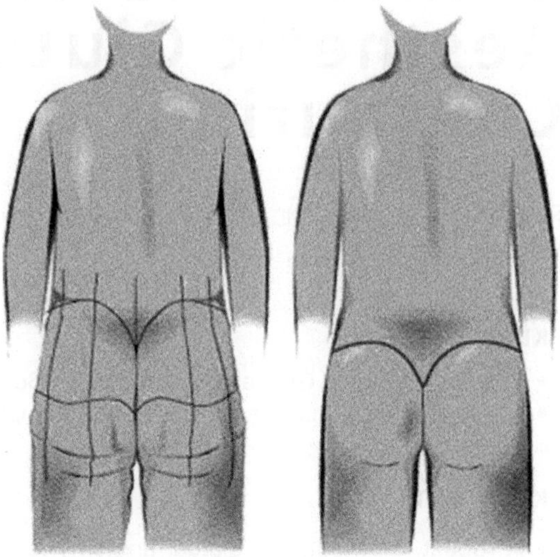

Fig. 3. Preoperative markings and postoperative position of the "inverted dart" modification to the posterior circumferential body lift incision.

body contouring procedures.[10] The sacral triangle should also be marked before augmentation with implants and serves as the medial borders of the dissection (**Fig. 5**). The positions of submuscular, intramuscular, and subfascial implants in relation to fascial and muscular structures are shown in **Fig. 6**.

Another important topical landmark is the lateral trochanteric depression formed by the greater trochanter and insertions of thigh and buttocks muscles, including the gluteus medius, vastus lateralis, quadratus femoris, and gluteus maximus. This depression is important in the aesthetics of an athletically toned buttock, although some ethnic groups (eg, African Americans and US Hispanics) prefer that the trochanteric depressions not be emphasized or even filled if pronounced.

The infragluteal fold serves as the inferior border of the buttock proper and is formed by thick fascial insertions from the femur and pelvis through the intermuscular fascia to the skin. These structures

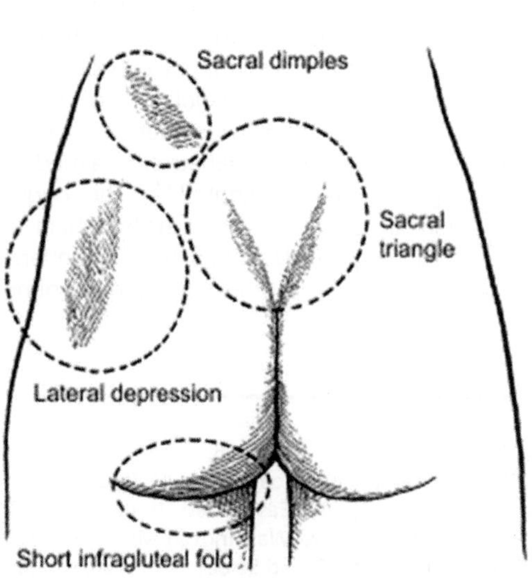

Fig. 2. The sacral dimples, sacral triangle, lateral depression, and a short infragluteal crease and important gluteal aesthetic landmarks.

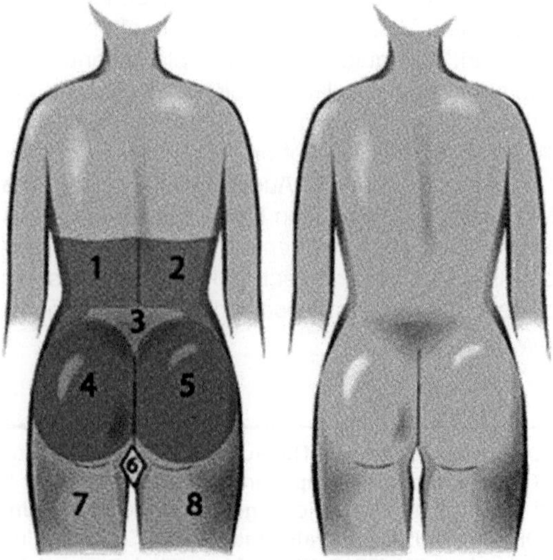

Fig. 4. The following are the eight gluteal aesthetic units: two symmetric flank units (1 and 2), one sacral triangle unit (3), two symmetric buttock units (4 and 5), one infragluteal diamond unit (6), and two symmetric thigh units (7 and 8).

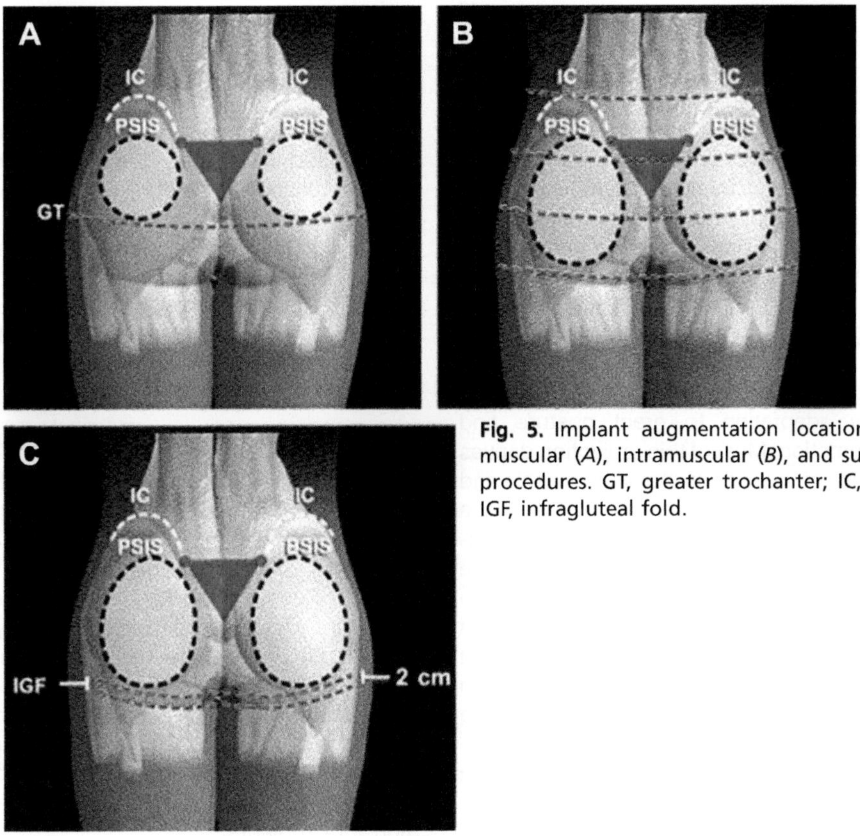

Fig. 5. Implant augmentation locations for submuscular (*A*), intramuscular (*B*), and subfascial (*C*) procedures. GT, greater trochanter; IC, iliac crest; IGF, infragluteal fold.

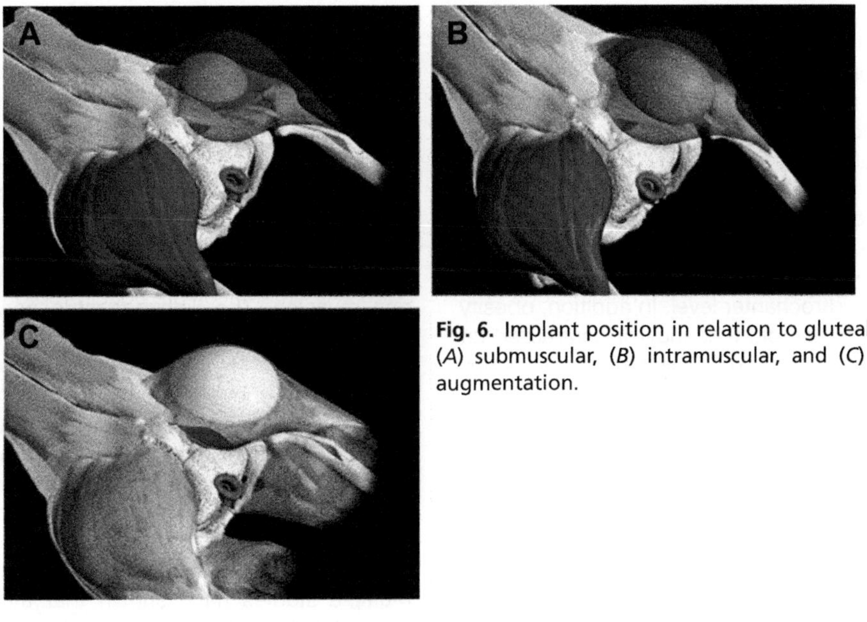

Fig. 6. Implant position in relation to gluteal anatomy: (*A*) submuscular, (*B*) intramuscular, and (*C*) subfascial augmentation.

create the fixed, well-defined subgluteal sulcus.[12] The length and definition of the infragluteal fold play important roles in aesthetically pleasing buttocks. A longer infragluteal fold suggests an aged, ptotic, and deflated-looking buttock with skin and fascial excess. In contrast, a shorter infragluteal fold contributes to a full, taught, and youthful buttock.[13] The ischial tuberosities, although not a part of the buttock proper, are the bony prominences on which people sit.

SUBCUTANEOUS FAT DISTRIBUTION

Projection of the buttocks in humans was likely an evolutionary adaptation to erect posture and bipedal locomotion. Most of this projection derives from the mass of the gluteus maximus muscle and associated lumbar lordosis of the spine. The amount of subcutaneous fat content also contributes to buttock projection and accounts for the round shape of the buttocks. This fat, along with its fascial investments, forms the lower border of the buttock proper. Subcutaneous fat content in the buttock region is usually greater in women versus men, infants versus adults, and in some ethnic groups. It is postulated that these differences in subcutaneous gluteal fat play a role in padding the buttock region for sleeping in the supine position and evolved as an adaptive mechanism for heat dissipation while maintaining sufficient adipose stores critical to normal physiology.[14]

Fat distribution has been studied using various methodologies in men and women. Generalized body types have been described and include the android, gynoid, and intermediate body types. The impact of weight loss, aging, and gender on these various body types have also been investigated. As women age and reach menopause they tend to develop a more centralized fat distribution, both intra-abdominally and subcutaneously, and the more gynoid body type develops more android characteristics.[15] The greatest differences in subcutaneous fat distribution between young compared with older women occur at the waist and midtrochanter level. In addition, obesity increases the android tendency or centralized fat distribution of both sexes. This helps explain why body type and overall fat distribution patterns are consistent among people with rapid and significant weight loss.[16]

Fat distribution changes in the buttocks associated with aging and weight gain have been studied anthrometrically and radiologically. One investigation of 115 randomly selected women ranging in age from 17 to 48 found statistically significant changes in several measurement parameters.[13] Weight gain causes an overall increase in buttock height and width, lengthens the intergluteal crease, and shortens the infragluteal fold. Aging, independent of weight gain, causes an increase in buttock height and lengthens the intergluteal crease and infragluteal fold. Aging and weight gain are associated with drooping of the infragluteal fold. Whereas weight gain alone increases buttock width, this measurement decreases with aging regardless of weight. Changes in subcutaneous adipose content and distribution in association with skin and fascial laxity are thought to explain these findings.

FASCIAL ANATOMY

In addition to volume loss and skin laxity, relaxation of the fascial apron contributes to gluteal ptosis. This fascial apron (**Fig. 7**) is analogous to the superficial fascial system described by Lockwood.[17] Resection and tightening of the skin and this superficial fascial apron not only improve gluteal ptosis but are a major component of the CBL procedure, with or without AGA. The deep gluteal fascia, or investing fascia of the gluteus maximus muscles, is critically important in AGA as a fixation point. It also serves as a strong retaining fascia in the subfascial approach to augmentation with implants.

The superficial fascial apron and the deep gluteal fascia fuse and become tightly adherent to form the infragluteal fold. This serves as the most caudal border of the buttock proper and is a difficult structure to replicate surgically.[12,18,19]

NEUROVASCULAR ANATOMY

The integrity of superficial anatomic structures of the lateral trunk, posterior trunk, and gluteal region are most at risk of injury during the posterior portion of a CBL or buttock-flank lift. The iliohypogastric and ilioinguinal nerves are branches of the L1 nerve root and originate in the sacral plexus (**Fig. 8**). These nerves travel inferiomedially between the transversus abdominis and internal oblique muscles. The iliohypogastric nerve divides into lateral and anterior cutaneous branches to supply skin overlying the lateral gluteal region and the area above the pubis on the anterior surface. Three-point or quilting sutures are used laterally to close dead space. Anatomic variations of the ilioinguinal, iliohypogastric, and lateral femoral cutaneous nerves (LFCN) are of clinical significance when contouring the lateral and anterior trunk and thighs during body contouring surgery. Multiple studies have shown that these nerves are subject to significant variation. In a fresh

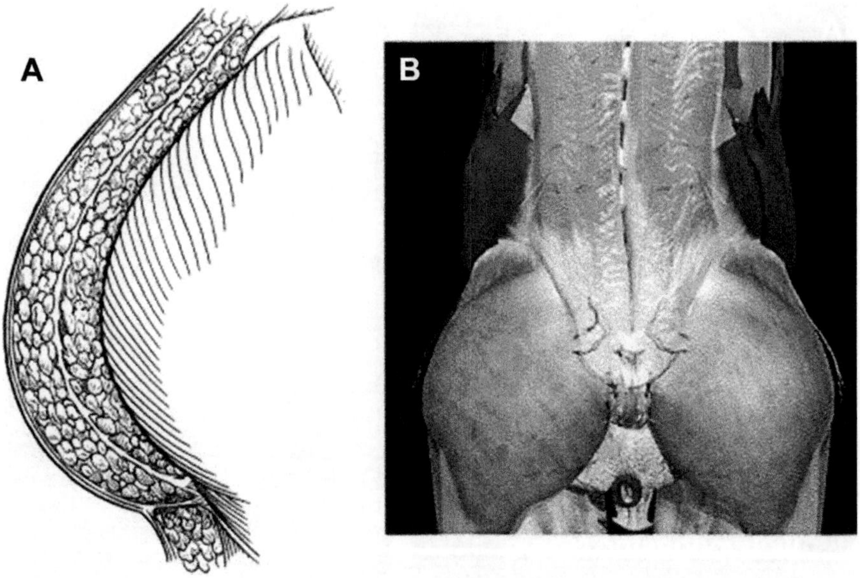

Fig. 7. Gluteal and superficial fascial system fascial anatomy. (*A*) Cut-away view of the structure of the superficial fascial system fascial apron and (*B*) the lumbosacral and gluteal fascia.

cadaveric study, Whiteside and colleagues[20] determined that, on average, the ilioinguinal nerve enters the abdominal wall 3.1 cm medial and 3.7 cm inferior to the anterior superior iliac spine (ASIS) and terminates 2.7 cm lateral to the midline and 1.7 cm above the pubic symphysis. The iliohypogastric nerve enters the abdominal wall musculature 2.1 cm medial and 0.9 cm below the ASIS and ends 3.7 cm lateral to the linea alba and 5.2 cm above the pubic tubercle.

Another study of human cadavers found that the position of the iliohypogastric nerve in relation to the ASIS can vary by 1.5 to 8 cm on the right side and 2.3 to 3.6 cm on the left side. The ilioinguinal nerve and its relation to the ASIS vary by 3.0 to 6.4 cm on the right and 2.0 to 5.0 cm on the left.[21] A study of 110 patients undergoing hernia repair determined that the course of both nerves was consistent with descriptions in anatomy texts in 41.8% of cases but varied significantly in 58.2% of patients.[22] Most variations related to take-off angles, bifurcations, aberrant origins, or CBL incisions made at or below the inguinal crease can put these nerves at risk. The lateral cutaneous branch of the iliohypogastric and the intercostal nerves also can be entrapped laterally during surgery. This may occur if aggressive lateral plication of the external oblique muscle is performed to enhance waist definition or if accessory branches occur at deeper layers of the abdominal wall. However, in 18 of 64 cases, the ilioinguinal nerve was superficial to the external oblique aponeurosis and the superficial inguinal ring.

The LFCN and its injury were described in 1885. Meralgia parasthetica is the clinical syndrome caused by LFCN compression or injury and is characterized by anesthesia, causalgia, and hypesthesias in its dermatomal distribution. Typically the nerve is described as coursing anterior to the ASIS and inferior to the inguinal ligament. Aszmann and colleagues[23] showed that in 4% of cadavers dissected, the nerve exited posterior to the ASIS and across the iliac crest. In another cadaveric study, Grothaus and colleagues[24] demonstrated that the LFCN is susceptible to injury as far as 7.3 cm medial to the ASIS and 11.3 cm below the ASIS on the sartorious muscle.

Sensation to the gluteal region and lateral trunk comes from several sources: the dorsal rami of sacral nerve roots 3 and 4; the cutaneous branches of the iliohypogastric nerve arising from the L1 root; and the superior cluneal nerves that originate from the L1, L2, and L3 roots and then pass over the iliac crest (see **Fig. 8**; **Fig. 9**). The protective cutaneous sensation transmitted by these nerves is temporarily disrupted during a CBL and AGA. Patients should be counseled about the need for frequent positional changes and avoidance of heating pads and electric blankets to prevent pressure necrosis or burns.

Perfusion to the skin overlying the gluteal region is supplied by perforating branches of the superior and inferior gluteal arteries, both of which branch from the internal iliac artery (**Fig. 10**). The lumbosacral region is also supplied by lumbar perforators. Some of these perforators must be sacrificed

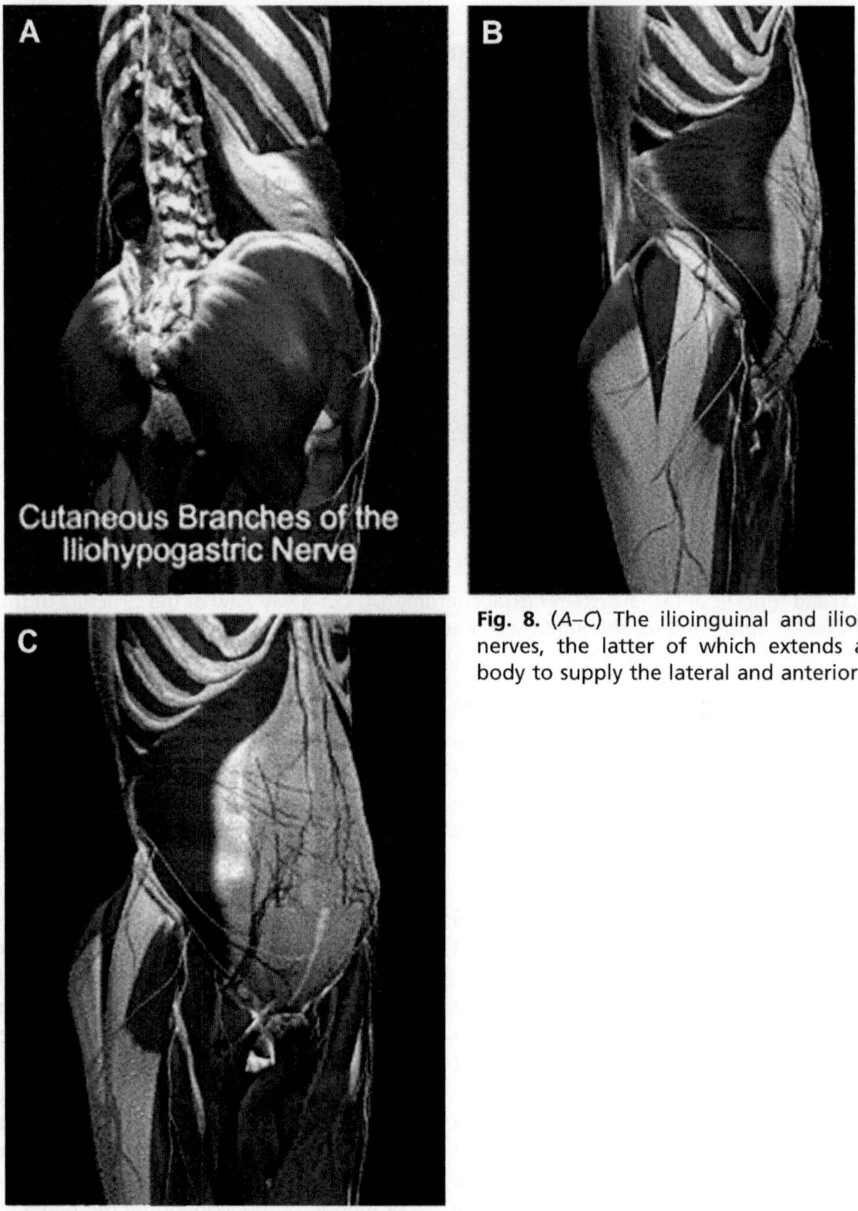

Fig. 8. (*A–C*) The ilioinguinal and iliohypogastric nerves, the latter of which extends around the body to supply the lateral and anterior aspects.

during the posterior portion of a CBL, an AGA with CBL, or a buttock-flankplasty. Even with this loss, the abundant vascular supply in the region provides robust perfusion to surrounding tissue flaps.[25,26]

DEEP NEUROVASCULAR AND MUSCULAR ANATOMY

The gluteus maximus muscle is a powerful extensor of the flexed femur and provides lateral stabilization of the hip. This expansive muscle originates in the fascia of the gluteus medius, the external ilium, the fascia of the erector spinae, the dorsum of the lower sacrum, the lateral coccyx, and the sacrotuberous ligament (**Fig. 11**). It inserts on the iliotibial tract and proximal femur. Innervation of the gluteus maximus comes from the inferior gluteal nerve.

The gluteus medius originates on the external ilium and inserts on the lateral greater trochanter (**Fig. 12**). It abducts the hip and helps stabilize the pelvis during standing and walking. The gluteus minimus muscle originates on the external surface of the ilium and inserts on the anteriolateral greater trochanter (**Fig. 13**). This muscle abducts

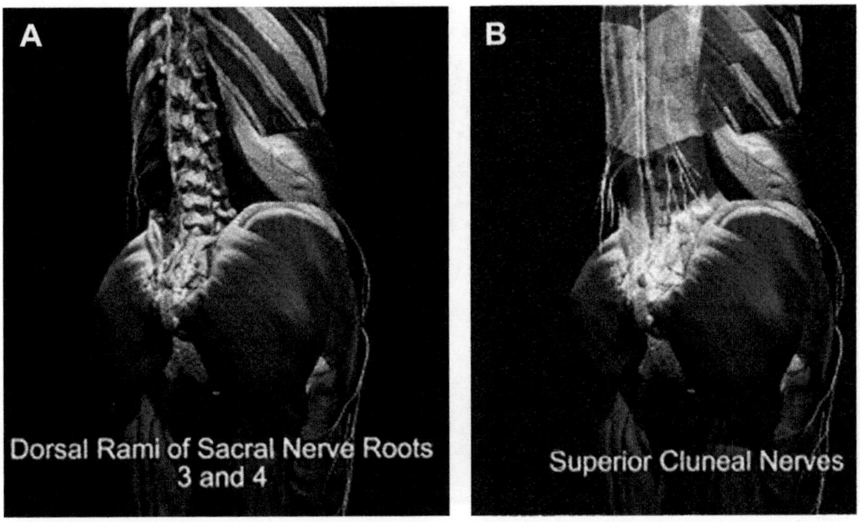

Fig. 9. Posterior cutaneous nerves: (*A*) dorsal rami of 53 and 54 and (*B*) the superior cluneal nerves.

the femur at the hip joint and serves as a pelvic stabilizer. Both the gluteus medius and gluteus minimus are innervated by the superior gluteal nerve. The superior gluteal artery and nerve exit the sciatic foramen above the piriformis muscle and travel through the plane between the gluteus medius and minimus. Both muscles are supplied by the superior gluteal artery and nerve (see **Fig. 10**).

The piriformis muscle is a lateral rotator and abductor of the femur and is innervated by branches of L5, S1, and S2. It originates at the anterior sacrum and inserts on the superior medial border of the greater trochanter (**Fig. 14**). This muscle serves as a landmark for the gluteal neurovascular structures, and the sciatic nerve. The piriformis marks the most inferior extent of an implant pocket for augmentation in the submuscular plane.

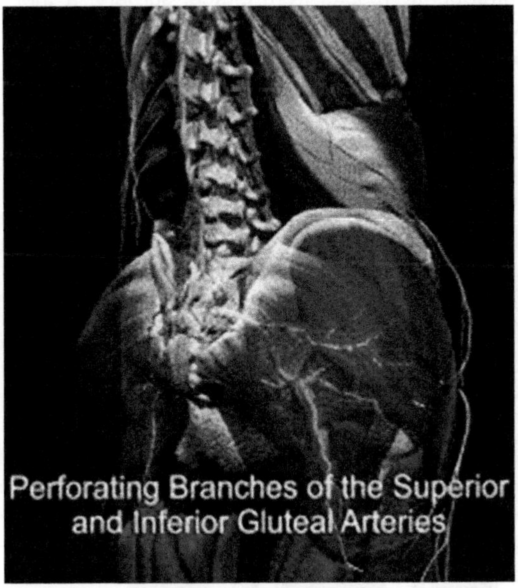

Fig. 10. Superior and inferior gluteal arteries and lumbosacral perforator arteries.

The superior gemellus, inferior gemellus, and obturator internus muscles are all lateral rotators and abductors of the femur and lie caudal to the piriformis. The tensor fascia lata muscle, which is the most anterior of the gluteal muscles, is superficial to the gluteus medius and minimus. Originating on the lateral iliac crest and ASIS, the tensor fascia lata inserts on the iliotibial tract (**Fig. 15**). It functions to stabilize the knee during extension. The terminal branch of the lateral femoral circumflex artery provides perfusion, with innervation supplied by the superior gluteal nerve, as are the gluteus minimus and medius.

The sciatic nerve is the largest nerve of the body and originates in the sacral plexus—at the nerve roots of L4 through S3. It has no gluteal branches except for one to the hip joint. The sciatic nerve leaves the gluteal region through the greater sciatic foramen below the piriformis muscle and above the superior gemellus muscle to enter the posterior compartment of the thigh (**Fig. 16**). Above the popliteal space, the sciatic nerve splits into the common peroneal nerve and the tibial nerve. Compression or injury of the sciatic nerve presents as loss of function of the posterior thigh compartment muscles, all muscles of the leg and foot, and loss of sensation of the lateral leg and foot and the sole and dorsum of the foot.[26] Anatomic studies have shown that the sciatic

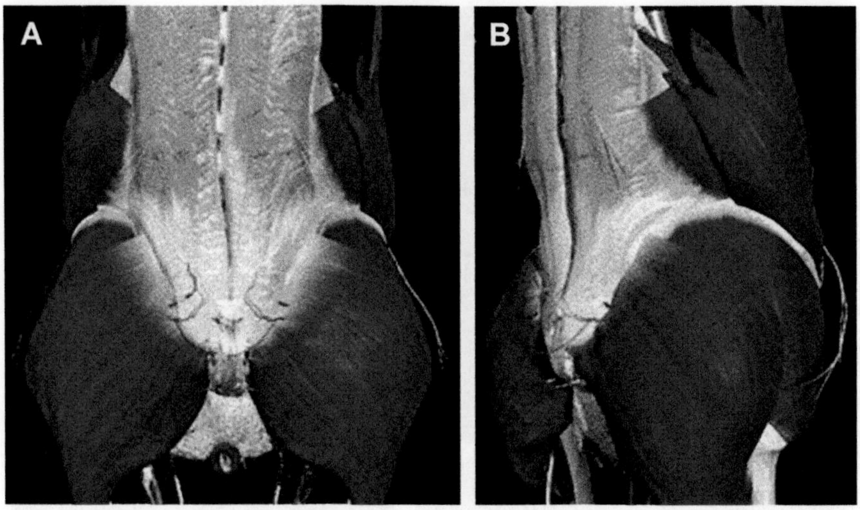

Fig. 11. (*A*, *B*) Gluteus maximus muscle and relationships to nearby anatomic structures.

nerve and its main branches (the tibial and common peroneal nerves) are subject to variability in relation to the piriformis muscle. The sciatic nerve leaves the pelvis through the infrapiriform foramen in 96% of cases. However, in 2.5% of cases the common peroneal branches away from the sciatic nerve early and exits through the piriformis muscle, whereas the tibial nerve exits below the piriformis. In another 1.5% of cases, the common peroneal nerve divides from the tibial nerve and exits the pelvis above the piriformis muscle, whereas the tibial nerve exits below the muscle.[27,28] Although uncommon, these anatomic variations must be looked for during gluteal procedures because their injury could lead to clinical complications during submuscular and intramuscular implant augmentation. Additionally, sciatic nerve axonomesis has been reported as a complication of autologous fat transfer procedures in the plastic surgery literature.

Gluteal compartment syndrome, although rare, has been reported in the literature. Possible causes include trauma, alcoholism, drug-induced coma, Ehlers-Danlos syndrome, sickle cell disease, gluteal artery aneurysm rupture, abdominal aortic aneurysm repair, orthopedic surgery, bone marrow biopsy, intramuscular injections, rhabdomyolysis, extreme physical overexertion, and prolonged surgical positioning the lateral decubitus or lithotomy positions.

Even though gluteal compartment syndrome infrequently results from gluteal surgery, a thorough knowledge of the gluteal compartments and the potential impact of different aesthetic

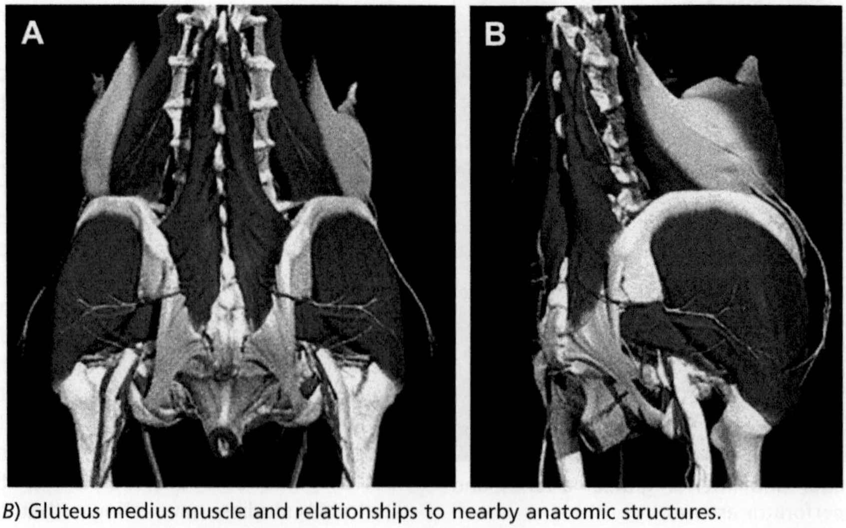

Fig. 12. (*A*, *B*) Gluteus medius muscle and relationships to nearby anatomic structures.

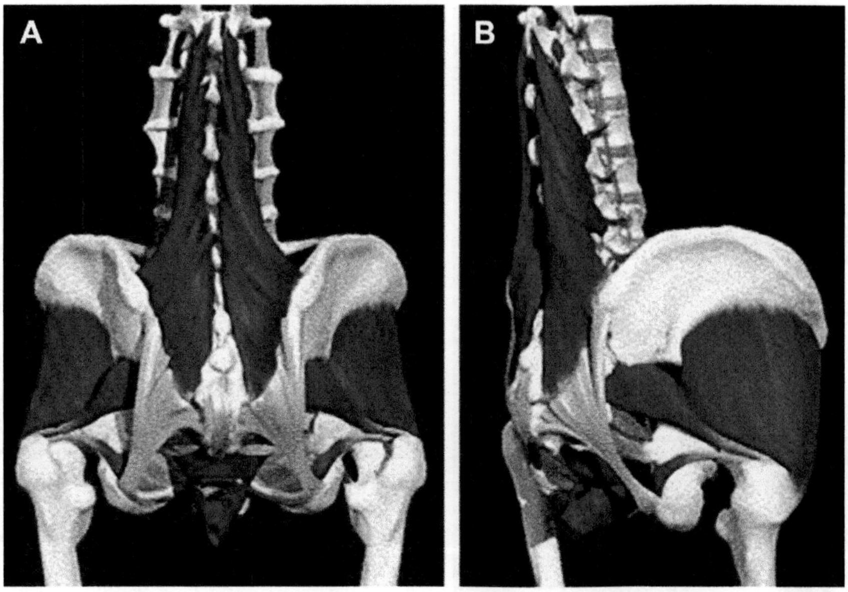

Fig. 13. (*A*, *B*) Gluteus minimus muscle and relationships to nearby anatomic structures.

procedures on these compartments is essential. A low index of suspicion and early intervention reduce any permanent negative sequelae of this potentially devastating clinical problem.

There are three gluteal compartments with inelastic boundaries: (1) the gluteus maximus compartment, (2) the gluteus medius-minimus compartment, and (3) the tensor fascia lata compartment. The gluteus maximus compartment is composed of the muscle plus its superficial and deep fibrous fascia, which is contiguous with the fascia lata of the thigh. This compartment attaches superiorly to the iliac crest and laterally to the iliotibial tract. Medially the superficial and deep gluteal fascia join the sacral, coccygeal, and sacrotuberous ligaments. The gluteus medius-minimus compartment is defined superiorly by the deep gluteal fascia, the tensor compartment, and the iliotibial tract laterally, with the ilium comprising the deep surface. The tensor fascia lata compartment is formed by the tensor fascia lata and the iliotibial tract. Most of the critical neurovascular structures are located in the gluteus medius-minimus compartment. Precise knowledge of these structures helps prevent operative injury and improve understanding of this rare compartment syndrome. The superior gluteal artery, vein, and nerve exit from above the

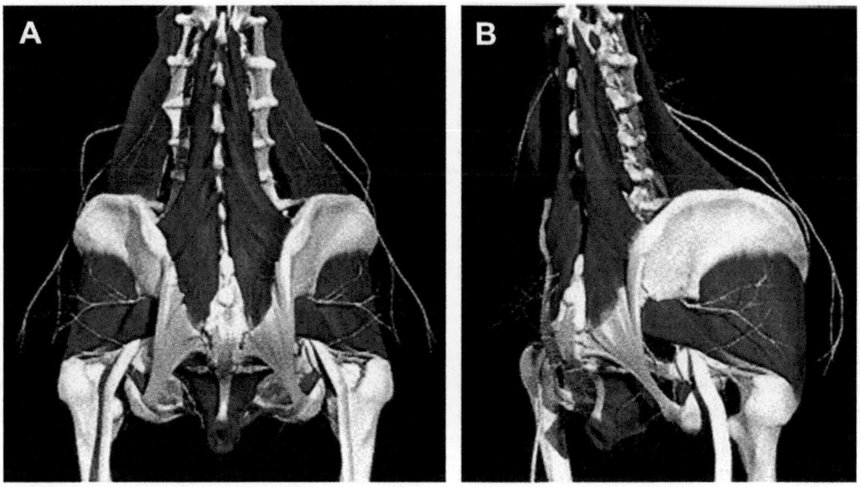

Fig. 14. (*A*, *B*) The location of the sciatic nerve, inferior and superior gluteal arteries, and veins in relation to the piriformis muscle.

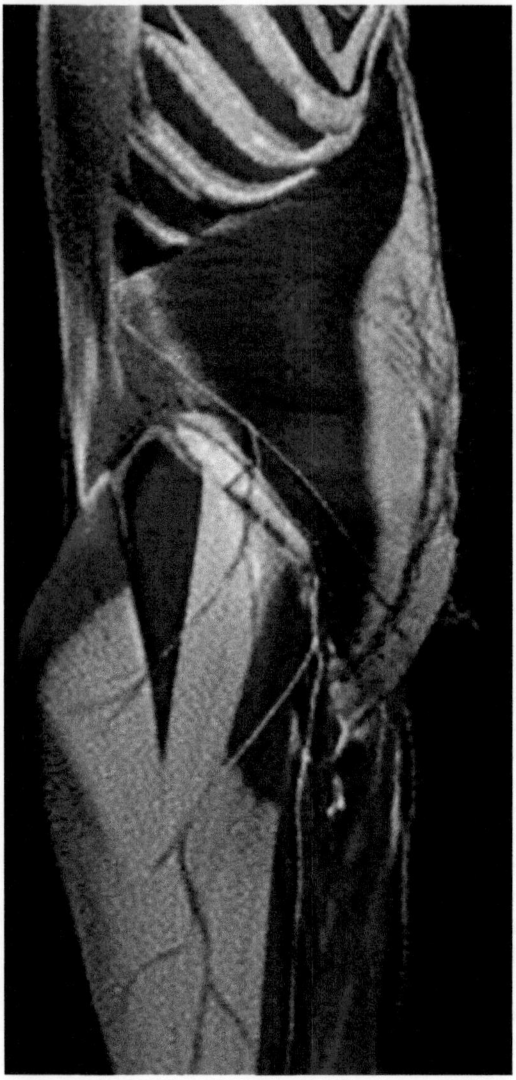

Fig. 15. Tensor fascia lata with gluteal-lumbosacral fascia removed.

piriformis muscle. The inferior gluteal artery, vein, and nerve exit beneath the inferior edge of the piriformis and above the superior gemellus muscle to penetrate the gluteus maximus muscle. The sciatic nerve, posterior femoral cutaneous nerve, pudendal nerve, nerve to the obturator internus, and nerve to the superior gemellus muscle also exit beneath the inferior border of the piriformis muscle.

Increased compartment pressures with diminished perfusion to the gluteal muscles and tensor fascia lata are caused by mass effect within these compartments. Damage to the vessels with bleeding and hematoma formation, or mass effect from a large implant, can theoretically increase compartment pressures beyond a safe limit. Although still disputed in the literature, a compartment pressure of greater than 30 mm Hg may cause necrosis of muscle in 4 to 6 hours and Wallerian nerve degeneration in 8 hours.[29–31]

Organized plastic surgery has recently focused on an increased risk of death associated with gluteal autologous fat transfer procedures reported in the plastic surgery literature and lay press. American Society for Aesthetic Plastic Surgery, American Society of Plastic Surgeons, and International Society of Aesthetic Plastic Surgery formed a task force to further evaluate the potential causes and preventive strategies. Traumatic macro fat embolization is one purported cause of these catastrophic outcomes. It is hypothesized that direct injection into the superior/inferior gluteal veins or associated varicosities as they exit above or below the piriformis muscle is the most likely mechanism. Alternatively, passive fat embolization into an injured vein along a negative pressure gradient was also hypothesized as another potential mechanism for gross fat embolization. This condition is distinct from micro fat embolization syndrome reported with liposuction. It is characterized by gross fat embolization and cardiopulmonary complications, which are detected at autopsy. Recommended preventive strategies include avoiding injecting fat into the deep muscular layer, injecting fat on withdrawal of the cannula, maintaining the cannula parallel to the buttocks surface when injecting, and using a 4.1-mm or larger cannula for injection. Knowledge of the neurovascular bundle anatomy and staying out of the danger zone defined by the borders reported by Rosique is vitally important to prevent this potentially tragic complication **https://journals.lww.com/plasreconsurg/Fulltext/2016/03000/Deaths_Caused_by_Gluteal_Lipoinjection___What_Are.65.aspx**. This emerging situation further supports the importance of familiarity with relevant clinical anatomy in improving patient outcomes and avoiding morbidity and mortality.[32–34]

SKELETAL CHANGES IN PATIENTS WITH MASSIVE WEIGHT LOSS

Aesthetic body contouring in patients with massive weight loss (MWL) is especially challenging. Residual lipodystrophy and skin laxity even after a CBL with or without an AGA often detracts from gluteal aesthetics. Furthermore, skeletal changes associated with obesity in several anatomic areas remain after weight loss and limit the effectiveness of body contouring efforts in the gluteal area. In particular, morbid obesity that precedes MWL produces postural changes that permanently affect the morphology of the skeleton.

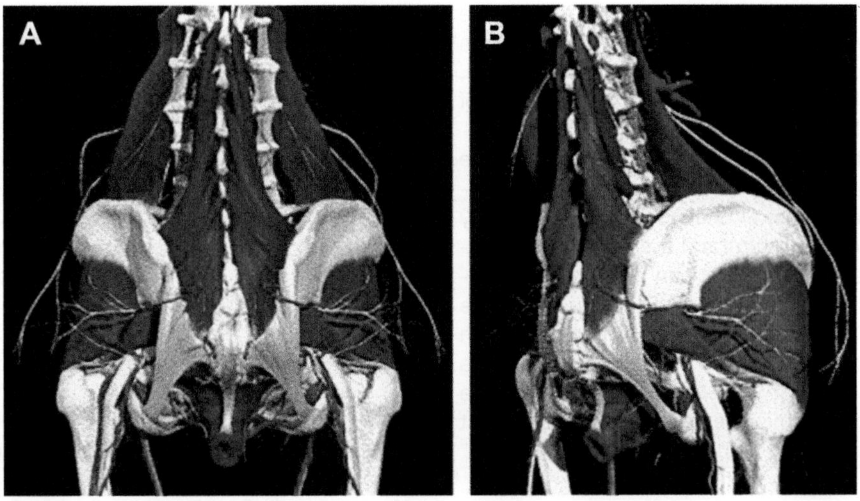

Fig. 16. (*A, B*) The sciatic nerve in relation to the superior and inferior gluteal arteries and veins.

Spinal column lordosis, vertebral compression, and/or pelvic rotation deleteriously affect gluteal projection.[35] The restrictive pulmonary disease associated with obesity and a postural obstructive component lead to pulmonary hyperinflation,[36] which causes permanent skeletal thoracic cage expansion. This barrel-chested appearance is also deleterious to gluteal aesthetics and cannot be corrected. MWL does not change these skeletal abnormalities and they may, in fact, be worsened. At the least, the appearance of these deformities is magnified. Poorly managed chronic hypocalcemia, vitamin D deficiency, and serum telopeptides that lead to osteopenia probably play a role in worsening these skeletal changes after surgical weight loss procedures.[37]

Although the skeletal changes that accompany obesity followed by MWL cannot be corrected, at least some of them can be disguised to some degree with gluteal procedures, especially AGA or fat transfer (please see Ashkan Ghavami and Nathaniel L. Villanueva's article, "Gluteal Augmentation and Contouring with Autologous Fat Transfer: Part I," in this issue). Knowledge of the anatomic abnormalities common in patients with MWL can help surgeons understand why the buttocks appear flattened after the posterior portion of a CBL or buttock lift. Understanding where and why more volume is needed to recreate gluteal projection also comes from familiarity with the anatomy of the gluteal and hip region.

POSITIONAL INJURIES

Intraoperative positioning for gluteal augmentation procedures presents many inadvertent opportunities for injuring patients. The prone and lateral decubitus positions common in gluteal procedures are fraught with risks to patients, including pressure sores, corneal abrasions, peripheral nerve compression, and traction injuries. Although the entire operative team is responsible for being vigilant and preventing these types of injuries, the surgeon possesses the most specialized knowledge of the impact that improper intraoperative positioning can have on a patient.

The lateral decubitus position, typically used for contouring liposuction of the flanks, back, and lateral thighs, or for a CBL, puts major peripheral nerve structures at risk. The use of an axillary roll protects the brachial plexus from compression against the clavicle while in this position. Protection of the common peroneal nerve is accomplished by using a gel mattress on the operative bed and avoiding compression against hard surfaces. Preoperatively, a gel mattress, "Roho," or "egg-crate" is useful in providing extra padding to prevent nerve injury or irritation, and decreasing the risk of developing a stage 1 pressure injury that may occur during and after long surgical procedures.

The prone position, as used in most gluteal procedures, also puts the patient at risk in several ways. The transition from the supine to the prone position should be a controlled process supervised by the surgeon. Protection of the airway by anesthetists, coordination of the team, and the presence of adequate personnel to make the turn effortless are all essential for safe positioning. The use of chest rolls to prevent hyperextension of the shoulder and brachial plexus compression is critical. Padding areas that include the ulnar nerve, knees, feet, and face is also important for preventing pressure sores or nerve injuries. Protecting the eyes with goggles is likely more effective than taping the eyes closed because tape can easily be displaced with movement and the moisture from lubricating ointment. If flexion of the hip is desired, a gel roll beneath the ASIS is a safe way of providing elevation.[38–40]

In patients who are overweight or obese, prone positioning can have hemodynamic and ventilatory consequences. Prone positioning also may decrease venous return and therefore affect preload and cardiac output. It can also have a negative impact on ventilation. For example, the weight of the patient on the chest wall can decrease expansion of the chest and manifest as increased ventilatory pressures. Careful vigilance and awareness diminishes the deleterious impact of these physiologic responses.[41,42]

SUMMARY

Surgeons cannot possess too much knowledge of anatomy. Although brief, this article describes some of the major anatomic issues that confront plastic surgeons when contouring and augmenting the gluteal region. Unless surgeons are experienced in gluteal procedures, they are encouraged to refresh their anatomic knowledge and the many types of nerve and vascular variations that occur. A better understanding of anatomy can improve the cosmetic results of gluteal augmentation. More importantly, it can also reduce the risks of complications, some of which, may be catastrophic or have long-term adverse effects on patients' lives.

REFERENCES

1. De la Pena JA. Subfascial technique for gluteal augmentation. Aesthet Surg J 2004;24:265–73.
2. Gonzalez-Ulloa M. Gluteoplasty: a ten-year report. Aesthetic Plast Surg 1991;15:85–91.
3. Mendieta CG. Gluteoplasty. Aesthet Surg J 2003;23(6):441–55.
4. Vergara R, Amezcua H. Intramuscular gluteal implants: fifteen years' experience. Aesthet Surg J 2003;23(2):86–91.
5. Cárdenas-Camarena L, Lacouture AM, TobarLosada A. Combined gluteoplasty: liposuction and lipoinjection. Plast Reconstr Surg 1999;104(5):1524–31.
6. Valero de Pedroza L. Fat transplantation to the buttocks and legs for aesthetic enhancement or correction of deformities: long-term results of large volumes of fat transplant. Dermatol Surg 2000;26(12):1145–9.
7. Pascal JF, Le Louarn C. Remodeling bodylift with high lateral tension. Aesthetic Plast Surg 2002;26:223–30.
8. Regnault P, Daniel R. Secondary thigh-buttock deformities after classical techniques: prevention and treatment. Clin Plast Surg 1984;11(3):505–16.
9. Cuenca-Guerra R, Quezada J. What makes buttocks beautiful? A review and classification of the determinants of gluteal beauty and the surgical techniques to achieve them. Aesthetic Plast Surg 2004;28:340–7.
10. Centeno RF. Gluteal aesthetic unit classification: a tool to improve outcomes in body contouring. Aesthet Surg J 2006;26:200–8.
11. Matarasso A, Wallach G. Abdominal contour surgery: treating all aesthetic units, including the mons pubis. Aesthet Surg J 2001;21:111–9.
12. Da Rocha RP. Surgical anatomy of the gluteal region's subcutaneous screen and its use in plastic surgery. Aesthetic Plast Surg 2001;25:140–4.
13. Babuccu O, Gozil R, Ozmen S, et al. Gluteal region morphology: the effect of the weight gain and aging. Aesthetic Plast Surg 2002;26(2):130–3.
14. Montagu A. The buttocks and natural selection. JAMA 1966;198:169.
15. Toth MJ, Tchernof A, Sites CK, et al. Menopause-related changes in body fat distribution. Ann N Y Acad Sci 2000;904:502–6.
16. Kopelman PG. The effects of weight loss treatments on upper and lower body fat. Int J Obes 1997;21:619–25.
17. Lockwood TE. Superficial fascial system (SFS) of the trunk and extremities: a new concept. Plast Reconstr Surg 1991;87:1009–18.
18. Lockwood TE. Transverse flank-thigh-buttock lift with superficial fascial suspension. Plast Reconstr Surg 1991;87:1019–27.
19. Lockwood T. Lower body lift with superficial fascial system suspension. Plast Reconstr Surg 1993;92:1112–22.
20. Whiteside JL, Barber MD, Walters MD, et al. Anatomy of ilioinguinal and iliohypogastric nerves in relation to trocar placement and lower transverse incisions. Am J Obstet Gynecol 2003;189(6):1574–8.
21. Avsar FM, Sahin M, Arikan BU, et al. The possibility of nervus ilioinguinalis and nervus iliohypogasticus injury in lower abdominal incisions and effects on hernia formation. J Surg Res 2002;107(2):179–85.
22. Al-dabbagh AK. Anatomical variations of the inguinal nerves and risks of injury in 110 hernia repairs. Surg Radiol Anat 2002;24(2):102–7.
23. Aszmann OC, Dellon ES, Dellon AL. Anatomical course of the lateral femoral cutaneous nerve and its susceptibility to compression and injury. Plast Reconstr Surg 1997;100(3):600–4.
24. Grothaus MC, Holt M, Mekhail AO, et al. Lateral femoral cutaneous nerve: an anatomic study. Clin Orthop Relat Res 2005;(437):164–8.

25. Taylor GI. The angiosomes of the body and their supply to perforator flaps. Clin Plast Surg 2003;30: 331–42.
26. Drake RL, Wayne V, Mitchell AWM. Gray's anatomy for students. Philadelphia: Elsevier, Churchill, Livingstone; 2005.
27. Babinski MA, Machado FA, Costa WS. A rare variation in the high division of the sciatic nerve surrounding the superior gemellus muscle. Eur J Morphol 2003;41(1):41–2.
28. Ugrenovic S, Jovanovic I, Krstic V, et al. The level of the sciatic nerve division and its relations to the piriform muscle. Vojnosanit Pregl 2005;62(1):45–9.
29. Prynn WL, Kates DE, Pollack CV Jr. Gluteal compartment syndrome. Ann Emerg Med 1994;24(6):1180–3.
30. Hill SL, Bianchi J. The gluteal compartment syndrome. Am Surg 1997;63(9):823–6.
31. Bleicher RJ, Sherman HF, Latenser BA. Bilateral gluteal compartment syndrome. J Trauma 1997; 42(1):118–22.
32. Mofid MM, Teitelbaum S, Suissa D, et al. Report on mortality from gluteal fat grafting: recommendations from the ASERF task force. Aesthet Surg J 2017; 37(7):796–806.
33. Cárdenas-Camarena L, Bayter JE, Aguirre-Serrano H, et al. Deaths caused by gluteal lipoinjection: what are we doing wrong? Plast Reconstr Surg 2015;136(1):58–66.
34. Rosique RG, Rosique MJF. Plastic & Reconstructive Surgery 2016;137(3):641e–2e.
35. Fabris de Souza SA, Faintuch J, Valezi AC, et al. Postural changes in morbidly obese patients. Obes Surg 2005;15:1013–6.
36. Ferretti A, Giampiccolo P, Cavalli A, et al. Expiratory flow limitation and orthopnea in massively obese subjects. Chest 2001;119:1401–8.
37. Giusti V, Gasteyger C, Suter M, et al. Gastric banding induces negative remodeling in the absence of secondary hyperparathyroidism: potential role of serum C telopeptides for follow-up. Int J Obes (Lond) 2005;29(12):1429–35.
38. Kroll DA, Caplan RA, Posner K, et al. Nerve injury associated with anesthesia. Anesthesiology 1990; 73:202–7.
39. Lincoln JR, Sawyer HP. Complications related to body positions during surgical procedures. Anesthesiology 1961;22:800–9.
40. Parks BJ. Postoperative peripheral neuropathies. Surgery 1973;74:348–57.
41. Watson RA, Pride NB. Postural changes in lung volumes and respiratory resistance in subjects with obesity. J Appl Physiol (1985) 2005; 98:512–7.
42. Brodsky J. Positioning the morbidly obese patient for anesthesia. Obes Surg 2002;12:751–8.

Classification System for Gluteal Evaluation
Revisited

Constantino G. Mendieta, MD[a], Aditya Sood, MD, MBA[b,*]

KEYWORDS

• Gluteal contouring • Buttock augmentation • Buttock reshaping • Gluteal fat grafting

KEY POINTS

- Buttock contouring and gluteal augmentation are 2 very different procedures that go hand in hand.
- The proposed classification system will help evaluate the anatomy of each patient and analyze the important contouring zones of the buttock.
- This system will standardize patient evaluation.

INTRODUCTION

The buttock area has received much media attention in recent years, which has produced increased patient demand for buttock reshaping or contouring and augmentation. Increasing patient demand has necessitated a more structured approach to evaluation of gluteal anatomy and the development of surgical procedures to enhance its beauty.

This phenomenon is reflected in statistics collected by the American Society for Aesthetic Plastic Surgery, which demonstrate more than 20,000 buttock augmentation procedures performed in 2016 (a 3267% increase compared with 2002).[1] More recently, the Aesthetic Surgery Education and Research Foundation formed the Gluteal Fat Grafting Task Force to investigate risks associated with fat grafting to the buttocks, and have published several recommendations.[2]

Although physician interest in gluteoplasty has been increasing, most plastic surgeons remain hesitant to perform the procedure because the operative techniques are not well understood, patient selection remains a mystery, and no evaluation system exists to standardize the approach. Although many gluteoplasty articles have been published in the past few years, they have primarily focused on technique and not on evaluation.[3–7] Thus far, with exception of the authors' previous publication, there have been few classification systems proposed for evaluating the different anatomic variations of the gluteal region.[8] This article presents a classification system that can be individualized for every patient to guide surgical planning for buttock contouring and gluteal augmentation.

The overall shape of the buttock is influenced by 4 different anatomic variables:

1. Underlying bony framework
2. Gluteus maximus muscle
3. Subcutaneous fat topography
4. Skin.

The interaction of these 4 variables gives the buttock an individualized and particular shape (**Fig. 1**A). To simplify this complex subject, imagine that the muscle is a removable structure. With the muscle detached, what remain are the bony

Disclosure Statement: No disclosures.
This article originally appeared in *Clinics in Plastic Surgery*, Volume 33, Issue 3, July 2006.
[a] Private practice, 2310 S Dixie Highway, Miami, FL 33133, USA; [b] Department of Plastic and Reconstructive Surgery, The Ohio State University Medical Center, Columbus, OH, USA
* Corresponding author. 4373 Times Square Boulevard, Dublin, OH, 43016.
E-mail address: asood17@gmail.com

Clin Plastic Surg 45 (2018) 159–177
https://doi.org/10.1016/j.cps.2017.12.013

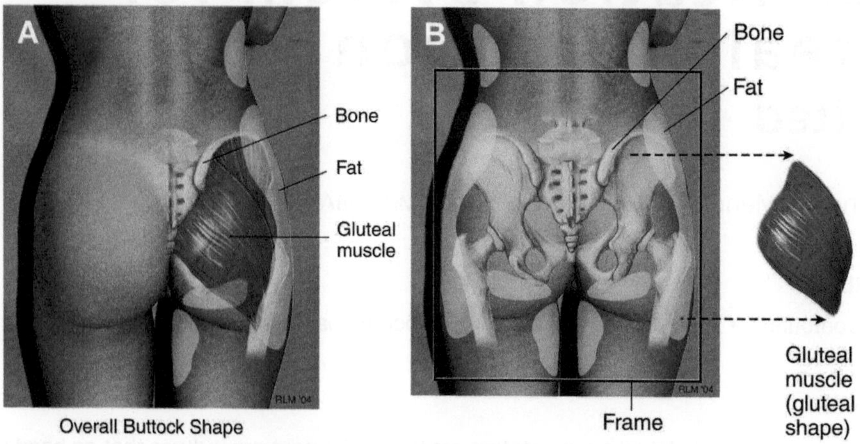

Fig. 1. (*A*) The overall shape of the buttocks depends on the bony framework, the gluteus maximus muscle, the location and amount of subcutaneous fat, and the tightness of the skin. (*B*) The buttock frame, with gluteus maximus muscle detached.

framework, fat, and skin, known collectively as the frame (**Fig. 1**B).

The proposed classification system for gluteal contouring focuses on evaluating and identifying the different frame types, gluteal aesthetic units, gluteal muscle types, and the relationship between the muscle and the frame. Finally, a ptosis classification system is presented.

THE FRAME (FAT, BONE, SKIN) AND GLUTEAL AESTHETIC UNITS

With the muscle out of the way, the surgeon must understand how the variables that compose the frame (bone, skin, and fat) interact to create a particular shape and affect the gluteal aesthetic units.

- The underlying bony framework influences the shape; however, because this structure cannot be surgically changed, it does not play a major role in the classification system other than to refer to it as a tall, short, or intermediate pelvic height.
- The skin plays a role when determining whether an upper buttock lift, inferior gluteal crease excision, or inner gluteal fold excision is necessary.
- Fat topography is the most important component of the frame and the easiest to modify. The subcutaneous fat has the greatest impact in establishing the overall shape of the frame that the gluteus muscle rests on.

The gluteal aesthetic units are most helpful when addressing this component of shape. Understanding the gluteal aesthetic units and their relation to the frame are of paramount importance before undertaking gluteal augmentation. The gluteal units are used to orient and determine which areas may benefit from liposuction versus fat transfer, which undoubtedly affects the overall frame discussion. Previously published work has described 10 aesthetic units to the posterior region (**Fig. 2**),[9] and another has described 8 gluteal aesthetic units: 2 symmetric flank units, 1 sacral triangle unit, 2 symmetric buttock units, 1 infragluteal diamond unit, and 2 symmetric thigh units (**Fig. 3**).[10] Careful anatomic analysis and surgical technique, as well as devoted communication with patients to determine their aesthetic preferences, are encouraged.

HOW TO IDENTIFY THE DIFFERENT FRAME TYPES

Identifying the different frame types is done by comparing and contrasting the amount of fat present in 3 particular zones. The most protruding point in the upper lateral hip is marked point A, the most protruding point in the lateral thigh is marked point B, and the lateral midbuttock is point C (**Fig. 4**).

The connection of points A and B on each side (left and right) of the body leads to identification of the 4 basic frame types: A-shaped, V-shaped, square, and round (**Fig. 5**).

Point C has 2 functions. The first is to help differentiate a round versus a square buttock. The round buttock has excess fat at point C, whereas the square buttock has equal amounts or is deficient (see **Fig. 5**). The second and most important function of point C is to help assess the degree of depression present at point C in the square, A-shaped, or V-shaped buttock. This depression

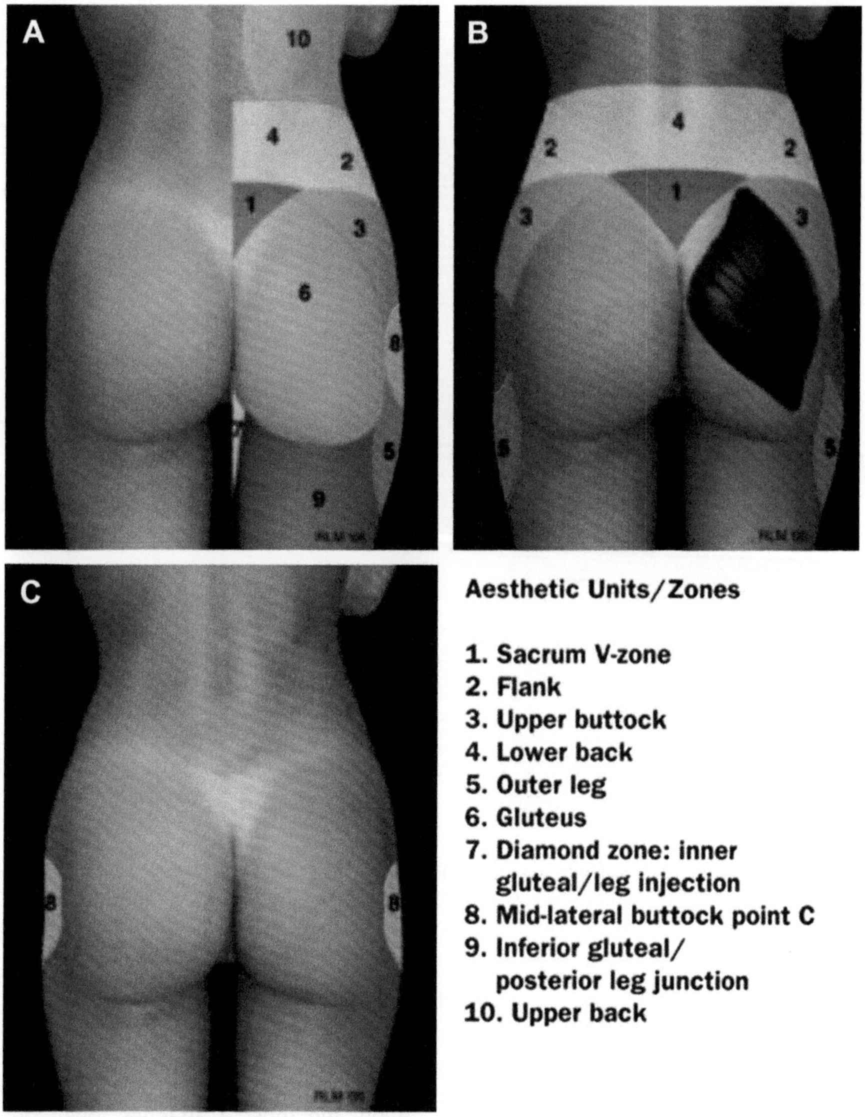

Fig. 2. (*A*) 10 aesthetic units to the posterior region are described. (*B, C*) Six important zones truly define the buttock frame or shape; including zones 1 to 5 and zone 8. (*C*) Zone 8 may require fat transfer to smooth contour. (*From* Mendieta CG. Gluteal reshaping. Aesthet Surg J 2007;27(6):641–55; with permission.)

is categorized as none, mild, moderate, or severe (**Fig. 6**).

The clinical significance of point C is that mild to moderate depressions usually do not require fat transfers because tremendous contour improvement is obtained through liposuction of the upper buttock, outer leg, or both. With a severe depression, however, the surgeon should consider fat transfers to this area.

CHARACTERISTICS OF THE 4 FRAME TYPES

Square Shape

The square buttock is the most common, seen in about 40% of patients. Equal volumes at point A and point B characterize the square-shaped buttock so that when these points are connected a square shape emerges (**Figs. 7** and **8**). Point C can have varying degrees of fat deficiency. This shape is the most malleable of the 4 types because any variations at points A, B, or C can turn it into a different shape.

This shape is unique in that it can be tall, intermediate, or short (see **Figs. 7** and **8**). To understand this concept, it must be remembered that the frame is composed of skin, fat, and bone. The bony framework is useful only for defining the pelvis as tall, intermediate, or short. The upper limit of the bony framework is the upper border of

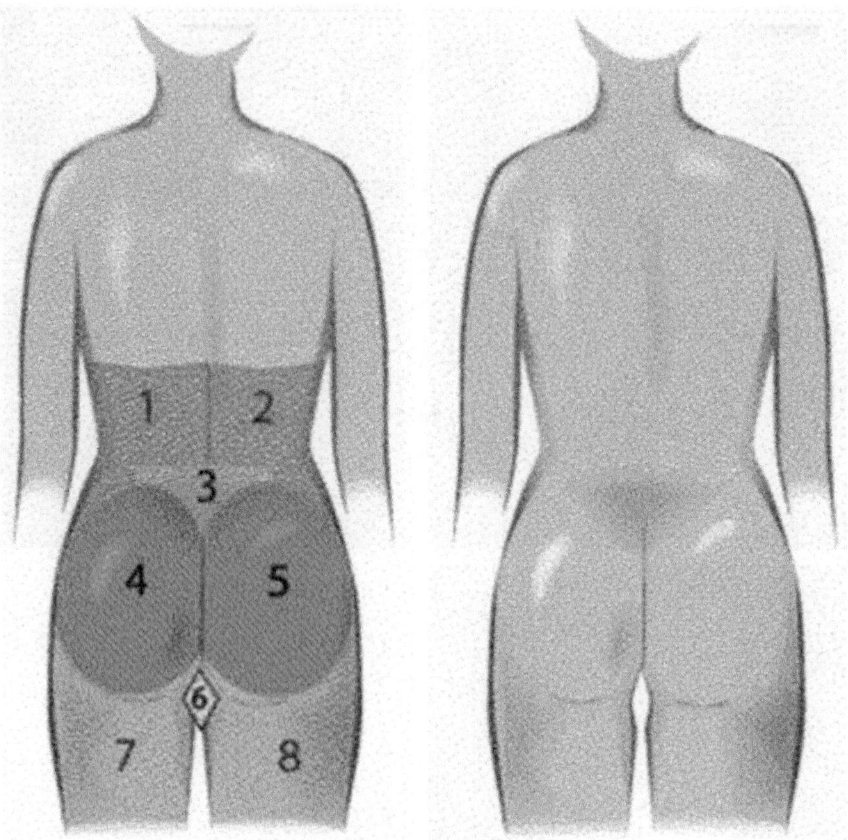

Fig. 3. The 8 gluteal aesthetic units include 2 symmetric flank units (1 and 2) 1 sacral triangle unit, 2 symmetric gluteal units (4 and 5), 2 symmetric thigh units (7 and 8), and 1 infragluteal diamond unit (6). (*From* Centeno RF. Gluteal aesthetic unit classification: a tool to improve outcomes in body contouring. Aesthetic Surg J 2006;26(2):200–8, with permission.)

the posterior iliac crest. There are 3 different height options for placement of the gluteus maximus on the bony frame. The first variation is attachment of the upper border of the gluteus muscle along the upper border of the entire iliac crest, which leaves very little space between the superior muscle edge and the iliac crest. This produces a short pelvic height in which the muscle usually has a 1:1 height-to-width ratio. In the second variation, the muscle attaches lower on the pelvic frame so that the superior edge of the muscle is about a half muscle-length away from the posterior iliac crest. This produces a tall pelvis (see **Fig. 8**). In this type, the muscle usually has a 2:1 height-to-width ratio.

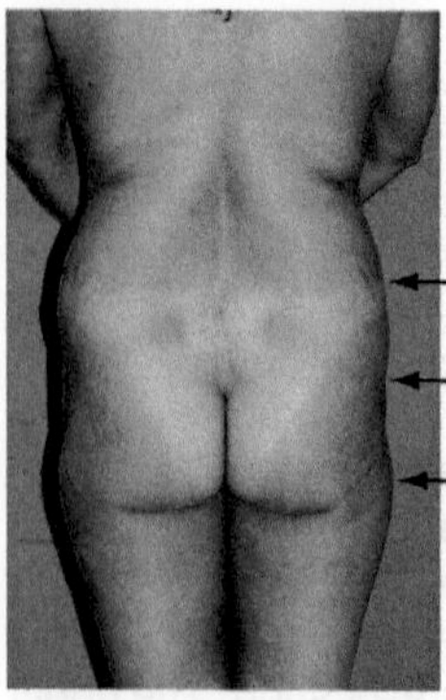

Fig. 4. Points A, B, and C, to be considered when evaluating frame type.

The intermediate variation between a tall and a short pelvis is classified as medium height. The muscle has a height-to-width ratio between 1:1 and 2:1. The square-shaped buttock is most often improved with liposuction of points A and B. Point C may require fat transfers, depending on the degree of depression at this point (**Fig. 9**).

Round Shape

The round buttock is seen in about 15% of patients. The round shape is characterized by having excess fat at point C. When all 3 points (A, B, and

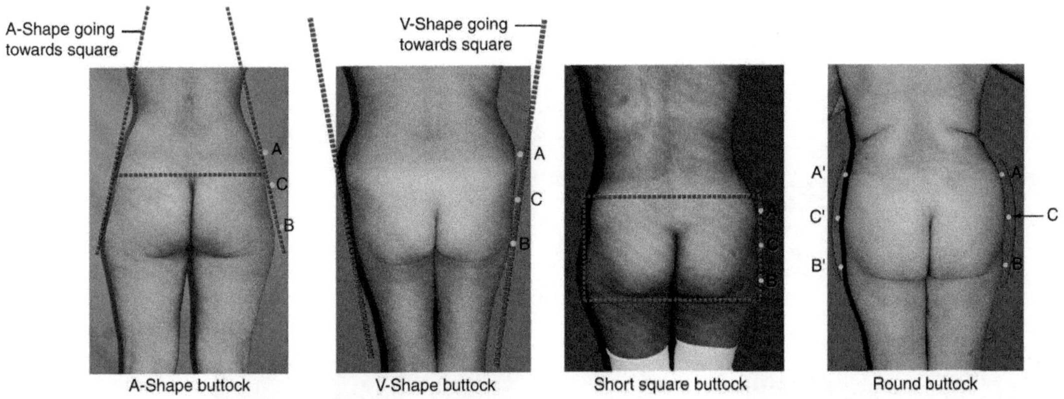

Fig. 5. The 4 buttock shapes: A-shaped, V-shaped, square, and round.

C) are connected, a gentle C-shaped curve becomes apparent (**Fig. 10**). Point C is crucial because it differentiates a round from a square shape. As point C diminishes, the buttock begins to take on a square shape.

Patients with round-shaped buttocks have a tendency to be heavier than those with a square shape. In the round shape, the gluteus maximus muscle may have a wide or normal gluteal base width; however, it most often has a narrow base. The height-to-width ratio of the muscle is usually 1:1.

This shape also may have a deformity that consists of excess fat or skin in the lower-inner (transition between the intergluteal and infragluteal folds) gluteal fold area. This fullness gives the buttock a so-called dirty diaper look that is not aesthetically pleasing.

A-Shaped (Pear-shaped)

The A-shaped buttock is present in about 30% of patients. When points A and B are connected, an A shape is apparent (**Fig. 11**). This shape is characterized by having more fat in the lateral upper thigh (point B) and less fat in the lateral upper hip area (point A). Ideally, point A should protrude more than other hip areas. As the fat at point B diminishes, the buttock begins to take on a square shape. Point C can be severely deficient but in most cases the depression is mild to moderate.

The A-shaped buttock is usually improved with liposuction of point B and occasionally of point A or lateral thigh (**Fig. 12**). Point C may require fat transfers, depending on the degree of depression. Excessive liposuction of point B should be avoided to prevent a sharp demarcation of the transition

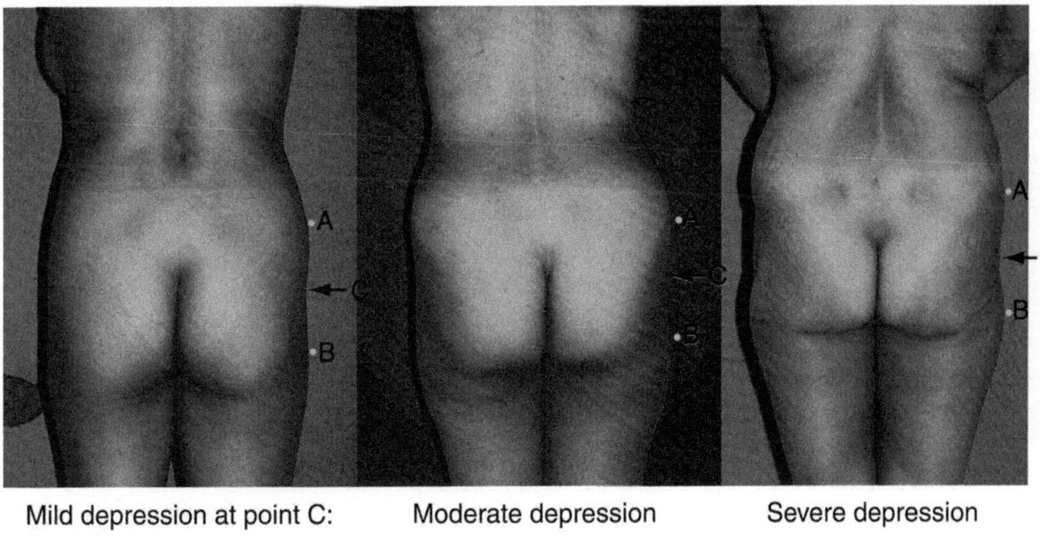

Fig. 6. Gluteal depressions seen in square buttocks.

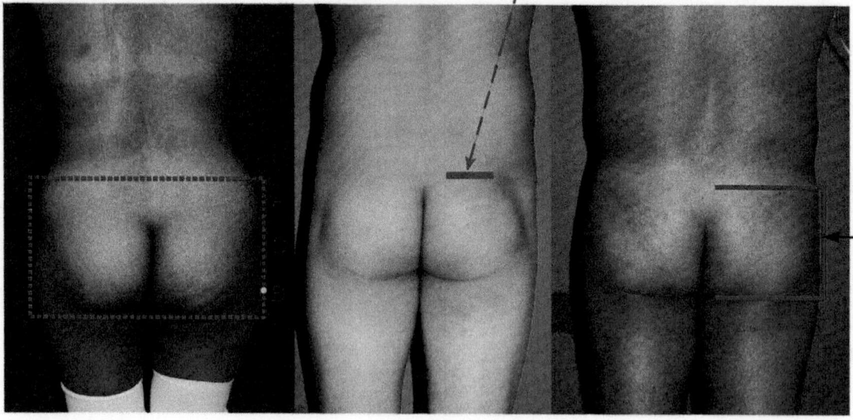

Fig. 7. Characteristics of the short square buttock. The gluteus muscle has a height and width ratio of 1:1.

zone from the gluteal muscle to the lateral thigh region.

V-Shaped (Apple-shaped)

The V-shaped buttock is seen in about 15% of patients. When points A and B are connected, a V shape can be appreciated, along with gluteal base width (**Fig. 13**). Most of the fat is located in the upper lateral hip area (point A) and very little in point B. Deficiency in the area of point C is rarely a problem. As point A diminishes, the buttock takes on a more square shape.

This shape is unique in that patients tend to have a tall pelvis, very thin legs, and a tendency toward central obesity. The pelvic anatomy is worth mentioning because a tall pelvis with a V shape gives a deceptively long appearance to the buttock; however, in reality, the muscle lies low on the pelvis and is often short, with a 1:1 height-to-width relationship. The intergluteal crease line also appears to be short and low-lying (**Fig. 14**). This appearance is created by 2 factors: (1) there is no gluteal volume above the top of the intergluteal fold and (2) the sacral height is 2 to 3 times taller than the intergluteal crease length.

In the ideal buttock, the sacral space is defined as the area between the L5-sacral junction and the upper end of the intergluteal crease length; this should be 50% to 100% of the intergluteal crease length. In **Fig. 14**, the intergluteal crease length is ideally considered to be half the gluteus muscle height,

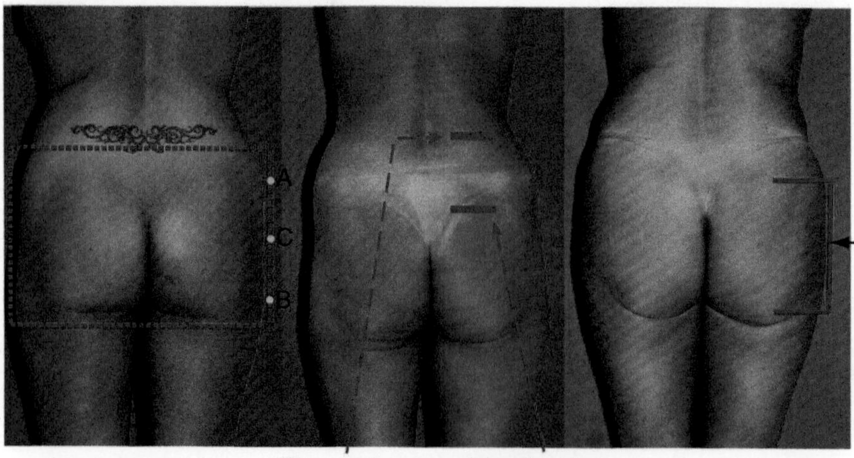

Fig. 8. The tall square buttock. The muscle height is about twice its width, for a 2:1 ratio.

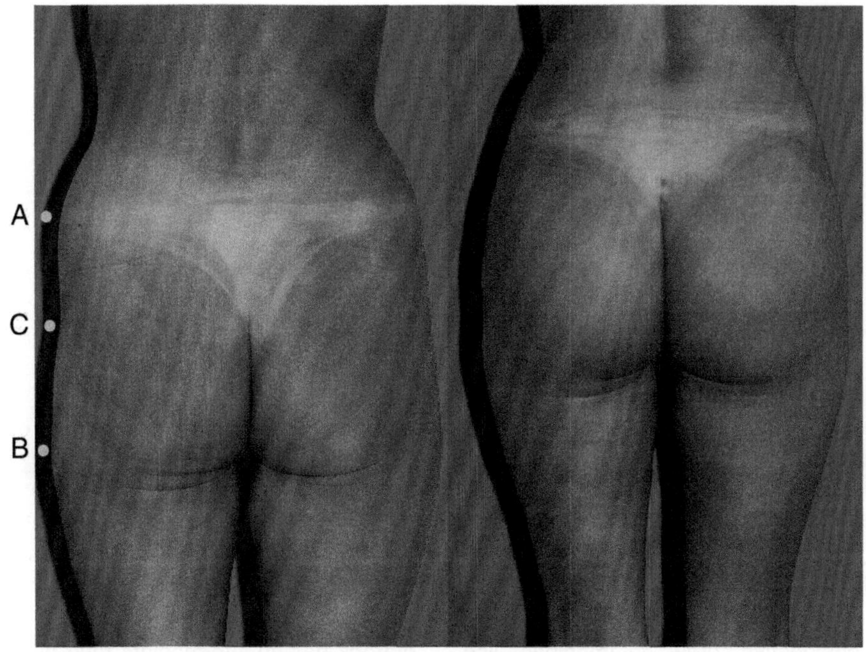

Fig. 9. A tall square buttock before (*left*) and after (*right*) gluteoplasty.

with one-fourth to one-third of the gluteal volume above the upper end of the crease and one-fourth to one-third of the volume below the inferior end of the line. The inferior end of the intergluteal crease is that take-off point from which the infragluteal fold deviates from the intergluteal crease. In patients with a V-shaped frame, the height of the gluteus muscle seems to be comparable to the short intergluteal crease, which creates the illusion that the upper half of the gluteus muscle is missing.

The clinical significance of the V-shaped buttock is that this shape is the hardest to recontour. The V shape is not very attractive; however, it can be improved with liposuction of point A and the flank area. Implants and secondary fat transfer to the upper inner muscle area are often required to

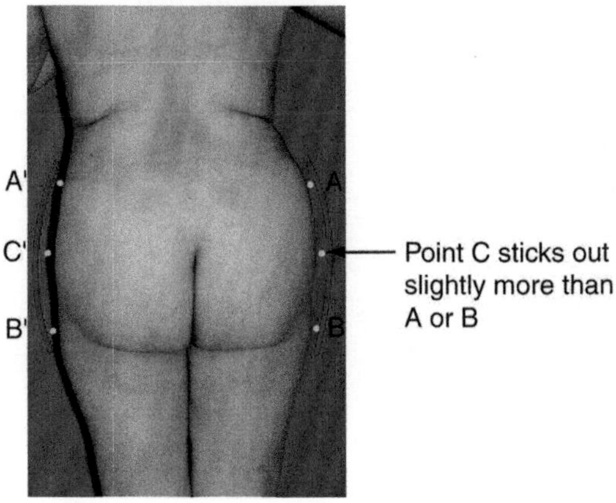

Fig. 10. Characteristics of the round-shaped buttock.

improve the V shape (**Fig. 15**). Lateral thigh and point C fat transfer can also help to improve the aesthetic outcome.

In-Between or Intermediate Shapes

Although most patients can be neatly categorized into 1 of the 4 frame types, others may not be as clear. Because each half of the body is not a mirror image of the contralateral side, asymmetry always exists. In some cases, however, the asymmetry is so obvious that the glutei appear to be from different families. In these cases, each buttock needs to be categorized separately (**Fig. 16**).

In some patients, the differences between each buttock may so subtle that they initially appear relatively symmetric. However, closer evaluation reveals that the overall composite buttock shape resembles or falls between 2 types. In these cases, the shape it most resembles, as well as the shape it leans toward (ie, V going toward square) must both be described before the optimal treatment can be determined.

THE GLUTEUS MAXIMUS MUSCLE

The gluteus maximus muscle may be classified according to its anatomy and its volume.

Gluteus Maximus Muscle Anatomy

Muscle height-to-width ratio

Imagine holding the gluteus maximus muscle in the hand. While looking at it from a posteroanterior

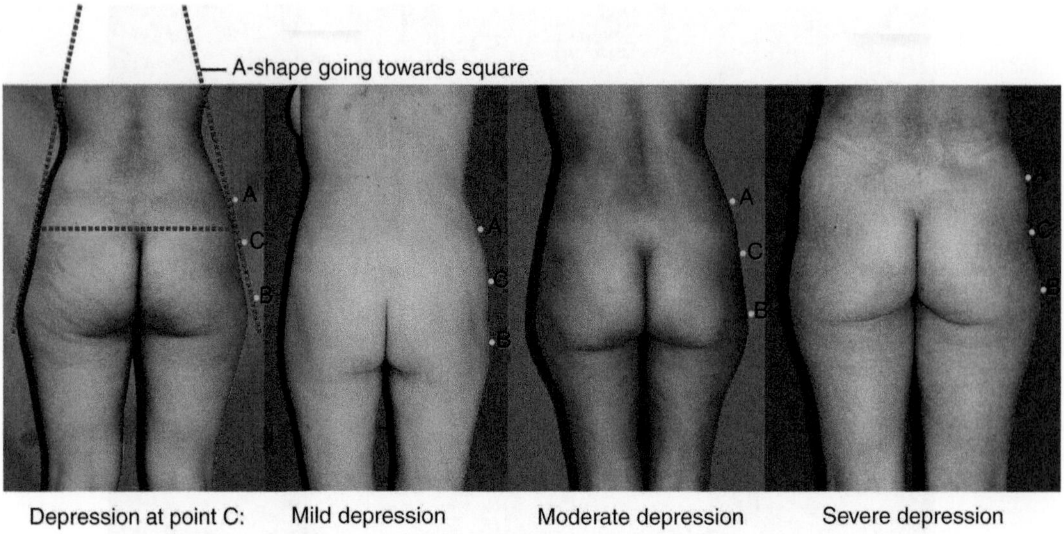

Fig. 11. Characteristics of the A-shaped buttock with mild, moderate, and severe depressions at point C. Point A should be the most protruding point of the hip area, which can be addressed with liposuction of point B.

(PA) view perspective, draw an imaginary line down the middle of the muscle (**Fig. 17**). Identify the superior and inferior points of the gluteus muscle, as well as the most medial and lateral points. The height-to-width relationship is readily apparent and will fall into 1 of 3 ratio categories: a short muscle has a 1:1 ratio, a tall muscle has a 2:1 ratio, and an intermediate muscle has a ratio between 1:1 and 2:1 (see **Figs. 7** and **8**). The ideal buttock has an intermediate ratio but leans more toward a 2:1 height to width ratio (see **Fig. 1**A).

In gluteal augmentation with implants, the height-to-width ratio is critical. The short muscle is best augmented with round implants because they have similar ratios (1:1), and the tall muscle (2:1 ratio) is best augmented with an anatomic implant.[3] The intermediate muscle has the most flexibility and easily accommodates the 3 implant shapes:

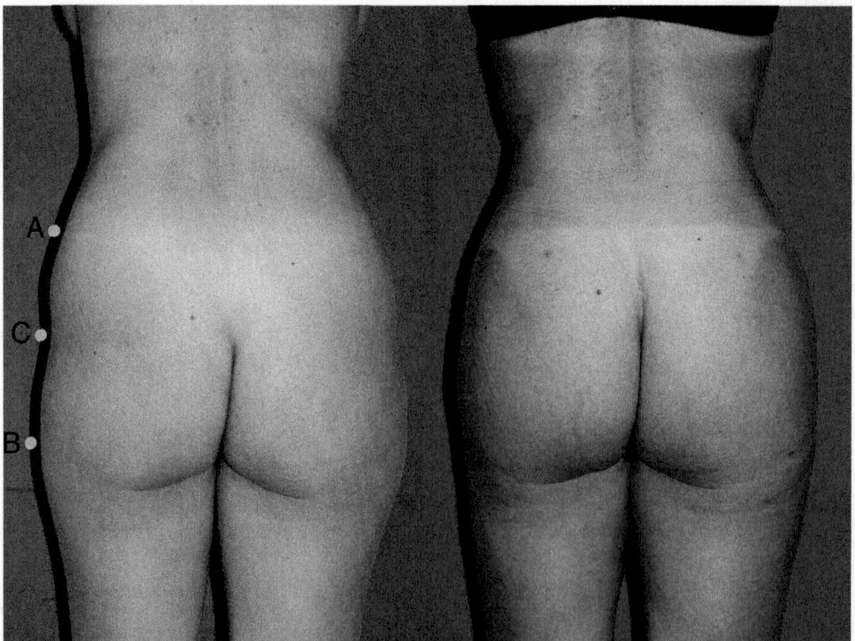

Fig. 12. A tall A-shaped buttock before (*left*) and after (*right*) gluteoplasty.

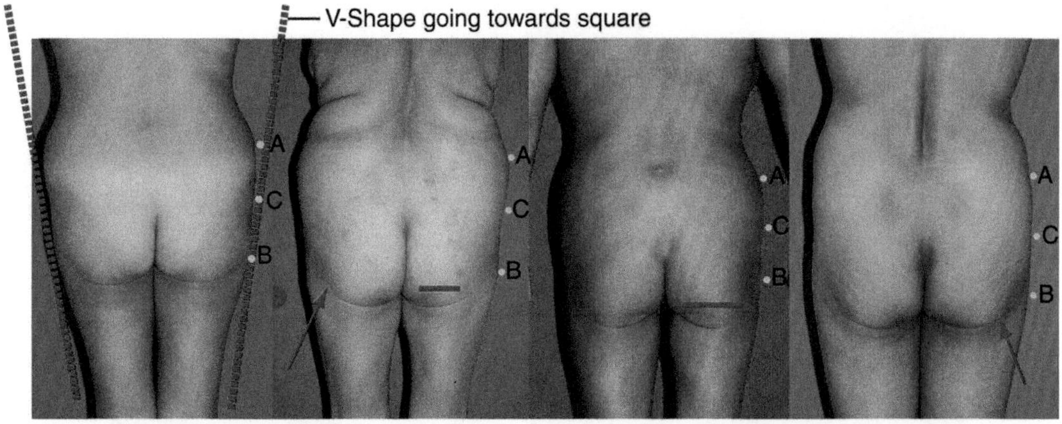

Fig. 13. Characteristics of the V-shaped buttock. Red arrow indicates lower lateral gluteal/leg junction sharp demarcation line: best treated with fat transfers. Solid line indicates gluteal base width demonstrating narrow and normal width.

round, anatomic, or oval. However, to make the final decision on implant shape, the lateral view usually needs to be considered (see later discussion).

Inferior gluteal base width (narrow, normal, or wide)

To determine the gluteal base width, draw a vertical, central reference line down the center of 1 of the buttocks (a midbuttock line, not a midmuscle line; see **Fig. 17**). Then identify the width of the gluteus muscle base and measure from the midline of the body. If the muscle base extends no further than the central midbuttock line, it is called a narrow base width. If it extends past the line by 10% to 30%, it is called a normal base width. If the gluteus muscle base extends 40% to 50% beyond the central midbuttock line, it is considered a wide base width. The youthful aesthetic buttock has a normal base width, and the inferior gluteal fold ends at the center or just lateral to the midbuttock line (see **Fig. 1**A).

Gluteus Maximus Muscle Volume

Gluteal muscle volume needs to be evaluated using 2 different photographic views: PA and lateral. This volume evaluation is used for 2 very different purposes.

Gluteus muscle volume on posteroanterior view

Imagine the gluteus muscle on the frame with the vertical, central midbuttock line drawn. In the ideal buttock, the gluteus maximus has equal volumes on either side of this line and has the shape of a football. To further evaluate volume,

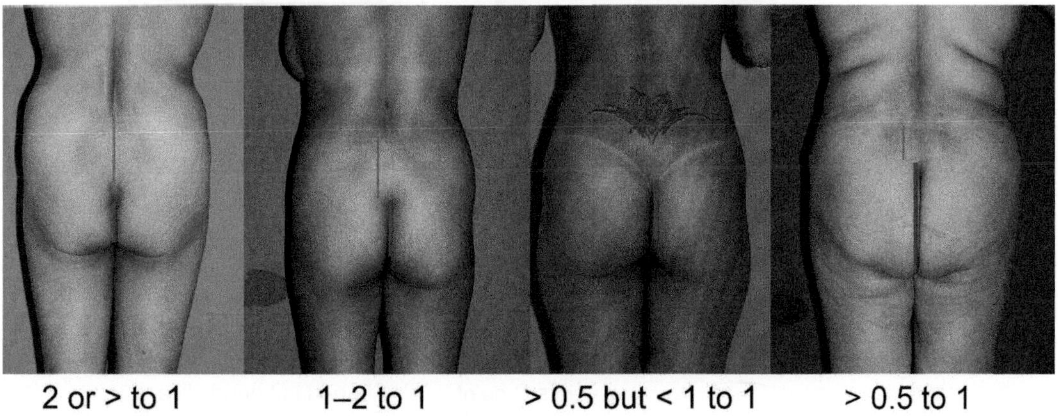

Fig. 14. The variety of ratios between the sacral height to gluteal crease length. To determine sacral height, measure from the lower back dimple area (L5-sacral junction) to the end of the superior aspect of the intergluteal crease (*blue line*). The ideal relationship is greater than 0.5 but less than 1 to 1. A gluteal crease with a less than 0.5:1 ratio appears excessively long, whereas a crease with a 2:1 ratio appears very short.

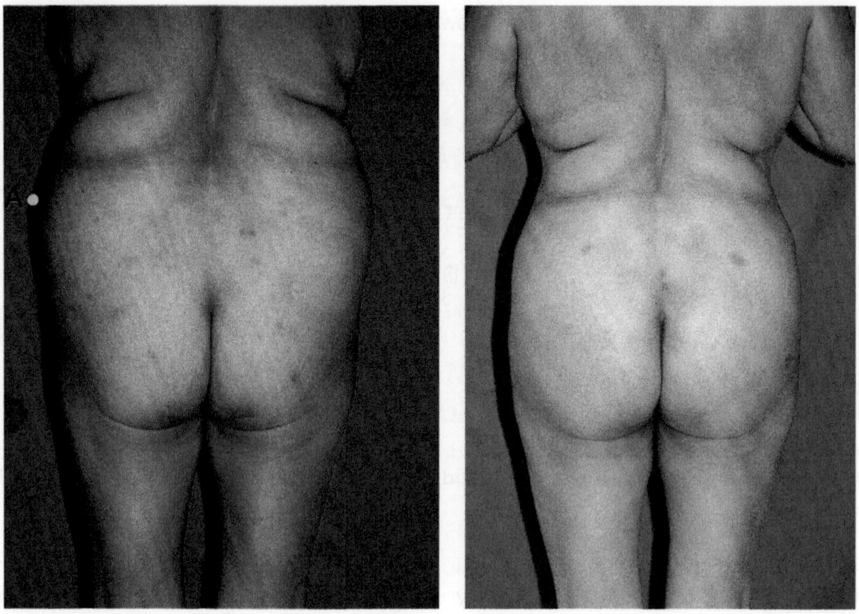

Fig. 15. A tall V-shaped buttock with a short muscle is seen before (*left*) and after (*right*) gluteoplasty.

add another horizontal midbuttock line (**Fig. 18**). This permits dividing the buttock into 4 quadrants: inner upper, outer upper, inner lower, and outer lower. The ideal buttock has equal volumes above and below this horizontal line, as well as to the left and right of the vertical line. When evaluating the PA view of the gluteus muscle, each of the 4 quadrants should be rated according to whether it has sufficient or deficient volume.

Gluteus muscle volume on lateral view

The presacral zone and the gluteus muscle are evaluated on the lateral view. The presacral area should have a nice inward sweeping curve that resembles a lazy S shape when followed from the midback to below the buttock (**Fig. 19**). If this area has too much fat, the S shape loses its crisp sweep and becomes blunt, which makes the buttock appear flat, at least in its superior aspect. If fullness in the superior aspect exists, the buttock

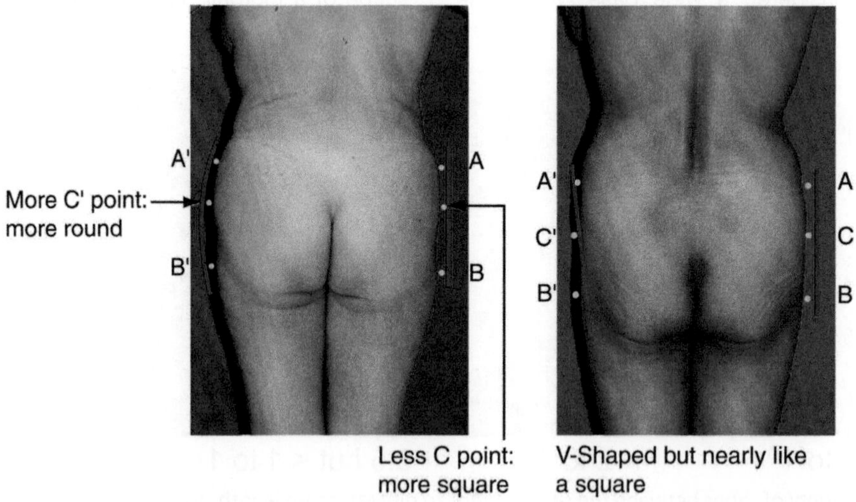

Fig. 16. The types of asymmetrical buttock shapes that may be encountered in a single individual. In the photo on the left, 1 buttock is round and the other more like a square. In the photo on the right, 1 buttock is V-shaped and the other more like a square.

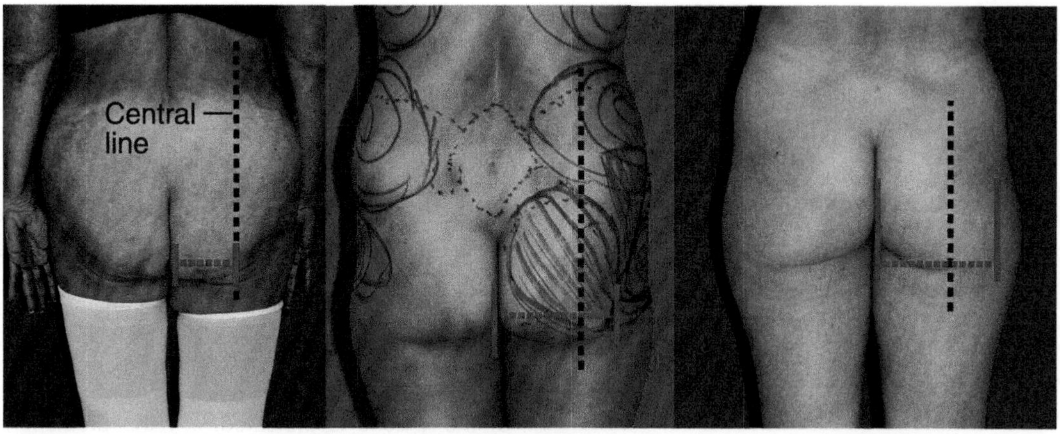

Fig. 17. Defining the inferior gluteal base width as narrow, normal, or wide.

contour can be tremendously improved with liposuction.

The lateral buttock view may be divided into 3 zones: upper, central, and lower (see **Fig. 19**). This division helps determine where most of the buttock bulk or volume is located. In the aesthetic buttock, most of the volume is in the central zone and the remainder of the bulk is equally distributed in the upper and lower zones. The overall impression is one of a C-shaped curve (see **Fig. 19**, this C is backward). It has been suggested that the point of maximum projection should be at the level of the pubic bone.[6]

Working from the zones seen in the lateral view, determine where most of the volume is located: lower, central, or upper buttock zones (**Fig. 20**). This determination is important when deciding what type of procedure or implant will most closely emulate the volume of the ideal buttock. If most of the volume is in the lower buttock, a round intramuscular implant will look best because it adds most of its projection in the upper and central zones and will, therefore, equalize the volumes throughout the buttock. If most of the volume is at the level of the midbuttock (central), any type of intramuscular implant will look good because the buttock is already well balanced. The authors prefer the oval or the round implants in these cases. If most of the volume is in the upper buttock, an anatomic implant will produce the best result because the anatomic shape adds most of its volume inferiorly. In these cases, a round implant will accentuate the already full upper buttock, which in turn emphasizes the volume deficiency in the lower buttock region.[11] The result is a contour that looks disproportionate.

When considering whether to use a round or an anatomic implant, the contour seen on the PA view takes precedence over the contour seen on the lateral view. The PA view determines if the gluteus muscle is tall (2:1 height-to-width ratio), intermediate (greater than 1:1 but <2:1 ratio), or short (1:1 ratio). In the intermediate cases, the lateral view is helpful for making the final determination about implant shape.

Relationship of the Gluteus Maximus Muscle to the Surrounding Frame

For the evaluation of the relationship of the gluteus maximus muscle to the surrounding frame, envision

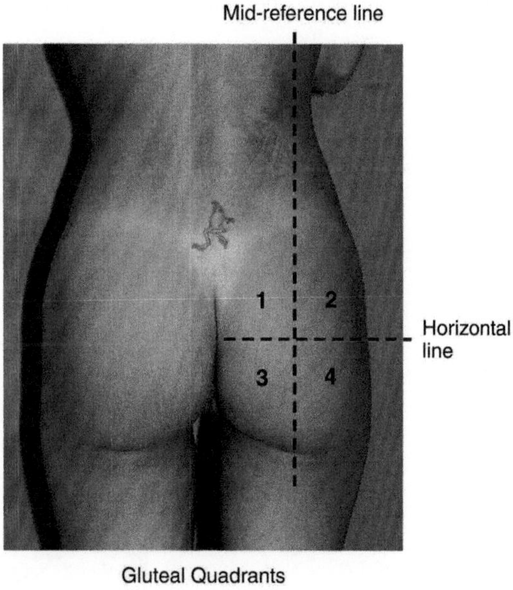

Fig. 18. The 4 gluteal quadrants: 1, inner upper quadrant; 2, outer upper quadrant; 3, inner lower quadrant; and 4, outer lower quadrant. Each quadrant should be evaluated as sufficient or deficient.

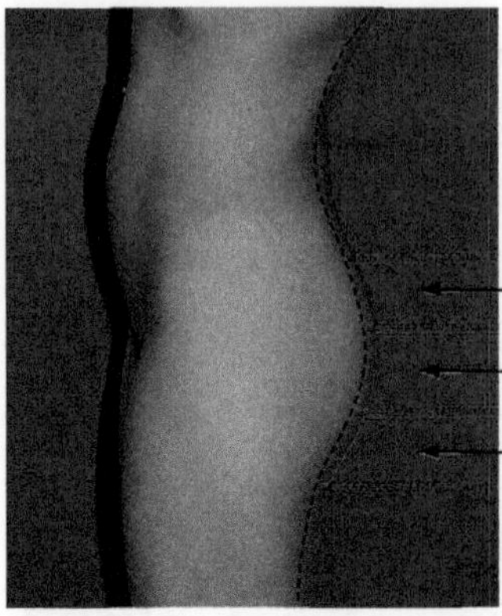

Fig. 19. The 3 zones of the buttock.

the gluteus muscle on the frame but critically examine whether the transition points between the gluteus muscle and the frame junction are smooth. These transitions are best visualized as the points at which the gluteus maximus muscle attaches to the bony framework. There are 4 attachment points that must be evaluated: the upper inner gluteal or sacral junction, the infragluteal fold-thigh junction, the lower lateral gluteal-thigh junction, and the midlateral gluteal-hip junction.

The gluteus muscle in relation to the upper inner gluteal-sacral junction: upper gluteal cleavage

In the upper gluteal cleavage attachment zone, the junction between the intergluteal and sacral space needs to be well-defined so that a V-shaped depression is apparent. This area is called the V-zone.[11] As this zone becomes more defined, the muscle has a greater aesthetic appeal. In the ideal buttock, the gluteal muscle edges should be well-defined and have a semicircular upward turn (**Fig. 21**). The superior edge of the muscle should culminate one-fourth to one-third the distance above the intergluteal crease line. If this space or the muscle edge is not well-defined, the buttock has a blunt and flattened appearance, especially on the lateral view. To improve the V-zone, evaluate whether the bluntness is caused by excess fat, lack of volume in the upper-inner muscle, or both. If the problem is fat, liposuction of the V-zone is indicated.[11] If the problem is lack of muscle volume, then augmentation with either implants or fat transfer is warranted.

The gluteus muscle in relation to the infragluteal fold-thigh junction: lower gluteal cleavage

To describe the gluteus muscle in relation to the infragluteal fold-thigh junction, the intergluteal crease serves as the midline. The upper end of the crease is easily identified; however, the inferior end requires definition. The inferior end of the intergluteal crease is the point where the buttock begins to separate from the midline. In the ideal buttock, this occurs at the lower two-thirds or three-quarters of the muscle (**Fig. 22**). The separation widens until it meets the inner thigh junction. At this point the infragluteal fold takes off from the intergluteal crease at a 45° angle.

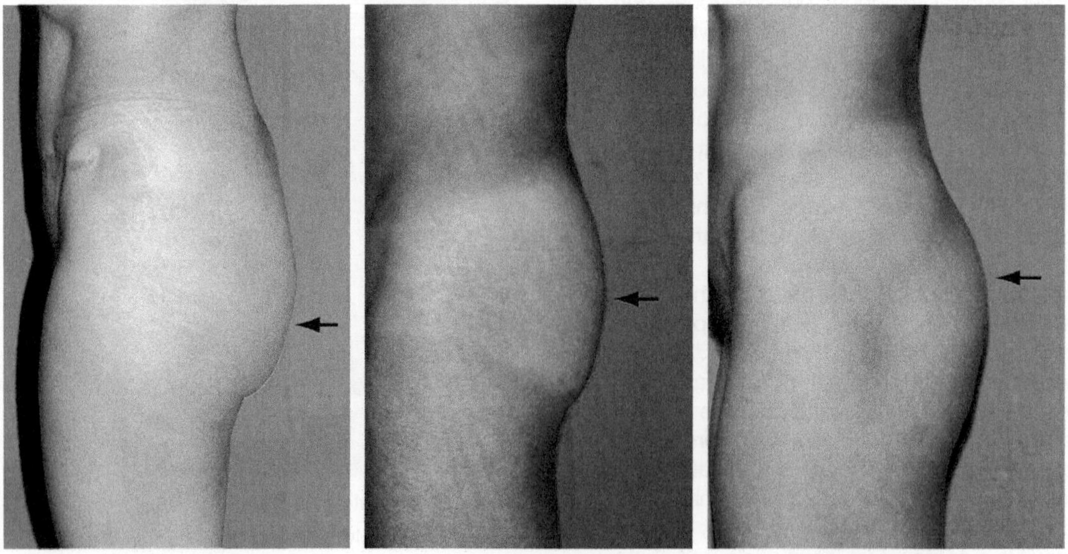

Fig. 20. Most of the buttock volume is located in the lower, central, or upper buttock zone.

In the ideal gluteal aesthetics, the relationship between the infragluteal fold and the inner thigh should create a diamond-shaped space (see **Fig. 22**). A fuller infragluteal fold and inner thigh make the fold more horizontal and the diamond-shaped space turns into a straight line, which is less aesthetically appealing. As the fullness at the junction increases more, the fold develops an inverse relationship and assumes an upward slope (negative angle). For purposes of evaluating the buttocks, the infragluteal fold slant may be defined as a downward slope (in degrees), a horizontal line, or an upward inverse slope.

Improvement of this zone depends on the severity of the fullness. When the infragluteal fold line is horizontal (see **Fig. 22**), liposuction of the inner thigh and infragluteal area may be indicated. For a negative upward slant (see **Fig. 22**), consider infragluteal, as well as inner thigh liposuction, and possible resection of infragluteal fold skin excess (**Fig. 23**). In the ideal buttock, the infragluteal fold should end at the midbuttock or slightly lateral.

The gluteus muscle in relation to the lower lateral thigh and midlateral hip

The last 2 gluteus muscle attachment points that must be evaluated are its relationships to the lower lateral gluteal-thigh junction and the junction of the lateral midbuttock and lateral thigh. In the aesthetic buttock (**Figs. 24** and **25**), the gluteus muscle edges are not seen because the transitions are smooth and produce what appears to be a single unit. In some patients, however, the muscle edge is well-delineated, which creates a sharp demarcation line (see **Figs. 24** and **25**).

These transition zones should be evaluated and graded as a smooth transition (no muscle edge seen), moderate demarcation (muscle edge barely visible), or sharp demarcation (muscle edge well-visualized) (see **Figs. 24** and **25**). As the moderate demarcation becomes more severe, fat transfers should be considered to help soften the transition.

SKIN LAXITY

The main reasons for assessing skin quality is to determine if an upper buttock lift or an excision of excess skin in the infragluteal fold is needed to recontour the buttocks. Skin laxity is seen most often in the patient with massive weight loss (**Fig. 26**). If skin wrinkling is present at points C or B, a buttock lift may be indicated. Another indication for a buttock lift is a severe depression at point C; however, fat transfers may also be required to correct a depression deformity. Always keep in mind that the greater the depression at point C, the greater the likelihood that the patient will benefit from an upper buttock lift.

GLUTEAL PTOSIS

The last step of the buttock evaluation is to determine if any buttock ptosis exists. To make this assessment, the lateral view is used to categorize buttock ptosis into no-ptosis and ptosis groups, both of which have 3 classes or subcategories. This categorization is important for choosing the best buttock reshaping procedure to perform.

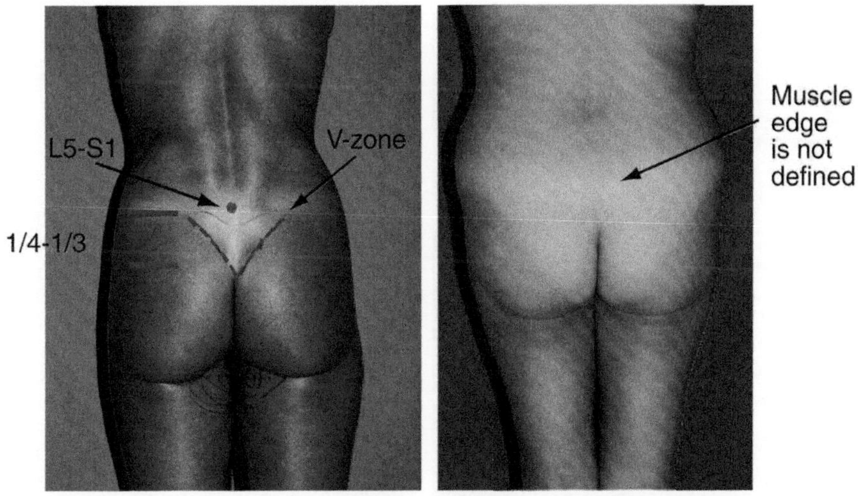

Fig. 21. Evaluating the relationship between the gluteus muscle and the upper inner gluteal-sacral junction. On the left, the dot marks the L5-S1 location, the solid line marks the end of the intergluteal crease line, and the dotted line marks the end of the upper muscle edge. The patient on the left has a well-defined V-zone with visible muscle fullness. The patient on the right has no visible V-zone because of the lack of muscle volume and the presence of presacral fat. The buttocks, therefore, appear flat.

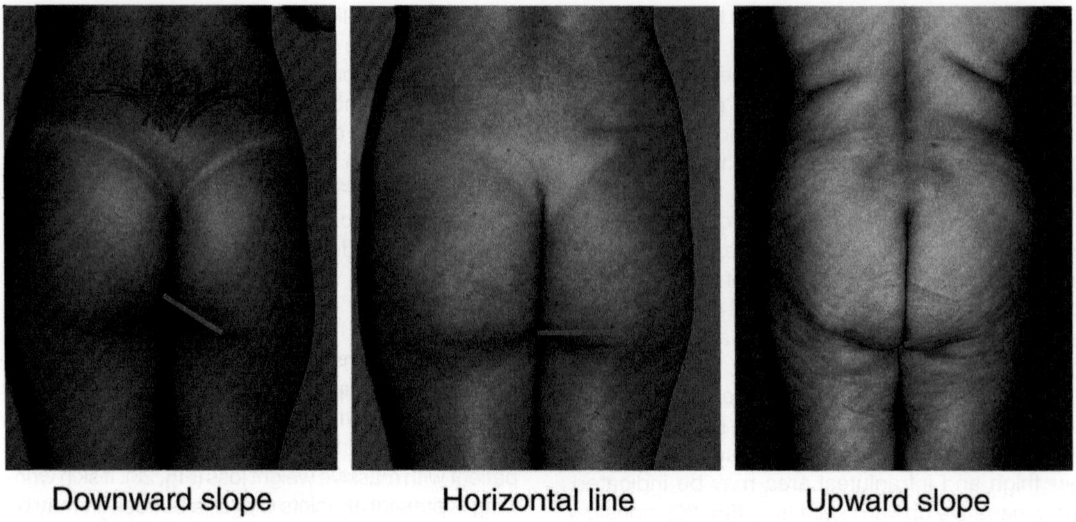

Fig. 22. The infragluteal fold (*red lines*) may have a downward slope (ideal with a well-defined diamond zone), be horizontal, or have an upward slope.

No-Ptosis Categories

In patients with no ptosis, the buttock volume is above the infragluteal fold and there is no drooping skin below the fold. However, the location of most of the buttock volume will vary and assists in categorizing patients with no ptosis into class A, B, or C (**Fig. 27**).

No ptosis: class A

In the no-ptosis class A, most of the buttock volume is centrally located with equal fat distribution in the upper and lower buttock zones. On the lateral view, no ptosis or depressions are evident, and the contour has a smooth C shape. Class A is the ideal shape, with aesthetically pleasing proportions when viewed laterally. Patients with no-ptosis class A require augmentation only.

No ptosis: class B

In the typical appearance of this class, there is no ptotic skin below the infragluteal fold but there is a deficiency or depression in the lower part of the central buttock zone (see **Fig. 27**). For this class, fat transfers should accompany buttock augmentation to the depression, although an anatomic

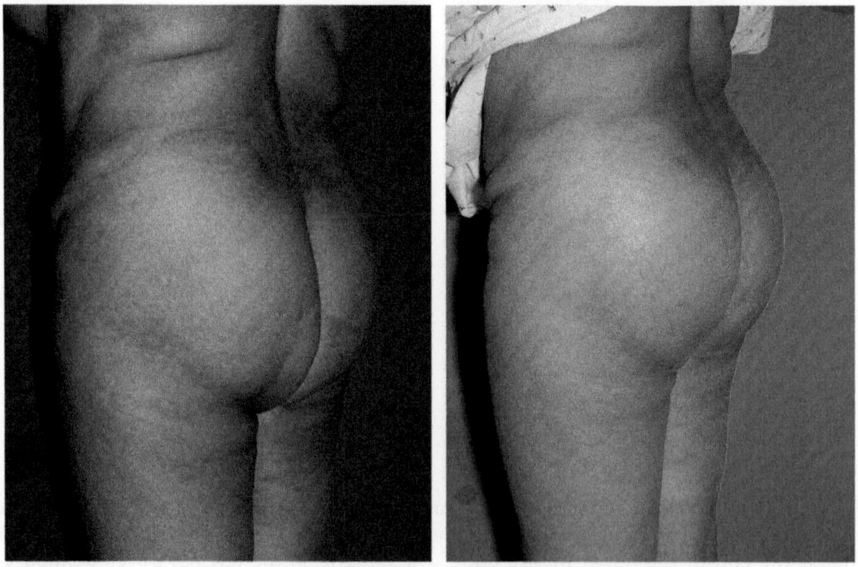

Fig. 23. Before (*left*) and after (*right*) photos of a patient who had augmentation with a large round implant, an infragluteal fold excision, and liposuction of the upper buttock and infragluteal area.

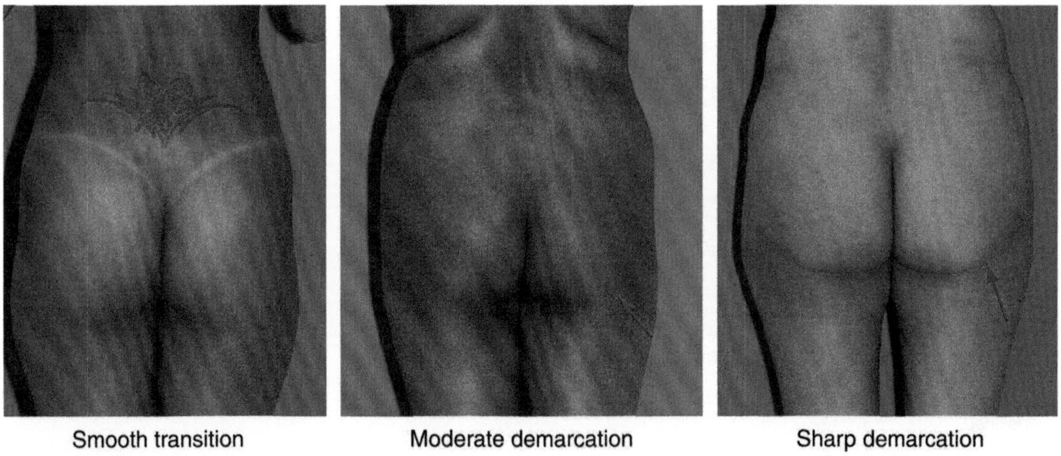

Fig. 24. Evaluating the lower lateral gluteal-thigh junction. The ideal junction is characterized by a smooth transition. Less than ideal transitions may have a moderate or sharp demarcation. Red arrows identify lower lateral gluteal/leg junction.

implant also helps in some cases. Fat transfers can be done at the time of surgery or as a second-stage procedure. Limited, conservative liposuction is another possibility for improving the contour of the lower gluteal area. For surgeons who prefer placing implants in the subfascial plane, a patient with no-ptosis class B is the ideal candidate because a subfacial implant has a more direct impact in this zone.[6]

No ptosis: class C

In the class C category, the skin does not droop below the infragluteal fold but neither is the fold appreciated. The fat is well-distributed throughout the buttocks, and no depressions are seen on the lateral view. An augmentation is usually sufficient for patients with no-ptosis class C.

Ptosis Categories

The ptosis classification applies when skin droops over the infragluteal fold and a skin fold is appreciated. The degree of overhang is divided into grades I, II, and III (**Fig. 28**).

Ptosis: grade I

Grade I ptosis is very similar to no-ptosis class C; however, some buttock volume and skin fall slightly below the infragluteal fold. On the lateral view, a fold of skin is apparent as a horizontal

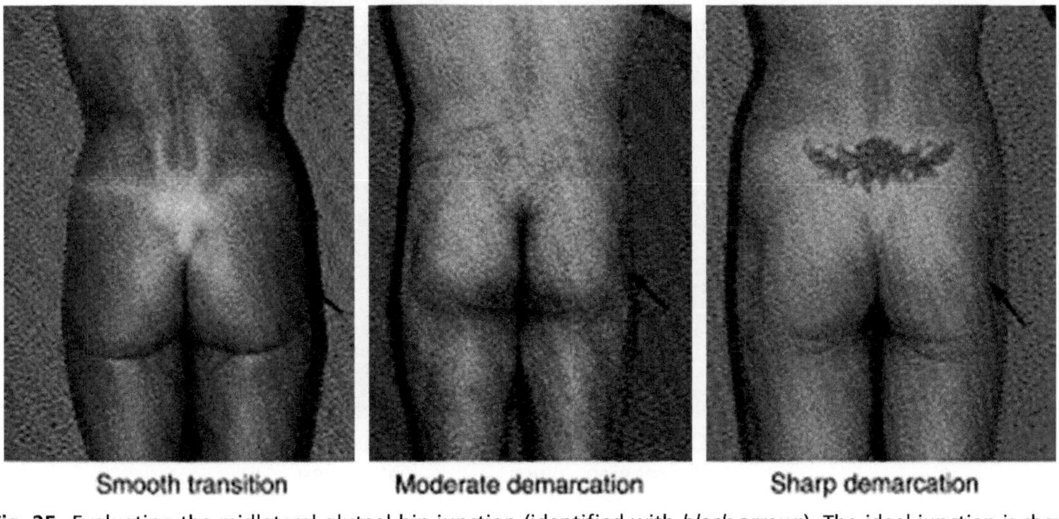

Fig. 25. Evaluating the midlateral gluteal-hip junction (identified with *black arrows*). The ideal junction is characterized by a smooth transition. Less than ideal transitions may have a moderate or sharp demarcation. In all 3 patients, point C has no depression.

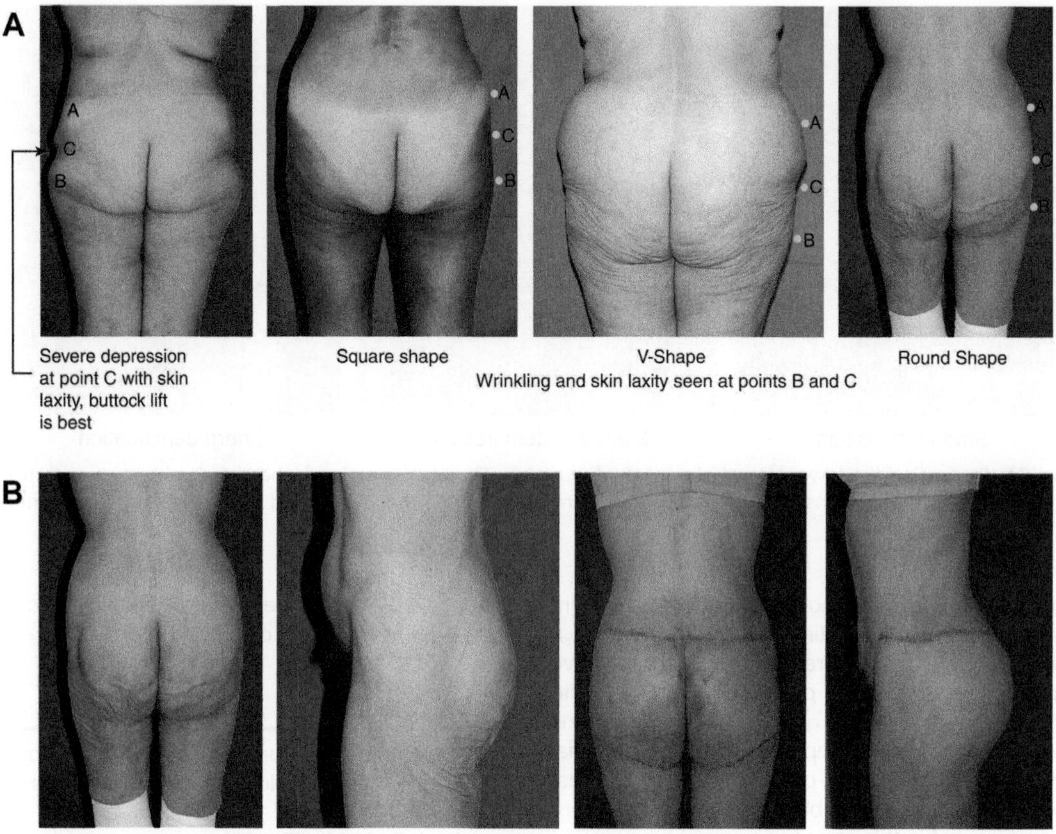

Fig. 26. (*A*) Evaluating skin laxity in buttocks with different shapes. The patient on the left has a severe depression at point C in addition to skin laxity. She is best treated with a buttock lift. The other 3 patients have skin laxity and wrinkling at points B and C. (*B*) The patient in the far right photo of Fig. 26A after undergoing an upper buttock lift with dermal flap. In a second-stage procedure, she had an infragluteal fold lift plus augmentation with an implant.

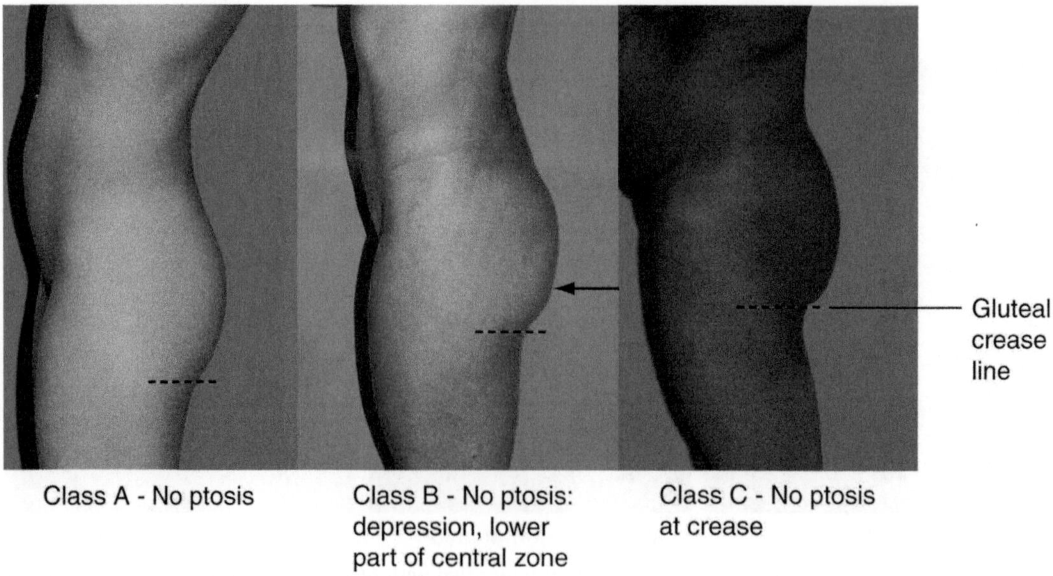

Fig. 27. Characteristics of patients with no gluteal ptosis and their classification into class A, B, or C. Dotted lines represent the infragluteal fold line (sometimes called a crease).

line. In these cases, an augmentation is usually sufficient and an upper buttock lift is rarely needed. In a very small group of patients with ptosis, grade I, excision near the inferior intergluteal crease may be considered but this is extremely rare. The authors recommend performing the augmentation first and then reevaluating the contour after 3 to 6 months.

Ptosis: grade II

In grade II ptosis, the infragluteal fold is apparent and skin droops below it. Whereas a grade I gluteal fold is horizontal, a grade II ptosis fold is more angular. With grade II, there is typically a depression in the upper portion of the lower gluteal zone (see **Fig. 28**). A loss of skin elasticity and presence of stretch marks are other characteristics. If skin wrinkling exists at point C or B, an upper buttock lift is indicated; however, most cases with grade II ptosis receive sufficient improvement with augmentation alone. These patients also may require excision near the inferior intergluteal crease. The authors' recommendation is to perform a gluteal augmentation first and then wait 3 to 6 months to see if excision is indicated.

Ptosis: grade III

Grade III ptosis has the most skin laxity, with the skin drooping well below the infragluteal fold on the lateral view. The fold extends laterally toward the middle of the thigh and its angle is greater than 30°. Also typical is a depression at the lower portion of the central gluteal zone (see **Fig. 28**). Skin wrinkling is common at point B, and the skin has poor elasticity with a fair amount of stretch marks. Treating grade III ptosis requires an upper buttock lift, an infragluteal fold excision, and a gluteal augmentation. Which procedure is performed first is the surgeon's preference.

PUTTING IT ALL TOGETHER

To achieve the best aesthetic buttock, shape buttock contouring and gluteal augmentation must be addressed concomitantly because they are interrelated. When approaching these patients, surgeons should think in terms of contour first and augmentation second. For simplicity, look at the buttock as 2 separate removable structures: the frame and the detachable gluteus maximus muscle. Then divide the evaluation into 4 tasks.

Evaluate the Frame and Gluteal Aesthetic Units

1. Determine if the pelvis is tall, intermediate, or short.
2. Determine the frame type as round, square, A-shaped, or V-shaped, and evaluate the gluteal aesthetic units. Understanding the frame type and status of each gluteal aesthetic unit will help identify which areas may benefit

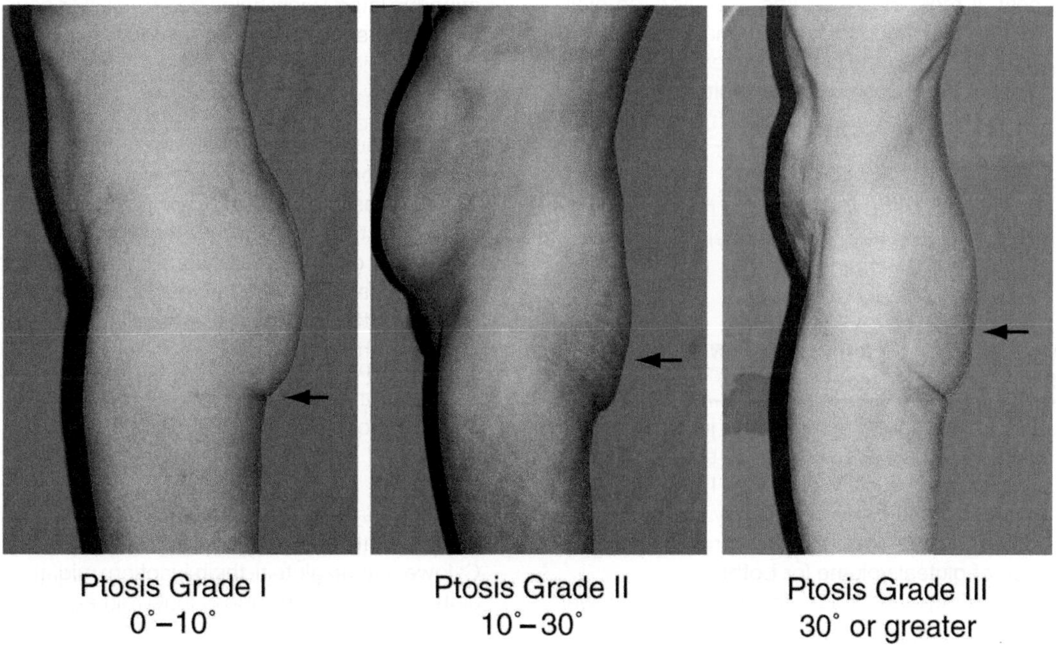

Fig. 28. Grades I, II, and III of gluteal ptosis. In grade I, the angle of the skin fold is less than 10°. In grade II, the angle of the skin fold is between 10° and 30°. Grade III is characterized by a skin fold angle of 30° or more; extension of the lateral fold into the midportion of the thigh is not uncommon with grade III ptosis.

from fat augmentation or liposuction, excision patterns, or surgical incision placement.

3. Determine whether the degree of depression at point C is none, mild, moderate, or severe. The amount of depression will determine if fat transfers are warranted. At this time, also evaluate the presence and amount of skin wrinkling at points A, B, and C.
4. Identify the sacral height as compared with intergluteal crease length. The sacral height should be less than one-third of the crease length. If the sacral height is equal to or greater than the crease length, the intergluteal crease may need to be visually lengthened by adding volume to the upper inner buttock or defining the V-zone with liposuction.

Evaluate the Gluteus Muscle

1. Determine whether the patient has a tall, intermediate, or short gluteus maximus muscle; this will help in implant selection. If the muscle is tall (2:1 ratio) use an intramuscular anatomic implant; if the muscle is short (1:1 ratio) use a round implant. Most patients will have a muscle that falls between tall and short (between 1:1 and 2:1 ratio); in these intermediate cases, a second criterion is needed. Using the lateral photographic view, identify where most of the gluteal volume lies (upper, middle, or lower zone of the buttock). If most of the volume is in the upper buttock, an anatomic implant is best. If most of the volume is central, an oval, round, or anatomic implant may be used. If most of the volume is in the lower zone, a round implant produces the best results.
2. Evaluate the inferior base width of the gluteus muscle to determine whether it is narrow, normal, or wide.
3. Evaluate the 4 quadrants of the muscle (upper-inner, upper-outer, lower-inner, and lower-outer) and determine whether the volume of each is sufficient or deficient.

Evaluate the 4 Junction Points Between the Muscle and the Frame

1. The upper inner gluteus-sacral junction (upper gluteal cleavage) often requires some definition to look aesthetically pleasing. If the area appears flat and blunt, there may be excess fat in the V-zone (intergluteal-sacral space) or a lack of gluteal volume (or both).
2. The infragluteal fold- thigh junction (lower gluteal cleavage) also requires definition. If too much fullness exists, the area that should be a diamond-shaped space is instead a straight line, which is much less appealing. Also evaluate the angle of the infragluteal fold. Does it have a downward 45° angle, run horizontally, or have an inverted upward slope? If excess fat exists, consider liposuction of the inner thigh and inner gluteal fold. Excision of infragluteal fold skin may also be beneficial if there is excess skin in this area.
3. Evaluate the other 2 attachment zones: the lower lateral gluteal-thigh junction and the lateral midbuttock-lateral thigh junction. Is there a smooth transition, moderate demarcation, or sharp demarcation? If there is a moderate or severe demarcation, consider fat transfers.

Evaluate Ptosis (Lateral View)

1. If ptosis exists, is it grade I, II, or III? This information (along with the information obtained from the PA view evaluation of skin laxity or wrinkling at points A, B, or C) will help the surgeon inform patients if they will need either an upper buttock lift (helpful for grades II and III) or a later excision of the inferior intergluteal crease.
2. If no ptosis is present, determine whether the buttock is class A, B, or C. This information will help identify whether fat transfers to the mid-lower gluteal area (class B) or liposuction of the infragluteal area is needed. Ptosis class also is a major factor in deciding whether to use an anatomic or round implant (an anatomic device will better fill in this area). Finally, evaluating the lateral view helps determine if liposuction of the sacral area is indicated.

SUMMARY

Buttock contouring and gluteal augmentation are 2 very different procedures that go hand in hand. This proposed classification system helps evaluate the particular anatomy of each patient and analyzes the important contouring zones of the buttock. In addition, this system standardizes evaluation and helps answer the following questions:

1. Is liposuction needed and, if so, in which gluteal aesthetic units: the flank, sacral area (V-zone), upper buttock (point A), lateral thigh (point B), infragluteal fold, or lower lateral gluteal-thigh junction?
2. Are fat transfers needed and, if so, in what gluteal aesthetic units or transition zones: point C; lower lateral gluteal-thigh junction; midlateral gluteal-hip junction; upper inner gluteal-sacral junction; or lower, central, or lower gluteal zone?
3. Is buttock augmentation needed with fat transfer or with implants?

a. If fat transfer, what volume, to which tissue plane, and to augment which portion of the frame or gluteal aesthetic units?
b. If implants, what shape and size, and what tissue plane (intramuscular, submuscular, or subfascial)?

4. Are any accessory or adjunctive procedures needed for contouring and, if so, which is most beneficial: buttock lift, lower gluteal cleavage crease excision, or infragluteal fold excess excision?

The procedure to perform is up to each individual plastic surgeon's comfort level and sense of aesthetics.

REFERENCES

1. ASERF outlines recommendations to increase safety of gluteal fat grafting procedures. Available at: https://www.surgery.org/media/news-releases/aserf-outlines-recommendations-to-increase-safety-of-gluteal-fat-grafting-procedures. Accessed December 19, 2017.
2. Mofid MM, Teitelbaum S, Suissa D, et al. Report on mortality from gluteal fat grafting: recommendations from the ASERF task force. Aesthet Surg J 2017;37(7):796–806.
3. Mendieta CG. Gluteoplasty. Aesthet Surg J 2003;23:441–55.
4. Robles JM, Tagliaprieta JC, Grandi M. Gluteo- plastia de aumento: implante submusculares. Cir Plast Iberolatinoamericana 1984;10(4):365–9.
5. González-Ulloa M. Gluteoplasty: a ten-year report. Aesthetic Plast Surg 1991;15:85–91.
6. De la Pena JA. Subfascial technique for gluteal augmentation. Aesthet Surg J 2004;24:265–73.
7. Vergara R, Marcos M. Intramuscular gluteal implants. Aesthet Plast Surg 1996;20:259–63.
8. Mendieta CG. Classification system for gluteal evaluation. Clin Plast Surg 2006;33(3):333–46.
9. Mendieta CG. Gluteal reshaping. Aesthet Surg J 2007;27(6):641–55.
10. Centeno RF. Gluteal aesthetic unit classification: a tool to improve outcomes in body contouring. Aesthet Surg J 2006;26(2):200–8.
11. Roberts TL III, Mendieta CG. Buttocks augmentation by micro fat grafting or implants. Presented at the ASAPS Aesthetic Surgery Meeting. Vancouver, Canada, April 15–21, 2004.

Complications in Gluteal Augmentation

Bivik Shah, MD[a,b,*]

KEYWORDS

• Buttocks • Gluteal augmentation • Autologous fat grafting • Complications

KEY POINTS

- Buttock augmetation.
- Buttock augmetation implant complications.
- Overview gluteal fat grafting complications.

Buttocks have always been important aesthetically to the overall torso aesthetics. Dating back to the first or second century BC, the Venus Callipyge statue is famous partly for the bare bottom. Since then, there has been a dramatic increase in the importance and allure of the attractive bottom. This has occurred primarily in the past 2 decades. The confluence of celebrity self-promotion, workout role models, and music videos that visually inspired millions have created a demand for beautiful bottoms.

Plastic surgery as a specialty has also played an important role. Until the past 2 decades, safe and consistent techniques were not well described or part of the mainstream of the specialty. With growing demand from patients and reliable techniques, buttock augmentation has become a staple procedure of many cosmetic plastic surgeons.

The popularity of buttock augmentation continues to rise. It continues to have one of the largest year-over-year increases of any surgical procedure. According to the American Society for Aesthetic Plastic Surgery (ASAPS) statistics, in 2013 there were 11,527 procedures buttock augmentation procedures. In 2016, there were 20,673 buttock augmentation procedures. Comparatively, the number of breast augmentation procedures in 2013 and 2016 were 313,327 and 310,444, respectively.[1,2]

Complications are also increasing. Unfortunately, the severity of the complications with buttock augmentation are significant and higher than in other common procedures in aesthetic plastic surgery.

BUTTOCK AUGMENTATION WITH FAT GRAFTING

Fat grafting for buttock augmentation has emerged as the primary technique used by a majority of plastic surgeons. In 2016, according to the ASAPS statistics, 92% of buttock augmentations were performed with fat transfer and only 8% with implants.[2] I think the explanation of the discrepancy between the number of cases between of the 2 main operations is that implant-based buttock augmentation is a more difficult operation with more immediate negative consequences. Fat grafting to the buttocks can be performed in a simpler fashion. Conceptually, it is not as daunting as implant surgery because there is not as great a worry about complications, such as implant migration, wound dehiscence, ptosis, palpability, and long-term reoperation.

Fat grafting for buttock augmentation began to take shape in the late 1990s and early 2000s.[3–6] It has been used for buttock contour and deformity correction as early as 1986 by Gonzalez and Spina.[7] Reports of complications, however, were lacking. Most of the early reports did not comment on complications or listed complications as "none." These early articles, however, usually included small numbers of patients, a small amount of grafted fat, or were often were used more for correction of deformity than for augmentation.[8,9] Restrepo[4] and Guerrerosantos[3] were probably the first to start reporting complications. Restrepo

[a] Private Practice, Columbus Institute of Plastic Surgery, Columbus, OH 43213, USA; [b] Department of Plastic Surgery, Ohio State University, Columbus, OH 43215, USA
* Private Practice, Columbus Institute of Plastic Surgery, Columbus, OH 43213.
E-mail address: drshah@instituteplasticsurgery.com

Clin Plastic Surg 45 (2018) 179–186
https://doi.org/10.1016/j.cps.2017.12.001

even reported 1 patient that developed sepsis but recovered well.[4]

After almost 2 decades of increasing popularity of the procedure, the notoriety of the procedure, and well-publicized complications, interest has shifted to meticulous documentation and understanding of the complications. There is a wide variation in the amount of fat grafted, graft preparation—high-speed centrifugation versus gravity versus low-speed centrifugation separation, and the anatomic location of the placement of fat.

Seroma

In a recent meta-analysis of all the studies to date, the seroma rate was 3.5%.[10] A seroma after fat grafting buttock augmentation usually occurs in the fat harvest site—the lumbosacral area. Specifically, the sacral triangle is most prone. Another literature review study by Oranges and colleagues[11] found the rate to be 3.1%. Both of these studies did not provide details on the use of suction drains or how aggressive the liposuction in the lumbosacral area was performed. To create the aesthetically pleasing shelf from the lower back to the upper buttock, aggressive liposuction needs to be performed in the lumbosacral area. From liposuction, it is known that seroma formation is dependent on the amount of fat left behind and the amount of denuded fascia. This is similar to the high rates of seroma from latissimus muscle flaps, which are already familiar. To help decrease and manage the impending seroma, some surgeons use a closed suction drain in this area. I now routinely use a closed suction drain and have not had a seroma since I started using a drain. The drain also helps give definition to the lower back upper buttock transition by decreasing the amount of fluid collection that happens in that area, which later seems to turn into fibrosis. Brunner and colleagues[12] looked at 261 fat grafting patients and found that after they started to use 2 drains (in the last 100 patients included in the study) they did not have any seromas.

Infection

Infection rates vary from 0.3% to 1.96% in the various studies published in the literature.[10,11] In 2 large meta-analyses, the infection rates were close to the 2% range.[11] Brunner and colleagues[12] were the first to describe fulminant sepsis with or without disseminated intravascular coagulation.[13,14] Brunner and colleagues reported an incidence of 0.4%. As expected, the most common bacteria were gram-negative (*Escherichia coli*, *Bacteroides fragilis*, Microaerophilic streptococci, *Pseudomonas aeruginosa*, and Enterococci). *Staphylococcus aureus* was one of the lowest, at only 1 of 150 patients. There were 1 patient with a slow-growing *Mycobacterium fortuitum chelonei* and 6 patients with an unknown pathogen.

A rare but consequential complication is the development of sepsis after fat grafting to the buttock. Most of the studies that discussed complications had small numbers of patients, which made it unlikely that sepsis was encountered. In their meta-analysis, Oranges and colleagues[11] found an incidence of 0.4% incidence. Restrepo and Ahmed[4] noted an incidence of 1 of 96 patients.

Bruner and colleagues[12] were also able to decrease the rate of infection from 13.3% initially to less than 2%. They believed this was due to the adoption of their protocol (**Table 1**).[12]

OTHER COMPLICATIONS

Due to the nature of fat grafting and the unpredictable nature of grafted fat resorption, there are a variety of complications that occur but are not quantifiable or measurable. Asymmetry and paraesthesia in the buttock skin and fat harvest sites are encountered. Various studies have put the incidence at 2% to 4%.[4,8,10–12]

FAT RESORPTION

One of the most frustrating aspects of fat grafting in the gluteal region is the amount of fat that does not survive and the lack of control over that process. Most surgeons seem to cite that 50% of the fat does not survive and, therefore, more than (double)

Table 1
Protocol used by Roberts and Bruner to help minimize infections

Preoperative	IV administration of ampicillin, gentamicin, and cefazolin
Preoperative	No shaving of pubic hair—only clipping
Intraoperative	Circumferential preparation
Intraoperative	Lap pad soaked in povidone/iodine placed in gluteal cleft
Intraoperative	Grafting cannula wiped with povidone/iodine before each syringe of fat is injected
Intraoperative	For each 200 cm^3 of fat harvested, add ampicillin 2g, sulbactam 1g, gentamicin 80 mg, and defazolin 2 g

Data from Bruner TW, Roberts TL, Nguyen K. Complications of buttock augmentation: diagnosis, management, and prevention. Clin Plast Surg 2006;33:449–66.

the estimated required volume should be grafted. This further reduces the pool of patients who are good candidates for this procedure. It is difficult to identify the specific origin of this frequently quoted percentage in the literature.

Streit and colleagues[15] recently published a study that showed decanting, centrifugation, and membrane filtration are all similar with some minor differences. One of the studies that best addressed this issue is from Castaneda and Ribeiro.[16] They looked at fat that was injected in the periumbilical area at 60 days, 30 days, 21 days, 15 days, 8 days, 5 days, and 2 days prior to a abdominoplasty. At the time of the abdominoplasty, they evaluated and removed the specimens. The results published in this study seem to be a potential source of the 50% graft survival estimate. They showed that the specimens that were injected at 60 days or 30 days had approximately 50% of the volume that was injected. The also noticed that the fat survived for approximately 1.5 mm from the periphery and the remaining central portion became a capsule/collagen/scar tissue matrix.[16]

To date, there are no published studies that objectively addressed fat survival in gluteal fat augmentation. Several studies have looked at fat survival in vitro, but they have all looked at survivability of fat cells overall, not from a volume standpoint.

OIL CYSTS, FAT NECROSIS, AND HYPERPIGMENTATION

The complications, oil cysts, fat necrosis, and hyperpigmentation, are not frequently discussed in the published series. Yet, they occur. Oil cysts and fat necrosis are difficult to detect because they are usually asymptomatic. If they are near the surface, they can drain spontaneously or only require a minor procedure to be treated. One study reported the incidence of fat necrosis at 4%.[12] In this study, it was a single patient who presented with oily drainage, who was treated with incision, drainage, and pigtail catheter placement.

FAT EMBOLISM

There are 2 potential mechanisms for fat embolization to cause a complication. The first is a mechanical obstruction of the lung vasculature through macroscopic fat particles. The second mechanism is a systemic and pulmonary inflammatory reaction resulting in reactive airway compromise. Mentz[17] describes a mortality rate of 15% with fat embolism with either mechanism. Generally, it is believed that any intraoperative event is most likely mechanical and any event that occurs postoperatively is most likely related to fat embolism syndrome (FES).

The focus currently has been on the mechanical obstruction mechanism through macroscopic fat embolization. There are 2 thoughts on the mechanism of entry of macroscopic fat particles into the vascular system. The first is a cannulation of the gluteal veins (superior or inferior) and the second is a traumatic transection of the gluteal vein by the grafting cannula. Most plastic surgeons lean toward the traumatic transection model for entry of the macroscopic fat particles into the vasculature system.[17–20] Mentz[17] and Wang and colleagues[20] separately came to the conclusion that fat emboli were more likely in individuals with varicosities of the gluteal veins. Wang and colleagues recommend screening for those varicosities.[20] Cardenas-Camarena and Colleagues[21] showed autopsy results of a transected gluteal vein.[22,23] Unfortunately, due to the small number of patients, these theories are difficult to prove or to show a statistically significant preponderance.

The mechanism of entry after a transected vein is by a pressure gradient. The high-pressure extravascular system (due to the introduction of fat into the area and the overall interstitial pressure of approximately 25 mm Hg) joins the low-pressure venous system. The venous system is especially low pressure in hypovolemic intraoperative or postoperative patients.

FAT EMBOLISM SYNDROME

The mechanism for FES is based on fat droplets and lipid globules entering the vasculature. This is usually related to the fat harvesting not the fat injection portion of the procedure. FES patients have been found to have fat droplets in bronchoalveolar lavage, urine, and serum. Diagnosis is usually based on a constellation of symptoms and treatment is only supportive. Gurd[24] delineated major and minor criteria for diagnosis of the syndrome. **Box 1** lists the criteria.

Usually, the neurologic symptoms are the first to appear and range from mild disorientation to a coma. Respiratory symptoms are the next to occur and can range from mild dyspnea to a clinical picture similar to acute respiratory distress syndrome. Approximately 50% of the patients also manifest a petechial rash.[20] The most frequent sign is tachycardia (similar to pulmonary embolism) but unfortunately it is a nonspecific sign. Wang and colleagues[20] published an excellent review of all the clinical and laboratory symptoms and findings related to FES.

The focus has intensified due to the increase in the number of reported deaths secondary to

Box 1
Criteria for fat embolism syndrome diagnosis by Gurd and Wilson

Major criteria
- Respiratory insufficiency
- Cerebral involvement
- Petechial rashes

Minor criteria
- Pyrexia
- Tachycardia
- Retinal changes
- Jaundice
- Renal changes

Laboratory findings
- Anemia
- Thrombocytopenia
- High erythrocyte sedimentation rate
- Fat macroglobulemia in the plasma

Data from Gurd AR, Wilson RI. The fat embolism syndrome. Br J Bone Joint Surg 1974;56:408–16.

gluteal fat grafting. This has also raised the awareness in the media, which has led to increased attention by the plastic surgery community.

An ASAPS Task Force survey evaluated 25 deaths related to gluteal fat grafting and Cardenas-Camarena evaluated 22 deaths from Mexico and Columbia. The ASAPS survey included Mexico and Columbia, so presumably some of these deaths that are reported may be reported in both studies. Based on these 2 studies, there are few important concepts[18]:

- The volume of fat does not correlate with risk of fat embolism.
- Location of fat grafting seems to correlate with risk of fat embolism. The deep gluteus maximus should be avoided. Presumably, becuase that is where the veins are located, they are at greater risk for transection.
- Injection of grafted fat should be limited to the superficial muscle and subcutaneous tissue.
- Cannula size should be 4.1 mm or greater.
- The cannula should be kept parallel to the plane of the buttock to avoid inadvertent deep intramuscular injection.

This risk of death has been calculated to be approximately 1:3000.[18] The ASAPS Task Force stressed that this is an inexact estimate due to the numerous limitations of the methodology of the study. They believe, however, that the estimate is significantly higher than for the other aesthetic procedures. For comparison, the overall mortality in an American Association for Accreditation of Ambulatory Surgery Facilities facility for any aesthetic procedure is 1:55,000 and many orders of magnitude higher than an abdominoplasty, which has been shown to be 1:135,000.[18]

BUTTOCK AUGMENTATION WITH GLUTEAL IMPLANTS

The first gluteal implant was described in 1969 by Bartels and colleagues[25] with a Cronin breast implant.[25,26] It became quickly evident that the mechanical forces of the gluteal region were too much for the thin-shelled silicone breast implants. They were quickly abandoned. At approximately the same time, patients experienced significant problems with wound dehiscence and implant exposure requiring removal.[27] Surgeons quickly moved to a thicker shell silicone gel implant. In the United States, a different route was taken. Due to the silicone gel breast implant moratorium and Food and Drug Administration regulations, these thicker-shelled silicone gel implants were never used in the United States. Instead, a solid silicone elastomer was used with and without a mild texturing on the surface. This mild texturing surface is completely different from the texturing process used in breast implants by the various manufacturers.

There are also significant variations in the aesthetic goals and requests by patients based on geography. These have resulted in significant differences in patient populations, average implant size, and type of implant in the various studies. Although the types of complications are similar, this places significant limitations on the ability to extrapolate the results to all geographic regions.

There are 3 main locations for placement of the implant in the gluteal region—subfascial, intramuscular, and submuscular. Based on a survey study by Mofid and colleagues[28] (19 respondents), 68% use the intramuscular technique.[28–30] A recent analysis of all recently published studies by Sinno and colleagues[10] showed a complication rate of 62.1% for the subfascial technique, 28.1% for the submuscular technique, and 8.8% for the intramuscular technique.

A significant limitation of all these studies is that most do not list the size of implants used. Different techniques have different limitations on the size of the implant that can be used. The subfascial technique allows for the largest implant to be used and is not protected by robust soft tissue coverage compared with intramuscular and submuscular techniques. There seems to be as a lower incidence of seromas with the 2 muscular techniques, perhaps because there is less subfascial dissection.

The overall complication rate also varied significantly between techniques. The overall complication rate ranged from the 30% range to some (with smaller numbers of patients) in the 8% to 10% range.[4,7,10,11] This is again probably due to the wide variation in technique, implants size used, and implant type used (silicone gel vs solid silicone). Some studies were based on surgeons using both techniques used throughout the study period. This article focuses on those risks that are universal to all 3 types of techniques.

INFECTION

The infection rate varies from 1% to 7%.[10,12,31–34] Senderoff[32] showed that he was able to decrease his infection rate down to 2% by using techniques used in breast augmentation, including an alcohol-based preoperative scrub by the patient, povidone/iodine soap scrub prior to the povidone/iodine preparation, a sterile towel on the skin to minimize contamination by skin flora, and minimal handling/skin contact of the implant.

The most common bacterium found was *Staphylococcus aureus* in 11 of 13 patients in Senderoff's study.[32] *Escherichia coli* was found in 1 of the 13 patients.[32] No other study noted the pathogen or even if cultures were obtained. There were no serious infections, similar to gluteal fat grafting.

SEROMA

The seroma rate varied from 3.7% to 19%.[4,5,8,12] Senderoff[32] was able to decrease the seroma rate from 9.09% to 2% with the use of quilting sutures in the subfascial patients. Not all studies had surgeons who used drains. This was especially true in the studies where the primary technique was intramuscular or submuscular. Senderoff[32] and Serra[37] were the only ones to describe the beneficial use of quilting sutures.

The studies from the United States consistently showed a higher seroma rate compared with South American and Central American counterparts. The limited number of patients and lack of detail about the implants make it difficult to pinpoint the root cause. There are certainly many differences, however. These include type of implant, size of implant, location of the implant, use of drains, and soft textured implants, and smooth implants.

Most studies agree that a seroma is the harbinger of wound dehiscence and, therefore, seroma management is critical to overall failure or success of the procedure. To that extent, Senderoff[32] proposes routine, scheduled aspiration at 1 week after the procedure. More aspirations are scheduled on a weekly basis depending on if any fluid was removed at 1 week.[32]

The studies with the lower seroma rates usually were based on patients who had the intramuscular or submuscular techniques.[34,35]

WOUND DEHISCENCE

Wound dehiscence rates are reported as high as 30% to 40%.[12,36] This is the most frustrating complication. It increases the chance for implant exposure and subsequent removal. Additionally, it makes it difficult for patients to manage their recovery and makes the resultant scar significantly worse. Mendieta[36] also agreed that this was his most significant frustration.

Again, there is large discrepancy between the US surgeons and the Central and South American surgeons. Consistently the US surgeons have a higher wound dehiscence rate than their counterparts to the south. The Central and South American surgeons have reported a rate of 2% to 5%.[33,34,37,38] One significant difference that is not often discussed in the literature is the size of the implants used. Serra and colleagues[37] believe that the size of the implant did not matter. Rather they believe that the development of a seroma was the harbinger of wound dehiscence.[37] In the article, however, no mention was made of the mean implant size used. All the patients in the article had implants of 300 cm^3. Also, he only performed intramuscular implants. This significantly limits the size of the implant that can be placed. The intramuscular technique also decreases the risk of implant exposure and subsequent removal. The lack of information about the implant sizes used makes it difficult to assess if there is any significant difference in the average implant sizes used in the United States compared with South and Central America. Mendieta[36] believed that the implants sizes used in the United States were larger and this played a significant role in the increased wound dehiscence rate.[36]

IMPLANT REMOVAL

The implant removal rate is equally varied as the wound dehiscence rate. The rate has been reported to be anywhere from 1.5% to 30%.[32,36] Most plastic surgeons believe this is due to implant size and type of implant. A large implant requires greater force for the retraction to insert the implant, resulting in greater tissue injury. Large implants have greater tissue tension. Also, in the United States, there are limits to firmer implants because the silicone gel implants are not available.

This further requires more forceful retraction and results in greater subsequent injury.

Most aesthetic surgeons have tried to manage this risk by matching patients to implant size, limiting sizes offered, and restricting activity for a longer period of time. Setting patient expectations with respect to what is achievable is also helpful. The possibility of dissatisfaction with the amount of volume augmentation as well as potential solutions should be discussed. A second operation to put a larger implant (after adequate time to allow tissue expansion) or fat grafting if patients have enough fat are possible alternatives.

CAPSULAR CONTRACTURE

Capsular contracture is a rarely seen complication with gluteal implant augmentation. Sinno and colleagues[10] reported a rate of 0.55% (1 patient who was seen 2 years after implantation). This was a composite based on a review of all the published articles at that point. This is a complication that has not been reported in virtually any other studies.

More research is needed to determine why there is such a difference between breast implants and gluteal implants. This is also true for Central and South American colleagues who are using silicone gel implants. These implants are similar to currently used breast implants. Another point of interest is that the location of the implant—submuscular, subfascial, or intramuscular—does not seem to affect the capsular contracture rate. Regardless of the location, the rate is barely detectable.

OTHER COMPLICATIONS

The usual complications of using implants all exist—hematoma 0.63%, sciatica 1%, asymmetry, implant malposition, implant rotation, and implant revision. These vary based on the location of implant. In general, intramuscular and submuscular techniques have less rotation but higher malposition.

LONG-TERM COMPLICATIONS

Unfortunately, there are no studies that have looked at any significant number of patients over a long period of time. The most common complications are implant ptosis and implant rotation with expansion of the pocket. Both of these are such a common yet unreported complications that there are a host of YouTube videos that show patients "flipping" their own implants. Although the incidence has not been reported for any long-term complications, there is a general consensus that they exist. The solutions to these long-term complications are often difficult. The best results are obtained with removal of the implant and delayed replacement 3 months to 6 months later. The literature suggests that this is more likely in the subfascial placement versus the intramuscular or submuscular placement.

AUTO-AUTOLOGOUS BUTTOCK AUGMENTATION

The first reports of using a patient's own tissue for augmentation seem to come from Pascal and Le Louarn in 2002.[39] This technique seems to have many benefits that elude the other primary techniques. With autologous (auto-augmentation), there is vascularized tissue that normally is discarded, tissue that is often in abundance, and tissue that is in the same area as the primary skin removal procedure. I believe its acceptance into mainstream buttock augmentation is limited for 2 reasons. First, this procedure can only be applied to a small subset of patients who require a true lower body lift, that is, not the majority of patients requesting buttock augmentation. Even among the patients who have significant excess skin and tissue in the lower truncal region, not all are good candidates for the procedure due to their anatomy and aesthetic preferences. Second, these procedures can become arduously long and have a gradual, lengthy learning curve, which prevented a more thorough adoption by massive weight loss surgeons.

COMPLICATIONS OF AUTOLOGOUS (AUTO-AUGMENTATION) BUTTOCK AUGMENTATION

Overall, I believe the primary complications are those ordinarily encountered from the primary skin reduction surgery. There does seem, however, to be an increase in some aspects.

Srivastava[40–42] retrospectively looked at his patients that had auto-augmentation versus those who did not have any augmentation, only skin removal. They found an increase in the total complication rate (42.5% vs 19.70%). This increase, however, was solely due to the significant increase in the wound dehiscence rate (30% vs 10.6%). All other complications—hematoma, seroma, infection, necrotic tissue, suture extrusion, and suture abscess—did not have any significant differences between the 2 groups. This seems appropriate given the increase in tension, undermining, and difficulty in preplanning the amount of skin resection.

Colwell and Borud[43] looked at autologous augmentation with a dedicated perforator for the flap. This, however, did not change the spectrum of complications. The most frequent complications continued to be wound dehiscence and some minimal fat necrosis.

Srivastava[40] found that increasing body weight, even when the body mass index was not significant, correlated significantly with increasing complications—wound dehiscence.

Schmitt[44] also looked at autologous auto-augmentation versus no augmentation. They had preponderance of augmentation patients (238 patients vs 42 patients). Also, their patients included implant and fat-based augmentation patients. A majority of the patients were autologous augmentation patients (76% vs 5% vs 4%). Again, there was no difference between the augmentation and the nonaugmentation groups for hematoma, seroma, infection, wound dehiscence, and all complications. This is different from Gusenoff[40], who found a significantly higher rate of wound dehiscence.

Overall, I believe the primary issues with auto-augmentation are wound dehiscence and the ability to achieve aesthetic ideals.

SUMMARY

Gluteal augmentation is rapidly gaining in popularity and this is driving aesthetic surgeons to quickly gain experience and develop techniques to meet patient expectations. Currently, the 2 main techniques—gluteal fat grafting and gluteal implant—for augmentation have significant limitations.

Autologous fat grafting seems to have a mortality rate that is75 times that of an abdominoplasty. This is not a sustainable rate of mortality. Society and individual surgeons are developing guidelines for the procedure based on theoretic etiologies. In a personal communication with a Columbian surgeon (Mauricio Herrera, MD, personal communication, 2017), he has stopped performing any gluteal fat grafting procedures due to the high mortality rate. Gluteal implant augmentation is also fraught with problems. Although it is rare to have the dire complication of gluteal fat grafting, it can be frustrating for surgeons and dissatisfying for patients. The risk of implant exposure limits the size of the implant, which requires a patient to settle for less. The placement of an implant in the intramuscular or submuscular location requires patient and surgeon to accept limitations in lower pole fullness, of a smaller pool of ideal patients for the procedure, and on which part of the buttock that is augmented.

REFERENCES

1. American Society for Aesthetic Plastic Surgery 2013.
2. American Society for Aesthetic Plastic Surgery 2016.
3. Guerrerosantos J. Autologous fat grafting for body contouring. Clin Plast Surg 1996;23:619–31.
4. Restrepo JC, Ahmed JA. Large-volume lipoinjection for gluteal augmentation. Aesthet Surg J 2002;22(1): 33–8.
5. Peren PA, Gomez JB, Guerrerosantos J, et al. Gluteus augmentation with fat grafting. Aesthetic Plast Surg 2000;24:412–7.
6. Cardenas-Camarena L, Lacouture AM, Tobar-Losada A. Combined gluteoplasty: liposuction and lipoinjection. Plast Reconstr Surg 1999;140(5):1524–31.
7. Gonzalez R, Spina L. Grafting of fat obtained by liposuction: technique and instruments. Rev Bras Cir 1986;76:243–50.
8. Pedroza LV. Fat transplantation to the buttocks and legs for aesthetic enhancement or correction of deformities: long-term results of large volumes of fat transplant. Dermatol Surg 2000;26(12):1145–9.
9. Monreal J. Fat tissue as a permanent implant: new instruments and refinements. Aesthet Surg J 2003; 23(3):213–6.
10. Sinno S, Chang JB, Brownstone ND, et al. Determining the safety and efficacy of gluteal augmentation: a systematic review of outcomes and complications. Plast Reconstr Surg 2016;137(4):1151–6.
11. Oranges CM, Tremp M, di Summa PG, et al. Gluteal augmentation techniques: a comprehensive literature review. Aesthet Surg J 2017;37(5):560–9.
12. Bruner TW, Roberts TL III, Nguyen K. Complications of buttocks augmentation: diagnosis, management, and prevention. Clin Plast Surg 2006;33:449–66.
13. Kamal M, El-Ali TG. Assessment of the risk of systemic fat mobilization and fat embolism as a consequence of liposuction: ex vivo study. Plast Reconstr Surg 2006;117(7):2269–76.
14. Condé-Green A, Kotamarti V, Nini KT, et al. Fat grafting for gluteal augmentation: a systematic review of the literature and meta-analysis. Plast Reconstr Surg 2016;138(3):437e–46e.
15. Streit L, Jaros J, Sedlakova V, et al. A comprehensive in vitro comparison of preparation techniques for fat grafting. Plast Reconstr Surg 2017;139:670e.
16. Carpaneda CA, Ribeiro MT. Study of the histologic alterations and viability of the adipose graft in humans. Aesthetic Plast Surg 1993;17:43–7.
17. Mentz HA. Fat emboli syndromes following liposuction. Aesthetic Plast Surg 2008;32:737–8.
18. Mofid MM, Teitelbaum S, Suissa D, et al. Report on mortality from gluteal fat grafting: recommendations from the ASERF Task Force. Aesthet Surg J 2017; 37(7):796–806.
19. Astarita DC, Scheinin LA, Sathyavagiswaran L. Fat transfer and fatal macroembolization. J Forensic Sci 2015;60(2):509–10.
20. Wang HD, Zheng JH, Deng CL, et al. Fat embolism syndromes following liposuction. Aesthetic Plast Surg 2008;32:731–6.
21. Cárdenas-Camarena L, Bayter JE, Aguirre-Serrano H, et al. Deaths caused by gluteal lipoinjection: what are

we doing wrong? Plast Reconstr Surg 2015;136(1): 58–66.
22. Coronado-Malagón M, Visoso-Palacios P, Arce-Salinas CA. Fat embolism syndrome secondary to injection of large amounts of soft tissue filler in the gluteal area. Aesthet Surg J 2010;30(3): 448–50.
23. Harrison D, Selvaggi G. Gluteal augmentation surgery: indications and surgical management. J Plast Reconstr Aesthet Surg 2007;60:922–8.
24. Gurd AR, Wilson RI. The fat embolism syndrome. Br J Bone Joint Surg 1974;56:408–16.
25. Bartels RJ, O'Malley JE, Douglas WM, et al. An unusual use of the Cronin breast prosthesis. Case report. Plast Reconstr Surg 1969;44(5):500.
26. Nolte WJ, Olofsson T, Scherstén T, et al. Evaluation of the Gurd test for fat embolism. J Bone Joint Surg Br 1974;56B(3):417–20.
27. Douglas WM, Bartels RJ, Baker JL. An experience in aesthetic buttocks augmentation. Clin Plast Surg 1975;3(3):471–6.
28. Mofid MM, Gonzalez R, de la Peña JA, et al. Buttock augmentation with silicone implants: a multicenter survey review of 2226 patients. Plast Reconstr Surg 2013;131(4):897–901.
29. Serra F, Aboudib JH. Gluteal implant displacement: diagnosis and treatment. Plast Reconstr Surg 2014;134(4):647–54.
30. Rosique RG, Rosique MJ, De Moraes CG. Gluteoplasty with autologous fat tissue: experience with 106 consecutive cases. Plast Reconstr Surg 2015; 135(5):1381–9.
31. Serra F, Aboudib JH, Marques RG. Reducing wound complications in gluteal augmentation surgery. Plast Reconstr Surg 2012;130(5):706e–13e.
32. Senderoff DM. Buttock augmentation with solid silicone implants. Aesthet Surg J 2011;31(3):320–7.
33. Andrade G, Coltro P, Farina Junior J, et al. Gluteal augmentation with silicone implants: a new proposal for intramuscular dissection. Aesthetic Plast Surg 2017;41(4):872–7.
34. Aboudib JH, Serra F, de Castro CC. Gluteal augmentation: technique, indications, and implant selection. Plast Reconstr Surg 2012;130(4):933–5.
35. Senderoff DM. Aesthetic surgery of the buttocks using implants: practice-based recommendations. Aesthet Surg J 2016;36(5):559–76.
36. Mendieta C. Intramuscular gluteal augmentation technique. Clin Plast Surg 2006;33:423–34.
37. Serra F, Aboudib JH, Cedrola JP, et al. Gluteoplasty: anatomic basis and technique. Aesthet Surg J 2010; 30(4):579–92.
38. Vergara R, Amezcua H. Intramuscular gluteal implants: 15 years' experience. Aesthet Surg J 2003; 23(2):86–91.
39. Pascal JF, Le Louarn C. Remodeling bodylift with high lateral tension. Aesthetic Plast Surg 2002; 26(3):223–30.
40. Srivastava U, Rubin JP, Gusenoff JA. Lower body lift after massive weight loss: auto-augmentation vs no augmentation. Plast Reconstr Surg 2015;135(3): 762–72.
41. Centeno RF. Autologous gluteal augmentation with circumferential body lift in the massive weight loss and aesthetic patient. Clin Plast Surg 2006;33: 479–96.
42. Centeno RF, Mendieta CG, Young VL. Gluteal contouring surgery in the massive weight loss patient. Clin Plast Surg 2008;35:73–91 [discussion: 93].
43. Colwell AS, Borud LJ. Autologous gluteal augmentation after massive weight loss: aesthetic analysis and role of the superior gluteal artery perforator flap. Plast Reconstr Surg 2007;119(1):345–56.
44. Schmitt T, Jabbour S, Makhoul R, et al. Lower body lift in the massive weight loss patient: a new classification and algorithm for gluteal augmentation. Plast Reconstr Surg 2017. [Epub ahead of print].

Practice-Based Patient Management Strategies in Gluteal Augmentation with Implants

Douglas M. Senderoff, MD*

KEYWORDS

• Gluteal implants • Gluteal augmentation • Buttock implants • Buttock augmentation
• Gluteal implant complications • Gluteal implant revision

KEY POINTS

- Address patients' expectations during the consultation to avoid postoperative dissatisfaction. Discuss benefits and point out risks associated with implants greater than 350 cm^3.
- Patient anatomy dictates implant selection. Implants vary in projection, diameter, and width and must be selected according to patient dimensions.
- Choose the appropriate insertion plane that will produce the best result with the least likelihood of aesthetic and surgical complications.
- Address complications early, and recognize when surgical intervention is required. Complications become more difficult to remedy when there is a delay in treatment.
- Revision surgery can be successfully performed to correct implant malposition or to replace implants removed because of infection.

HISTORY

Gluteal augmentation with implants (GAI) first appeared in the scientific literature in an article in *Plastic and Reconstructive Surgery* in 1969 by Bartels and colleagues[1] where he described placing a round breast implant into the left gluteal muscle to correct asymmetry of the muscle due to atrophy. This implant was inserted through an infragluteal incision, which is not the current surgical approach to gluteal implant placement. Cosmetic gluteal enhancement was first described in 1973 by Cocke and Ricketson[2] using a silicone breast implant placed subcutaneously. The results were suboptimal. Subcutaneous gluteal implant placement for the correction of "sad" buttocks was described by Gonzalez-Ulloa[3] using gel implants with fixation ears. Three surgical approaches to implantation were described, including bilateral supragluteal, infragluteal fold, and the intergluteal crease.

The first description of gluteal implant placement beneath the gluteus maximus and medius muscles was by Robles and Tagliapietra in 1984.[4] This approach reduced the incidence of capsular contracture but required positioning in the upper third of the buttocks to avoid the sciatic nerve.[5]

Intramuscular implant placement first appeared in the literature in 1996 in an article by Vergara and Marcos.[6] In this article, they described placement of gluteal implants 2 to 3 cm below the gluteus maximus muscle through an intergluteal incision. This approach avoided dissection near the sciatic nerve while providing adequate coverage of the implant. In an article by De la Pena[7] in 2004, the technique of subfascial implant placement was described. In this article, the

The author has nothing to disclose.
Mount Sinai Beth Israel Medical Center, New York, NY, USA
* Park Avenue Aesthetic Surgery, 461 Park Avenue South, New York, NY 10016, USA
E-mail address: aestheticdoc@aol.com

Clin Plastic Surg 45 (2018) 187–195
https://doi.org/10.1016/j.cps.2017.12.002

investigator discussed the benefits of subfascial implantation, including avoiding muscle dissection and potential sciatic nerve injury while providing a stable periprosthetic space. In a 2012 cadaver study by Hwang and colleagues,[8] the thickness and tension of the gluteal aponeurosis was evaluated and found to be of sufficient strength to hold subfascial gluteal implants in the proper position.

CURRENT SURGICAL APPROACH

The current approach to GAI is based on 3 variables: implant position, implant shape, and choice of incision. Subfascial and intramuscular are the two placements most widely used, whereas subcutaneous placement is not advisable. The choice of incision is either single intergluteal or bilateral paramedian. In a 2013 survey by Mofid and colleagues[9] of US and international surgeons, 53% preferred a single midline incision. In a 2015 survey by Mezzine, 84% of French surgeons preferred a single midline incision.[10] The author's preferred approach is a single midline intergluteal incision. Implants are available as either round or anatomic shapes with varying degrees of texturing. Surgeons in the United States have access only to soft-solid silicone elastomer implants. Cohesive gel implants are not approved by the Food and Drug Administration for use in the United States.

PATIENT SELECTION

The 5 main indications, precautions, and contraindications for buttock augmentation with implants were described in a 2016 continuing medical education article by the author.[11]

Indications for gluteal augmentation with implants

- Lack of volume
- Lack of projection
- Buttock asymmetry
- Contour deformity
- Limited fat for transfer

Precautions

- Body mass index greater than 30
- Prior buttock injections
- Poor wound healing
- Autoimmune disease
- Radiation to buttocks

Contraindications

- General or local infection
- Diabetes
- Psychological instability
- Inadequate soft tissue
- Unrealistic expectations

Once the decision is made to proceed with gluteal implant surgery, decisions regarding implant placement and implant shape need to be determined. These decisions are based on an understanding of the gluteal anatomy and the aesthetic considerations of an ideal buttock.

The aesthetic evaluation of buttock implant patients has been described by Mendieta[12] whereby he discusses importance of the contribution of muscle and fat specific to each patient.

An understanding of the surgical anatomy is essential to creating an attractive buttock.

The clinical anatomy of the buttock has been well described in a 2006 article by Centeno and Young.[13] A 2010 article by Serra and colleagues[14] discusses the surgical anatomy of the buttock emphasizing the variations in the exit of the sciatic nerve. Characteristics of beautiful buttocks have been well described in a 2006 article by Cuenca-Guerra and Lugo-Beltran,[15] including 4 consistent features.

Features of beautiful buttocks

- Lateral depressions
- Short infragluteal fold
- V-shaped crease of sacral triangle
- Supragluteal fossettes

Buttock implants are commonly placed in either the subfascial or intramuscular position (**Figs. 1** and **2**). Surgeons should be familiar with the advantages and disadvantages of these surgical approaches. Several surveys have shown a surgeon preference for intramuscular placement.[9,10]

There is no single-surgeon published study showing the superiority of either subfascial or intramuscular placement of gluteal implants. In the author's published series of 200 consecutive buttock implantations, there was no significant difference in infection rates between subfascial and intramuscular gluteal implants.[16] A 2013 review of 30 articles comparing different pocket locations by Flores-Lima and colleagues[17] determined intramuscular placement to have the lowest complication rate. There are several advantages and disadvantages to the intramuscular technique of GAI that surgeons need to be aware of.

Advantages of intramuscular placement

- Less palpability
- Less visibility
- Less infragluteal stretching

Disadvantages of intramuscular placement

- Indistinct dissection plane
- Lack of inferior fullness
- Proximity to sciatic nerve

In addition, the size of the implant that can be placed intramuscularly is limited by the width of

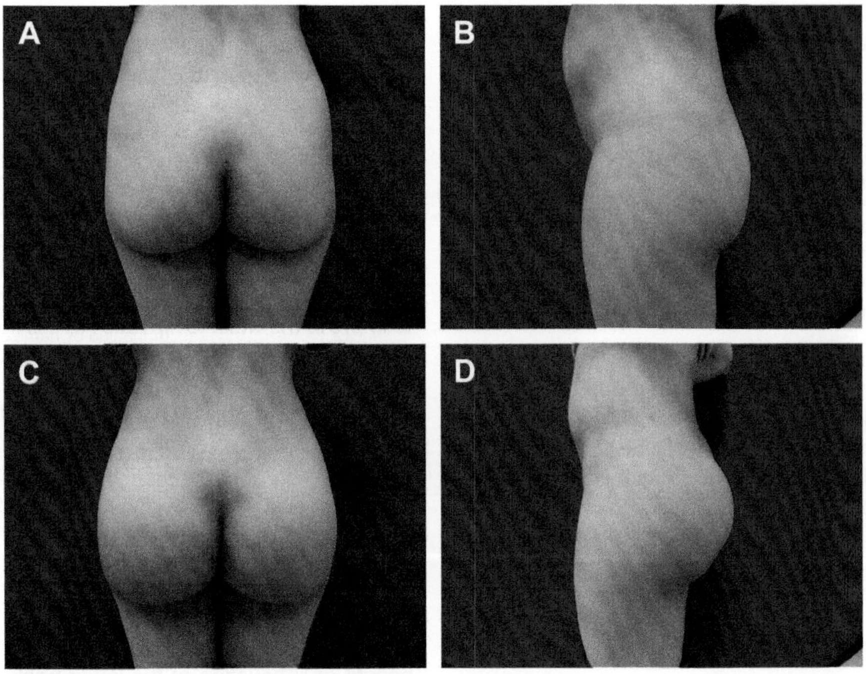

Fig. 1. A 35-year-old woman with buttock hypoplasia requesting increase in volume and projection. (*A, B*) Six months after subfascial gluteal augmentation with 276 cm^3 solid, round silicone implants. (*C, D*) Note improvement in volume and point of maximal projection.

the gluteal musculature and the ability to obtain a secure tension-free muscle approximation.[18,19] The question of implant-related changes to the gluteal musculature was addressed by Serra through volumetric evaluation using computed tomography (CT) scans and functional assessment studies. Intramuscular implantation resulted in atrophy of the gluteus maximus muscle between 2.6% and 6.4% with a subsequent return of strength and no physical limitations.[20,21] The intramuscular surgical technique has been well described in the surgical literature; although not the focus of this article, several key points should be noted. Dissection should be blunt and maintain a 2- to 3-cm muscle thickness over the implant with sizers being useful to determine the adequacy of dissection.[22–24] Palpable landmarks as described by Gonzalez[25,26] can be used to guide intramuscular dissection to optimize correct implant positioning and avoid superficial dissection and insufficient muscle coverage. The gluteus maximus is at risk for perforation as it curves downward laterally. The use of intraoperative ultrasonography has been reported to aid in dissection of the muscle to maintain sufficient thickness.[27]

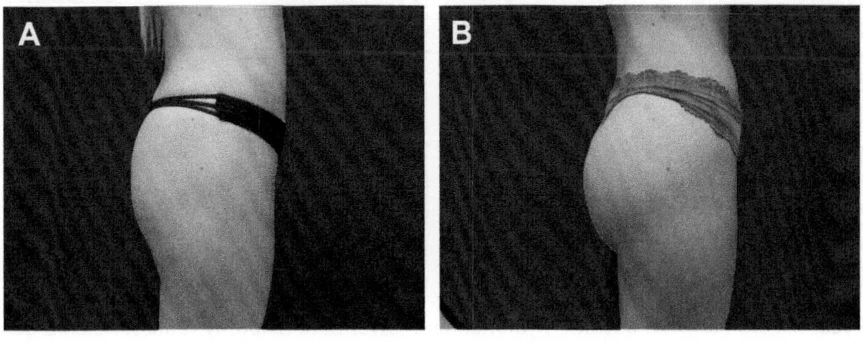

Fig. 2. A 28-year-old woman with buttock hypoplasia requesting increase in volume and projection. (*A*) Six months after intramuscular gluteal augmentation with 189-cm^3 solid, round gluteal implants. (*B*) Note improvement in volume and projection.

Subfascial gluteal augmentation has several advantages and disadvantages:

Advantages of subfascial implant placement

- Easier dissection
- Global enhancement
- Increased projection

Disadvantages of subfascial implant placement

- Palpability
- Visibility
- Infragluteal fold displacement

The subfascial approach can be useful in patients with thick soft tissue and minimal skin laxity. This technique can be learned quickly because of the distinct anatomic plane of dissection. Blood loss is less than with intramuscular dissection, and implants can be more easily positioned inferiorly when lower pole fullness is needed. The author has developed a simple algorithm to provide recommendations for implant shape and placement based on the length of the buttock and the amount of subcutaneous fat.[11]

Recommendations for implant shape and position

- Long buttocks: oval anatomic implant
- Short buttock: round implant
- Thick subcutaneous fat: subfascial or intramuscular placement
- Minimal subcutaneous fat: intramuscular placement
- Inadequate soft tissue: implantation not recommended

Adjunctive surgical procedures may be performed before or after GAI. The procedures described include liposuction of the lower back, fat transfer to the hips, and skin excision of the infragluteal fold. Liposuction of the lower back can be safely performed at the time of gluteal implantation to improve the waist to hip ratio (WHR). In articles by Singh[28] and by Roberts and colleagues,[18] the concept of WHR as an indicator of female attractiveness is discussed. This quotient is obtained by dividing the circumference of the waist by that of the hips with the ideal quotient of 0.7.[18,28] A 2016 study by Gupta and colleagues[29] suggests that the current ideal WHR is 0.6.[29] Liposuction of the infragluteal area or lower back with fat injections has been described by several investigators to fill in depressions and reduce contour irregularities.[30–32] The author recommends discussing the benefit of liposuction of the lower back and flanks to improve the results of implantation (**Fig. 3**). In patients with excess flank adiposity, the addition of an implant alone without additional contouring can result in a boxy and unpleasing shape. Gluteal lift can be combined with gluteal augmentation to

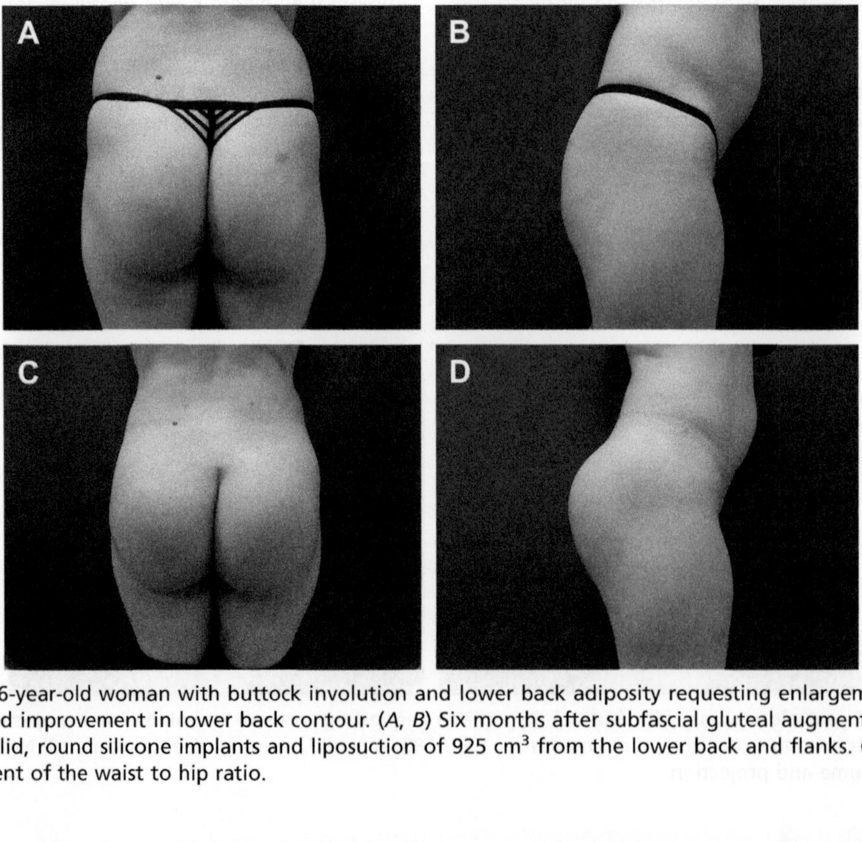

Fig. 3. A 36-year-old woman with buttock involution and lower back adiposity requesting enlargement of the buttock and improvement in lower back contour. (*A, B*) Six months after subfascial gluteal augmentation with 301-cm^3 solid, round silicone implants and liposuction of 925 cm^3 from the lower back and flanks. (*C, D*) Note improvement of the waist to hip ratio.

remove redundant skin and improve the buttock shape as described by De la Pena-Salcedo and colleagues.[33] In patients with severe laxity of the buttocks, a buttock lift can be performed before buttock augmentation as described in an article by Gonzalez.[34]

Ancillary contouring procedures

- Liposuction of back, flanks, hips, buttock
- Fat grafting to hips, buttock
- Infragluteal fold revision
- Buttock lift

The author prefers to stage excisional contouring procedures in association with gluteal implants. Infragluteal fold excision can be performed either before or after implantation (**Fig. 4**). The infragluteal area may be slightly improved after buttock augmentation resulting in less of a requirement for skin resection. Therefore, it may be preferable to wait several months after implantation to determine the amount of skin resection necessary. In cases of severe laxity, a buttock lift can provide a repositioning of the soft tissue in preparation for gluteal augmentation with an implant.

POSTOPERATIVE MANAGEMENT

Immediately after surgery, patients are placed on a stretcher in the prone position and a compression garment is applied. Patients are encouraged to wear the garment for 3 weeks and remain in the prone position as much as possible. Sitting is discouraged for 2 to 3 weeks. Exercise and strenuous activity may be resumed after 8 weeks. Early ambulation is encouraged to avoid venous thromboembolism. The author prescribes oral antibiotics for 5 days because of the risk of infection associated with gluteal implants. Muscle relaxants are not prescribed after subfascial augmentation but can reduce discomfort in intramuscular implant patients. Drains are not usually used after subfascial implantation. After intramuscular implantation, drains can be useful to accelerate healing and minimize edema. Drains are removed when less than 25 mL of fluid is obtained over a

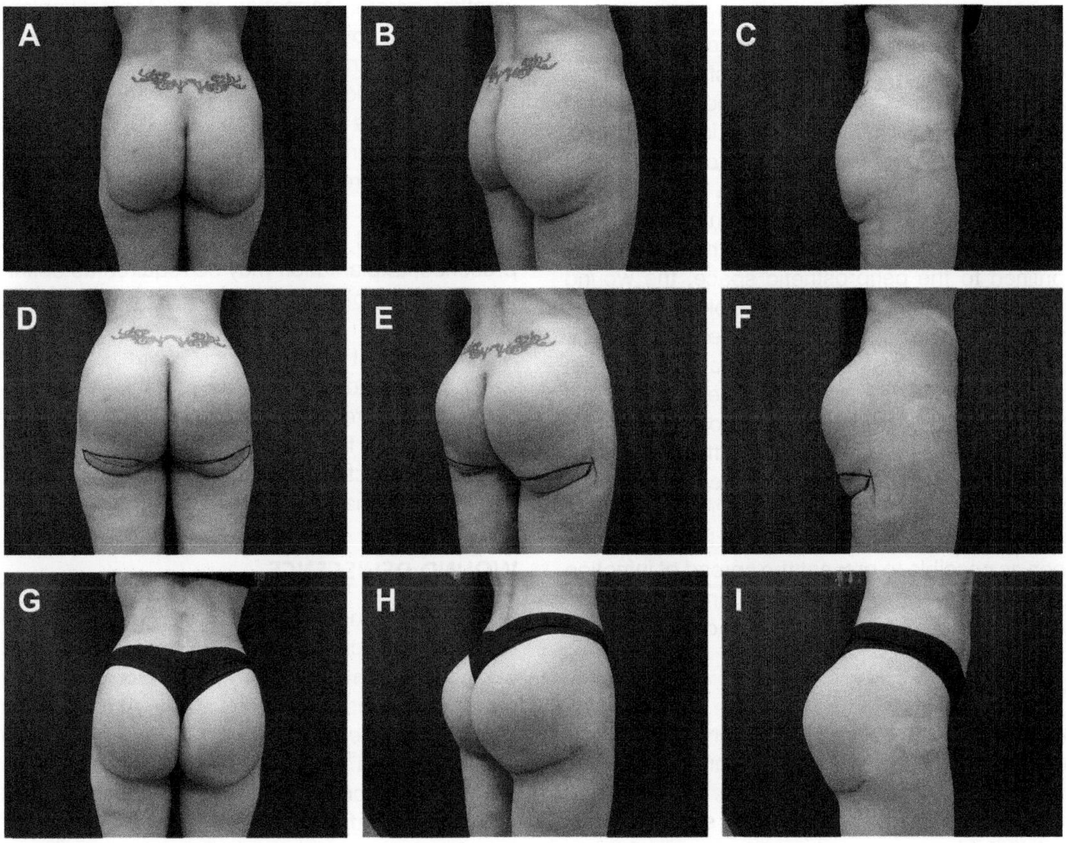

Fig. 4. A 46-year-old woman with buttock involution requesting restoration of volume and correction of skin laxity. (*A–C*) One month after subfascial buttock augmentation with 276-cm^3 solid, round silicone implants. Note preoperative markings for infragluteal fold revision. (*D–F*) Eleven months after gluteal augmentation and staged infragluteal fold revision (*G–I*).

24-hour period, which is usually 5 to 7 days postoperatively. Management of postoperative gluteal augmentation patients requires an awareness of the potential complications and the recommended interventions. It is important to intervene early when complications arise in order prevent further problems.

Postoperative recommendations

- Wear compression shorts for 3 weeks.
- Remain in the prone position as much as possible.
- Avoid exercise for 8 weeks.
- Recognize and treat infections early.
- Aspirate and send fluid for qualitative culture.
- Remove infected implants as soon as possible.

INFECTION

Infection may occur within the first week of surgery presenting with pain, swelling, and warmth. If drains are present, the fluid can be sent for gram stain and qualitative culture. Aspiration of the buttocks with an 18-gauge needle can yield fluid for culture. Antibiotics may be initiated and adjusted or discontinued after the culture results are obtained. It is unlikely that an infection of the periprosthetic space can be successfully managed with antibiotics alone. Once a diagnosis of surgical site infection is made, surgical intervention is required. The periprosthetic space should be explored and the implant removed. Intraoperative cultures are suggested. The wound is then irrigated with antibiotic solution. If the infection is confined to the periprosthetic space, the wound may be closed at the time of exploration. If the intergluteal incision becomes purulent or necrotic, wound closure is not advisable at the time of explantation. In no circumstances should an implant remain in an infected periprosthetic space. If the infection is unilateral, the unaffected implant may remain in place. Published infection rates for GAI range from 1% to 7%.[10,16,35,36] The author recommends removal of infected implants as soon as possible to prevent the spread of infection to the intergluteal area, avoiding an open wound after explantation requiring months of wound care.

SEROMA

Seroma formation after GAI occurs early in the postoperative period and is common after subfascial and intramuscular implantation. This accumulation of fluid in the periprosthetic space is often undetectable on physical examination until it becomes sizable, which is usually greater than 150 mL. Patients may complain of uncomfortable pressure in one or both buttocks 2 to 3 weeks postoperatively. The author recommends aspiration with an 18-gauge needle of the inferior aspect of the involved buttock when there is suspicion of seroma. The infragluteal area can be compressed manually to allow fluid to be aspirated effectively. This fluid should be sent for qualitative culture to check for possible infection. If the fluid is cloudy, antibiotics should be initiated. Serial aspiration of seromas should be performed weekly until there is 10 mL or less. Ultrasound can be useful in detecting and localizing seromas. Seroma rates have been reported at 2% by De La Pena[37] using textured cohesive gel implants in the subfascial position. Aboudib[36] reported a 4% seroma rate using smooth cohesive gel implants intramuscularly.[35] The author, using semisolid smooth and textured implants in both the subfascial and intramuscular position, reported a 28% seroma rate after the implementation or routine aspiration, which revealed seromas that were not detected on physical examination.[16] Although seroma rates have been reported to be higher in the United States where semisolid silicone elastomer implants are used instead of gel, it is still unclear in the literature whether seroma formation is related to implant size, texture, consistency, or placement. Seromas larger than 100 mL may become infected or lead to implant migration or extrusion as fluid dissects through tissue expanding the periprosthetic space. Persistent large seromas may require drain insertion until resolution. Seromas ranging from 200 to 300 mL that fail closed suction drainage require surgical exploration to evaluate for biofilm presence. Explantation may be required as definitive treatment of chronic seromas.

Management of seroma

- Compression shorts
- Serial aspiration
- Qualitative fluid culture
- Closed suction drain if persistent
- Open drainage with explantation

WOUND DEHISCENCE

Minimizing tissue tension through careful layered closure and securing each side of the intergluteal wound is recommended to avoid wound healing problems. Dehiscence rates after GAI have been reported between 6% and 30%.[24,34,35] Sinno and colleagues[38] reported wound dehiscence to be the most common complication of buttock augmentation after a review of 43 articles containing 2375 patients. Oranges and colleagues,[39] in a recent review of 52 studies on gluteal augmentation, also determined that wound dehiscence was the most common complication after GAI followed by seroma and infection. The author reported an incidence of 1.5% and found this complication to be rare and avoidable.[16] In a published series by Vergara,[40] there were no instances of wound dehiscence using implants between 250 and 350 cm^3. The author recommends avoiding implants greater than 350 cm^3 in primary gluteal augmentation. Minor wound separations can be managed with local care. Separation of the incision to the level of the subcutaneous tissue can be treated with dressing changes until the wound is suitable for closure. Wound dehiscence with exposure of the implant requires explantation. Intramuscular implants need not be removed if the periprosthetic space is not exposed. In an article by Serra and colleagues,[41] wound healing complications were reduced by using adhesion sutures to tack down the subcutaneous tissue to the midline.

Management of wound dehiscence

- Minor wound separation can be treated with local care.
- Deep wound separation is treated with local care until the wound can be closed.
- Dehiscence with implant exposure requires implant removal.

HEMATOMA

Serial aspiration of the buttock can be effective in treating small nonexpanding hematomas. Operative intervention with implant removal, irrigation of the periprosthetic space, and implant replacement with a drain is the recommended treatment of a firm, tender buttock in which hematoma is suspected. The author reported a hematoma rate of 2%.[16] Wound dehiscence, infection, and capsular contracture are risks of untreated hematomas.

CAPSULAR CONTRACTURE

The most likely cause of capsular contracture is inflammation of the periprosthetic space due to the presence of bacteria. It is possible that semisolid elastomer gluteal implants resist mild deforming pressure due to their density. Capsular contracture usually presents as a firmness to the buttocks with an implant that cannot be displaced within the periprosthetic space. Patients with capsular contracture often complain of a constant tightness and discomfort of the buttocks. The management of capsular contracture of the buttock depends on the degree of discomfort and may include exploration of the buttock with capsulotomy or implant removal if evidence of biofilm formation is observed.

SCIATICA

Unilateral or occasionally bilateral pain in the posterior thigh radiating to the calf is not uncommon in the early postoperative period, as swelling and inflammation exert pressure on the sciatic nerve. Complaints of sciatic nerve pain have occurred after both subfascial and intramuscular implant placement. This condition almost always resolves within several weeks and may be improved with the use of antiinflammatory medication.

AESTHETIC CONCERNS

The management of patients with poor aesthetic results requires obtaining a surgical history focusing on 3 key components: implant size, shape, and placement. Knowledge of these 3 pieces of information will allow for a successful plan for correction. Patients dissatisfied with the size of the buttocks may benefit from implant exchange to a larger size after 6 months when the periprosthetic space has stabilized. It is safer to insert an implant of appropriate size initially with exchange to a larger size later to avoid wound healing complications. Poor buttock shape characterized by inadequate projection of the inferior aspect of the buttock can be addressed by either exchanging the implant from round to oval in patients with long buttocks or by inferior repositioning of a high-riding poorly positioned implant. Oval implant rotation may contribute to buttock asymmetry, as the desired point of maximal projection can change as the implant rotates. In a study by Serra and colleagues,[20] CT evaluation of oval intramuscular implants revealed symmetric rotation from vertical to oblique in all patients at 3 months. The author recommends exchange of oval implants to round in cases of asymmetry due to implant rotation and to change the point of maximal projection as needed. Site change should be considered in patients with unacceptable palpability and visibility of subfascial implants. Intramuscular repositioning of superficial implants can reduce these concerns and improve the aesthetic result. Serra and Aboudib[42] described repositioning displaced intramuscular implants into a new deeper intramuscular space to correct malposition. In an article by Jaimovich and colleagues,[43] displaced intramuscular implants were stabilized and projection was improved by internal suturing of the capsule. In instances whereby patients have chronic pain and inflammation, explantation is recommended. Implant replacement can be performed after 6 months. Fat grafting to the explanted buttock can restore size and symmetry. Sympygia, defined by the author as communication of the buttocks in the midline with loss of the intergluteal crease, can be corrected by capsule resection and restoration of implant boundaries.[44]

Managing poor results

- Determine the implant size, shape, and position.
- Change to a larger size after 6 months.
- Consider changing the implant shape to oval or round.
- Change the site to an intramuscular or subfascial position.
- Remove chronically inflamed or infected implants.
- Replace the implant after 6 months.
- Consider fat grafting to restore size and correct asymmetry.

REFERENCES

1. Bartels RJ, O'Malley JE, Douglas WM, et al. Unusual use of the Cronin breast prosthesis: case report. Plast Reconstr Surg 1969;44:500.
2. Cocke WM, Ricketson G. Gluteal augmentation. Plast Reconstr Surg 1973;52:93.
3. Gonzalez-Ulloa M. Gluteoplasty: a ten year report. Aesthet Plast Surg 1991;5:85–91.
4. Robles J, Tagliapietra J. Gluteoplastia de aumento: implante submuscular. Cir Plast Iberolatinoamericana 1984;10:365–9.
5. De la Pena JA, Rubio OV, Cano JP, et al. History of gluteal augmentation. Clin Plast Surg 2006;33:307–19.
6. Vergara R, Marcos M. Intramuscular gluteal implants. Aesthet Plast Surg 1996;20:259–62.
7. De la Pena JA. Subfascial technique for gluteal augmentation. Aesthet Surg J 2004;24:265–73.
8. Hwang SW, Nam YS, Hwang K, et al. Thickness and tension of the gluteal aponeurosis and the implications for subfascial gluteal augmentation. J Anat 2012;221:69–72.
9. Mofid MM, Gonzalez R, de la Pena JA, et al. Buttock augmentation with solid silicone implants; a multicenter survey review of 2226 patients. Plast Reconstr Surg 2013;131:897–901.
10. Mezzine H, Khairallah G, Abs R, et al. Buttocks enhancement using silicone implants: a national practices assessment about 538 patients. Ann Chir Plast Esthet 2015;60:110–6.
11. Senderoff DM. Aesthetic surgery of the buttocks using implants: practice-based recommendations. Aesthet Surg J 2016;36:559–76.
12. Mendieta CG. Classification system for gluteal evaluation. Clin Plast Surg 2006;33:333–46.
13. Centeno RF, Young VL. Clinical anatomy in aesthetic gluteal body contouring surgery. Clin Plast Surg 2006;33:347–58.
14. Serra F, Aboudib JH, Cedrola JP, et al. Gluteoplasty: anatomic basis and technique. Aesthet Surg J 2010;30:579–92.
15. Cuenca-Guerra R, Lugo-Beltran I. Beautiful buttocks: characteristics and surgical techniques. Clin Plast Surg 2006;33:321–32.
16. Senderoff DM. Buttock augmentation with solid silicone implants. Aesthet Surg J 2011;31:320–7.
17. Flores-Lima G, Eppley BI, Dimas JR, et al. Surgical pocket location for gluteal implants: a systematic review. Aesthet Plast Surg 2013;37:240–5.
18. Roberts TL, Weinfeld AB, Bruner TW, et al. "Universal" and ethnic ideals of beautiful buttocks are best obtained by autologous micro fat grafting and liposuction. Clin Plast Surg 2006;33:371–94.
19. De La Pena JA, Rubio OV, Cano JP, et al. Subfascial gluteal augmentation. Clin Plast Surg 2006;33:405–22.
20. Serra F, Aboudib JH, Marques RG. Intramuscular technique for gluteal augmentation; determination and quantification of muscle atrophy and implant position by computed tomographic scan. Plast Reconstr Surg 2013;131:253e–9e.
21. Serra F, Aboudib JH, Neto JI, et al. Volumetric and functional evaluation of the gluteus maximus muscle after augmentation gluteoplasty using silicone implants. Plast Reconstr Surg 2015;135:533e–41e.
22. Hidalgo JE. Submuscular gluteal augmentation: 17 years of experience with gel and elastomer silicone implants. Clin Plast Surg 2006;33:435–47.
23. Mendieta CG. Intramuscular gluteal augmentation. Clin Plast Surg 2006;33:423–34.
24. Mendieta CG. Gluteoplasty. Aesthet Surg J 2003;23:441–55.
25. Gonzalez R. Gluteal implants: the "XYZ" intramuscular method. Aesthet Surg J 2010;30:256–64.
26. Gonzalez R. Augmentation gluteoplasty: the XYZ method. Aesthet Plast Surg 2004;28:417–25.
27. Gonzalez R, Mauad F. Intraoperative ultrasonography to guide intramuscular buttock implants. Aesthet Surg J 2012;32:125–6.
28. Singh D. Universal allure of the hourglass figure: an evolutionary theory of female physical attractiveness. Clin Plast Surg 2006;33:359–70.
29. Gupta CS, Wong WW, Motakef S, et al. Redefining the ideal buttocks: a population analysis. Plast Reconstr Surg 2016;137:1739–47.
30. Aiache AE. Gluteal recontouring with combination treatments: implants, liposuction, and fat transfer. Clin Plast Surg 2006;33:395–403.
31. Cardenas-Camerena L, Paillet JC. Combined gluteoplasty: liposuction and gluteal implants. Plast Reconstr Surg 2007;3:1067–74.
32. Cardenas- Camarena L, Silva-Gavarrete JF, Arenas-Quintana R. Gluteal contour improvement: different surgical alternatives. Aesthet Plast Surg 2011;35:1117–25.

33. De la Pena-Salcedo JA, Soto-Miranda MA, Vaquera-Guevara MO, et al. Gluteal lift with subfascial implants. Aesthet Plast Surg 2014;37:521–8.
34. Gonzalez R. Buttocks lifting: how and when to use medial, lateral, lower, and upper lifting techniques. Clin Plast Surg 2006;33:467–78.
35. Bruner TW, Roberts TL, Nguyen K. Complications of buttock augmentation: diagnosis, management, and prevention. Clin Plast Surg 2006;33:449–66.
36. Aboudib JH, Serra F, de Castro CC. Gluteal augmentation: technique, indications, and implant selection. Plast Reconstr Surg 2012;130:933–5.
37. De La Pena A. Subfascial buttock implant augmentation. Presented at The Annual Meeting of the American Society of Plastic Surgery. Chicago, September 27, 2005.
38. Sinno S, Chang JB, Brownstone ND, et al. Determining the safety and efficacy of gluteal augmentation: a systematic review of outcomes and complications. Plast Reconstr Surg 2016;137(4): 1151–6.
39. Oranges CM, Tremp M, Di Summa PG, et al. Gluteal augmentation techniques: a comprehensive literature review. Aesthet Surg J 2017;37(5):560–9.
40. Vergara R. Intramuscular gluteal implants: 15 years experience. Aesthet Surg J 2004;23:86–91.
41. Serra F, Aboudib JH, Marques RG. Reducing wound complications in gluteal augmentation surgery. Plast Reconstr Surg 2012;130:706e–13e.
42. Serra F, Aboudib JH. Gluteal implant displacement: diagnosis and treatment. Plast Reconstr Surg 2014;134:647–54.
43. Jaimovich CA, Almeida MW, Aguiar LF, et al. Internal suture technique for improving projection and stability in secondary gluteoplasty. Aesthet Surg J 2010;30:411–3.
44. Senderoff DM. Revision buttock implantation: indications, procedures and recommendations. Plast Reconstr Surg 2017;139(2):327–35.

Submuscular Gluteal Augmentation

Jorge E. Hidalgo, MD*

KEYWORDS

• Submuscular implants • Gluteal prostheses • Buttock implants • Body contouring

KEY POINTS

- In properly selected patients and with the right type of implants, submuscular plane augmentation offers softest tissue coverage and more natural results and a smooth transition from the lower back to the gluteal region.
- In order to avoid excessive upper pole fullness and determine the plane of implantation, preoperative markings are essential.
- Today fewer implant augmentations and lipo-transfers are performed because of an alarming increase in the very dangerous but much less expensive use of synthetic fillers.
- The author describes a very simple approach that he has developed to determine if patients are good candidates for a submuscular plane gluteal augmentation.

Video content accompanies this article at http://www.plasticsurgery.theclinics.com/.

Augmentation and contouring of the gluteal region have become extremely popular in the last few years with increased demand from our patients.

As plastic surgeons, we have the opportunity to use basically 2 methods of accomplishing this: using buttock implants or fat grafting. Both of them have their own considerations: implants in different planes (submuscular, intramuscular, or subfascial) and fat grafting in the subcutaneous and/or intramuscular plane.

Both techniques have their own associated complications: less serious but more common complications, such as wound dehiscence with implants and fat absorption with grafting, and more serious and less frequent complications, such as infections and hematomas with implants and fat embolism with autologous fat grafting.

ADVANTAGES OF THE SUBMUSCULAR PLANE

Placing the implant in the submuscular plane provides the most soft tissue coverage, less implant palpability, visibility, and a natural contour and transition from the lower back.

The restricted caudal undermining due to the presence of the sciatic nerve below the inferior border of the pyramidal muscle will not interfere with a satisfactory contour in properly selected patients, as described later.

The intramuscular space popularized by Vergara and Amezcua[1] and Gonzalez[2] is the author's second choice in patients who have a short pelvis and require having the implant placed in a more caudal position, below the pyramidal muscle.

This intramuscular plane described by Gonzalez as the "sandwich plane"[3] divides the gluteus maximus muscle thickness in half following his somewhat elaborate XYZ method. As he mentions in this article, intramuscular undermining at this plane is difficult; it is impossible to assess the thickness of the muscle preoperatively, and there is no anatomic undermining plane to be followed.

Despite these limitations, his excellent results speak for themselves.

Disclosure: The author has nothing to disclose.
Faculty of Medicine, University San Martin de Porres, Alameda del corregidor 1531 avenue, Los Sirius Urbanization, Las Viñas, La Molina, Lima 12, Peru
* Juvencia Aesthetic Surgery Center, Jr. Trujillo 343 - Magdalena, Lima 17, Peru.
E-mail addresses: drhidalgo@juvencia.com; drjorgehidalgo@gmail.com

Clin Plastic Surg 45 (2018) 197–202
https://doi.org/10.1016/j.cps.2017.12.003

Anatomy

The gluteal anatomy is described in Robert F. Centeno and colleagues' article, "Clinical Anatomy in Aesthetic Gluteal Contouring," in this issue, and has been previously reviewed by Mendieta[4] and Gonzalez.[5]

In addition, in the CD included with this article, there is a video of an excellent surgical cadaver dissection by Dr Barouidi[6] of the entire gluteal region (Video 1).

Preoperative markings and selection of patients

The author still uses as the inferior limit of dissection of 2 horizontal lines drawn from the tip of the coccyx to both greater trochanters.[7]

To avoid the appearance of either excessive elongation or shortening of the gluteal region, the author has incorporated, in the preoperative planning and patient selection, a simple measurement between the posterior iliac crest, the described horizontal line (distance A), and the subgluteal crease of fold (distance B) (**Fig. 1**).

To avoid the possibility of excessive upper fullness, distance A should be at least double the of distance B for a submuscular gluteal augmentation.

If distance A is shorter, the intramuscular should be used to facilitate lower placement of the implant to achieve an ideal aesthetic outcome.

Patients with a wide iliac crest, narrow and short pelvis, or with flaccid or ptotic buttocks are poor candidates for any plane of gluteal implantation and could be better managed and contoured with fat grafting (**Fig. 2**).

Surgical technique

The surgical technique was described first by the pioneer, late Dr Jose Robles and colleagues[8] from Argentina in 1984. The author began developing his technique in 1988, presented at the 1992 annual meeting of the Lipoplasty Society of North America in Washington DC[9]; it was filmed and available through the Plastic Surgery Educational Foundation of the American Society of Plastic Surgeons in 1993[10] and published in *Clinics in Plastic Surgery* in 2006.[7]

The surgical technique can be viewed in Video 1.

As proposed by Mendieta,[4] shaping the gluteal region should be prioritized over adding volume to increase size. In addition to doing liposuction of the waist and hips, the author is now doing simultaneous lipo-transfer to the lateral gluteal depressions to obtain rounder and pear-shape buttocks.

Because the submuscular plane described by Robles and colleagues[8] is not always easy to identify, in some cases, the author develops the pocket with at least 3 to 4 cm of muscle depth. Therefore, in some patients, the implants are probably placed in a deep intramuscular plane.

The author does not leave a midline intergluteal island of skin as proposed by Gonzalez.[3] He uses a midline incision; the intergluteal fold is recreated by taking bites in the presacral fascia, subcutaneous tissues, and skin margins at the time of wound closure.

Selection of implants

The author has always used the Silimed (Silimed, Inc, Rio de Janeiro, Brazil) round, moderate-profile silicone cohesive gel with thick, resistant shell implants developed by Dr Robles and collegues.[8]

High-profile implants are more prone to result in an unnatural pointy contour, even more when patients bend forward or lift up their thighs.

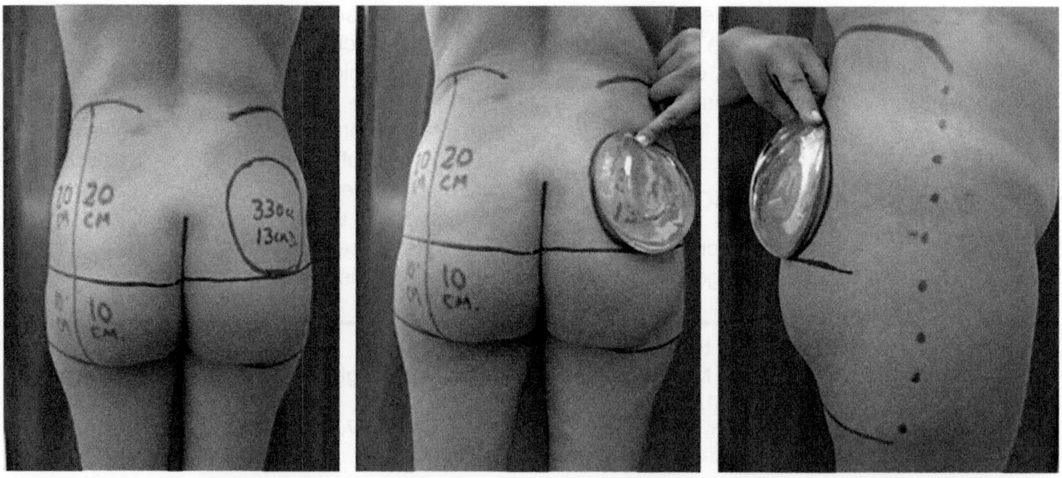

Fig. 1. Preoperative marking and measurements for the selection of patients and plane of augmentation.

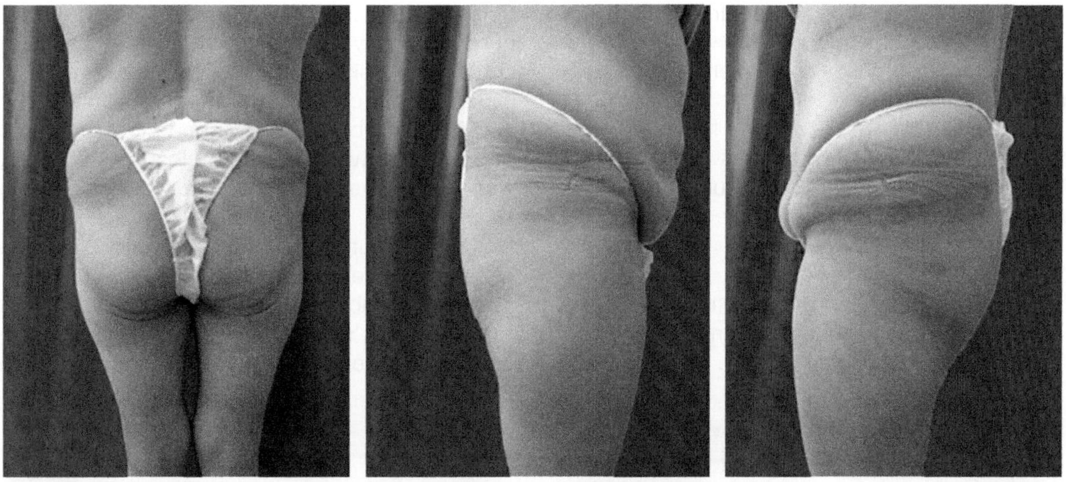

Fig. 2. Patients with wide and short pelvis are poor candidates for gluteal implants.

The author was initially using 240-, 270- and 300-cm^3 implants; but nowadays he more frequently uses implants between 300 cm^3 and 350 cm^3.

For the United States, when the silicone gel implants were banned by the Food and Drug Administration, the author developed the round silicone elastomer implants with Silimed–Sientra (Sientra Inc, Dallas, Texas) of 250-, 290- and 340-cm^3 volumes.

Several other companies manufacture elastomer gluteal implants, including Hanson Medical Inc, (Kingstone, WA), AART, Inc (Reno, NV), and Spectrum Designs Medical (Carpinteria, CA).

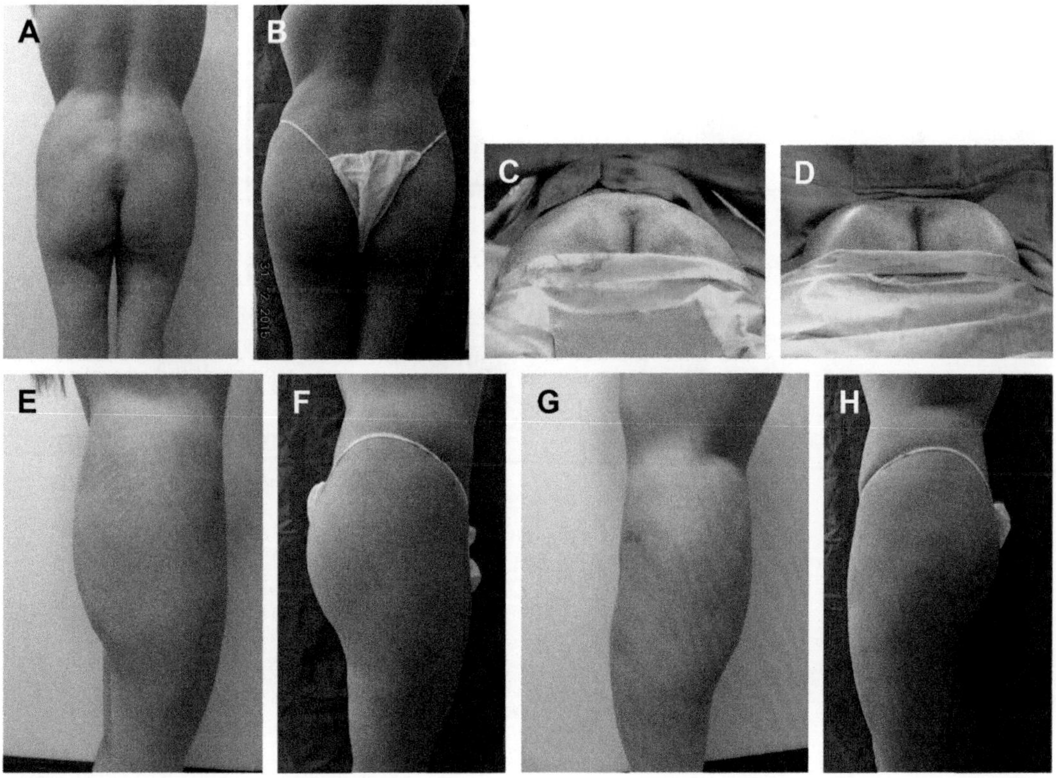

Fig. 3. (*A–H*) Preoperative, intraoperative, and 6-month postoperative pictures of a 38-year-old woman with 330-cm^3 implants.

The narrow tear-drop or anatomic implants should be reserved for patients with a narrow pelvis and for intramuscular augmentation to facilitate lower placement.

Results

The results of the surgical technique can be seen in **Figs. 3–5**.

Complications

In the author's experience, superficial infections and/or wound dehiscence continue to be the most frequent complications (**Fig. 6**). Superficial dehiscence is treated with cleansing and wound care to heal by secondary intention. In cases of complete dehiscence, proper wound care is initiated until clean granulation tissue is noted in the wound bed. Deep wound closure is then performed; 1 week later, the closure is finished, with approximation of the superficial layers and skin margins.

Since the author's last publication in 2006,[7] he has not experienced any clinically detectable hematomas or submuscular periprosthetic infections.

In the author's early experience, he had the opportunity to treat a patient who presented with

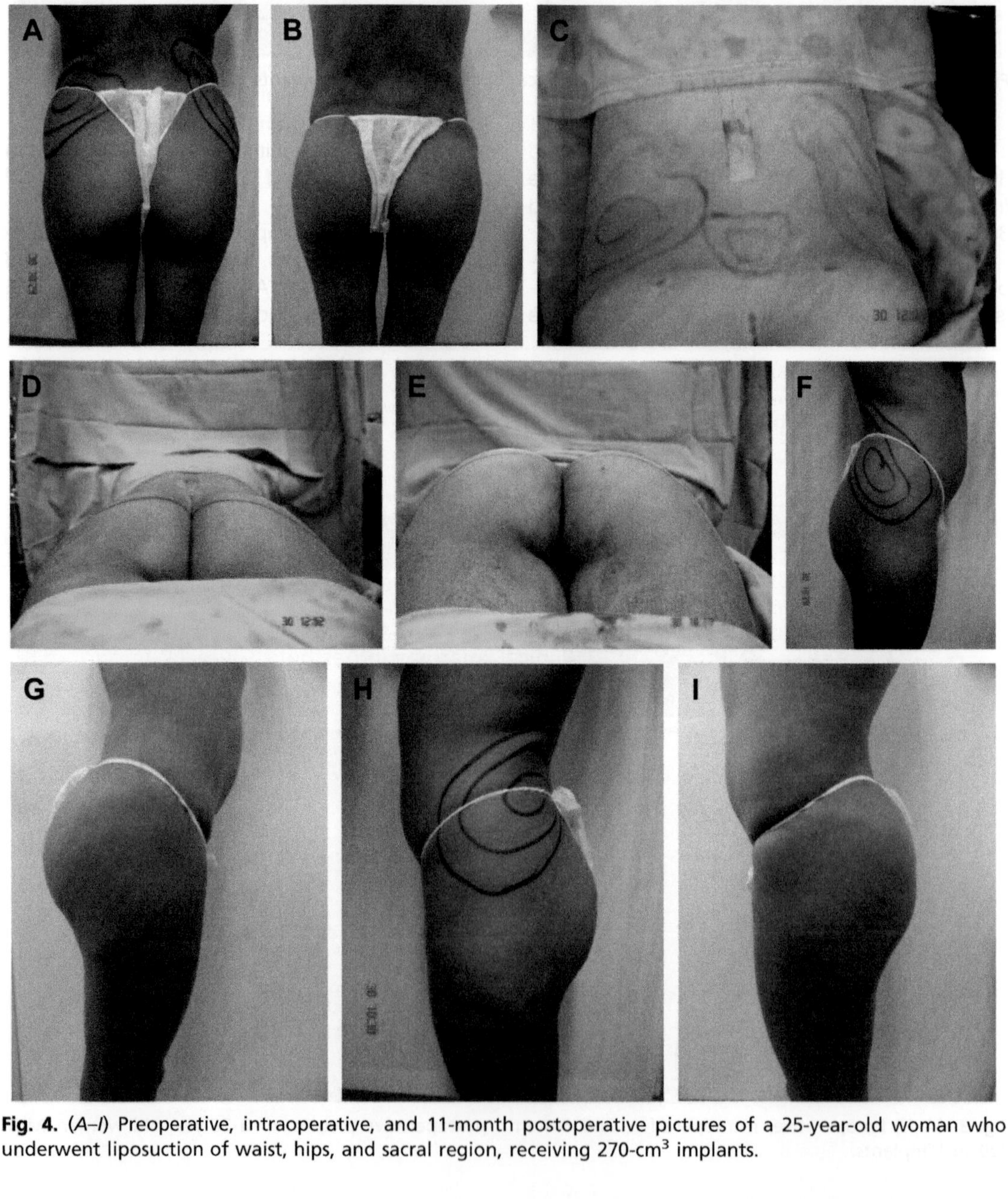

Fig. 4. (*A–I*) Preoperative, intraoperative, and 11-month postoperative pictures of a 25-year-old woman who underwent liposuction of waist, hips, and sacral region, receiving 270-cm³ implants.

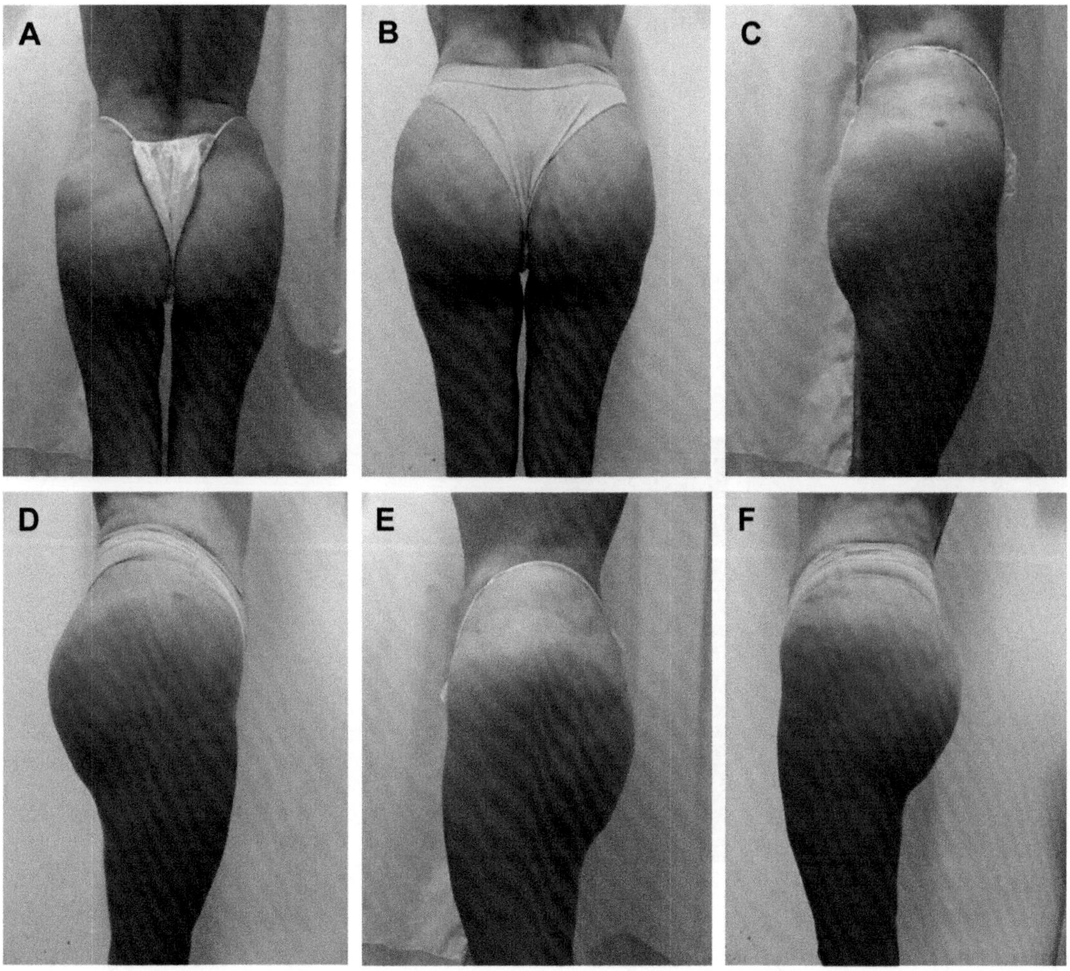

Fig. 5. (*A–F*) Preoperative and 4-month postoperative pictures of a 67-year-old woman with 300-cm^3 implants.

herniation of her implant of the left buttock (**Fig. 7**). At surgery, 220-cm^3 saline-filled silicone implants were found and replaced with 270-cm^3 silicone gel gluteal implants. The left buttock implant was herniated through a very thin muscle layer. A deeper pocket was developed below the deep layer of the implant pocket. The implant was replaced, and the center of the roof of the new pocket was reinforced with rotation of local muscular and underlying capsule flaps.

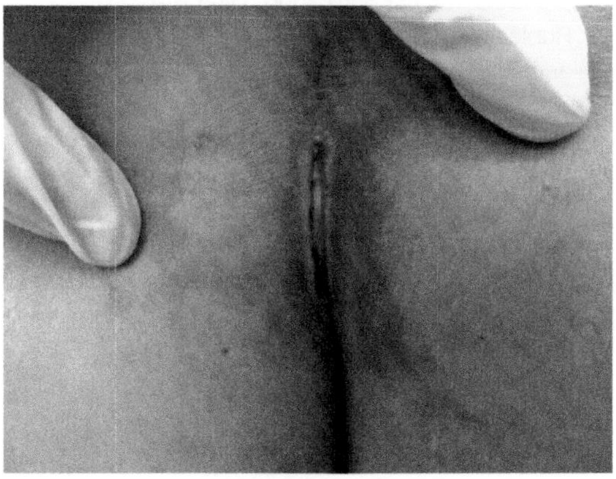

Fig. 6. Superficial wound dehiscence.

SUMMARY

Despite the availability of other choices of planes for buttocks implantation, the author thinks that, in properly selected patients, the submuscular technique remains useful and relevant. With the use of elastomer or silicone gel and round, moderate-profile implants, the submuscular augmentation can deliver softer, natural results.

Today we are performing fewer implant augmentations and lipo-transfers because of an alarming increase in the very dangerous but much less expensive use of synthetic fillers. These materials, some of which are illicit, are now being

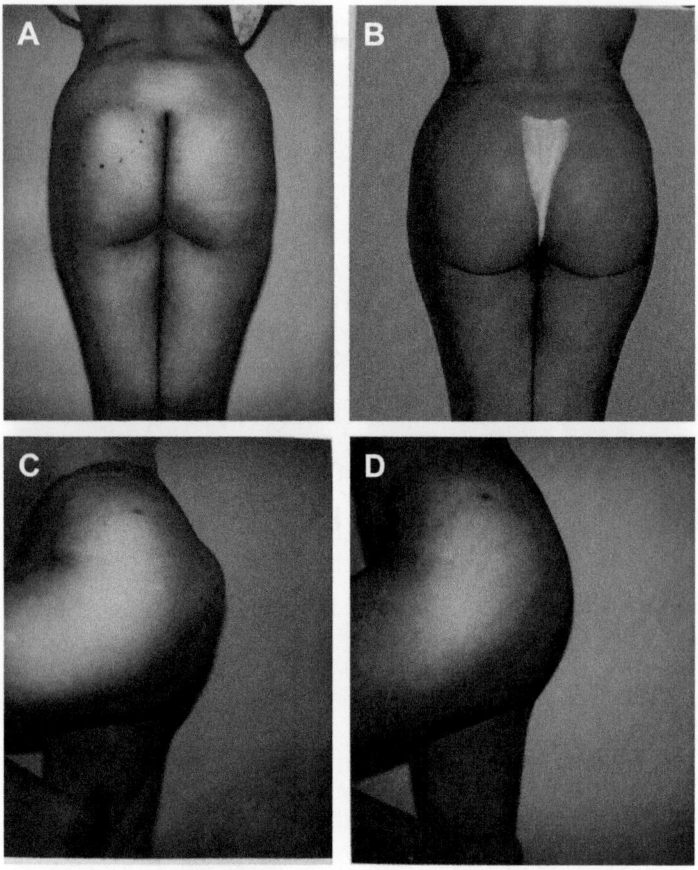

Fig. 7. (*A–D*) Preoperative and postoperative pictures of corrected left herniated implant.

injected deep intramuscularly. The resulting complications can be delayed for several years before they become apparent.

We will probably be facing them in the future and, as plastic surgeons, will be called in for treatment in the years to come.

SUPPLEMENTARY DATA

Supplementary data related to this article can be found online at https://doi.org/10.1016/j.cps.2017.12.003.

REFERENCES

1. Vergara R, Amezcua H. Intramuscular gluteal implants. Aesthetic Plast Surg 2003;23:86–91.
2. Gonzalez R. Buttocks reshaping and the posterior body contour: the XYZ intramuscular method. Rio de Janeiro (Brazil): Indexa Ed; 2006. p. 109–43.
3. Gonzalez R. Gluteal implants: the XYZ intramuscular method. Aesthet Surg J 2010;30(2):256–64.
4. Mendieta C. Gluteoplasty. Aesthet Surg J 2003;23: 441–55.
5. Gonzalez R. Buttocks reshaping and the posterior body contour: anatomy. Rio de Janeiro (Brazil): Indexa E.d; 2006. p. 77–91.
6. Baroudi R. Buttocks augmentatios. [Video # 61224] Lipoplasty Society of North America. 1991.
7. Hidalgo J. Submuscular gluteal augmentation: 17 years experience with gel and elastomer silicone implants. Clin Plast Surg 2006;33:435–47.
8. Robles J, Tagliaprieta J, Grandi M. Gluteoplastia de aumento; implantes submusculares. Clin Plastic Surg 2006;33:435–47.
9. Hidalgo J. Submuscular augmentation gluteoplasty. Presented at the 10th annual Meeting of the Lipoplasty Society of North America. Washington, DC, October 1992.
10. Hidalgo J. Submuscular augmentation gluteoplasty [Video # 9513] Plastic Surgery Educational Foundation. Aesthetic Body Contouring Series. 1993.

Intramuscular Gluteal Augmentation with Implants Associated with Immediate Fat Grafting

Paulo Miranda Godoy, MD[a,*],
Alexandre Mendonça Munhoz, MD, PhD[a,b,c,d,1]

KEYWORDS

- Gluteal augmentation • Silicone implant • Fat grafting • Intramuscular approach • Outcome
- Complications

KEY POINTS

- The latest generations of silicone implants and the introduction of surgical techniques, such as the intramuscular approach, have improved aesthetic outcomes after gluteal augmentation.
- The advantages of the intramuscular pocket are soft tissue coverage and avoidance of the limitations of the subfascial position. In the gluteal region, this technique is useful to minimize the appearance of the implant edges and provides an adequate support system.
- Autologous fat grafting is a more frequent procedure. Various clinical studies state that fat grafting may be an option to treat gluteal defects secondary to aesthetic deformities.
- Most candidates for primary and secondary gluteal augmentation can be successfully treated with this technique.
- Ideal primary candidates are those with significant gluteal deformities in terms of volume, skin laxity, and projection with less soft tissue to adequately cover the implant. Ideal secondary candidates are those with partial/total soft tissue deficiency with visible implant contours and patients with irregularities of the implant surface.

Video content accompanies this article at http://www.plasticsurgery.theclinics.com/.

INTRODUCTION

Gluteal augmentation is a well-known procedure and continues to be one of the most frequently performed aesthetic surgeries worldwide.[1–3] Gluteoplasty is one of the fastest-growing plastic surgeries in the field of aesthetic procedures.[4]

Disclosures: Dr A.M. Munhoz is a consultant to Allergan Corporations and Motiva/Establishment Labs. Dr P.M. Godoy has nothing to disclose.

Contributor's Statement: P.M. Godoy is principal investigator of this study. A.M. Munhoz is coinvestigator. The principal investigator made significant contributions to the conception and design of this study. A.M. Munhoz made substantial contributions to the acquisition, analysis, and interpretation of data. P.M. Godoy and A.M. Munhoz drafted the article. All authors revised the article for intellectual content, gave final approval of the version to be published, and have sufficiently participated in the work to take public responsibility for appropriate portions of the content.

[a] Hospital Moriah, São Paulo, São Paulo, Brazil; [b] Hospital Sírio-Libanês, São Paulo, São Paulo, Brazil; [c] Cancer Institute of São Paulo, University of São Paulo, São Paulo, São Paulo, Brazil; [d] Plastic Surgery Division, University of São Paulo School of Medicine, São Paulo, São Paulo, Brazil
[1] Present address: Rua Mato Grosso, 306 cj. 1706 – Higienópolis, São Paulo, São Paulo 01239-040, Brazil.
* Corresponding author. Rua Iguatemi 44, Itaim Bibi, São Paulo, São Paulo 01451-010, Brazil.
E-mail address: paulo@paulogodoy.com.br

Clin Plastic Surg 45 (2018) 203–215
https://doi.org/10.1016/j.cps.2017.12.004

In the United States, the number of gluteal augmentations, which include implants and lipofilling, increased by more than 20% between 2014 and 2015.[4,5]

The development of modern silicone implants as well as new surgical techniques has led to widespread acceptance of gluteal augmentation in recent years. Although gluteal augmentation has a high rate of patient satisfaction, some patients may present unsatisfactory results and require surgical revision.[2] In the authors' experience, many of these reoperations are required for problems related to soft tissue, such as implant visibility and palpability, not implant failure. Although subfascial implant placement can provide satisfactory postoperative recovery,[5,6] it may sometimes result in visibility of the implant edge and limited soft tissue coverage.[7–10] With the introduction of submuscular implant placement, reduced implant visibility and a lower incidence of complications, such as implant malpositioning, displacement, and extrusion, were observed in some series.[1,2,7–10] Undesirable shaping of the implant and the gluteal area, however, is sometimes observed in some groups of patients.[2] To avoid this outcome, fat injections around the implant may be used to achieve the desired contour and shape; this combination of options, using both implant and fat, has the potential to reduce the chance of exaggerated and less natural results.

Recently, implant placement using the intramuscular pocket associated with immediate fat grafting is gaining popularity as a result of the better results it yields compared with subfascial techniques. Like other investigators, the authors have found that satisfactory outcome and good results can be achieved in selected patients after intramuscular augmentation (**Box 1**).[8–10]

As with composite breast surgery, over the past 10 years there has been resurgence in the use of autologous fat grafting in gluteal shaping, for a variety of indications.[2,3,11–13] Autologous fat grafting has been performed more frequently since 2008, when new clinical recommendations were released.[14,15] Based on various clinical studies, the American Society of Plastic Surgeons concluded that fat grafting may be considered to treat breast defects associated with oncological diseases and aesthetic deformities.[15] Although refinement in fat grafting procedures has improved reproducibility, it has been the authors' impression that a standardized technique remains to be described.

Box 1
Advantages of intramuscular approach for gluteal augmentation

- Improved upper-pole contour
- Avoids implant edge visibility
- Helps keep the implant in place
- Reduces muscular dynamics over the implant

Given that implants and the intramuscular technique are effective and predictable procedures for aesthetic gluteal surgery,[8–10] a variety of unsatisfactory outcomes may result from the limited ability of the overlying soft tissue to adequately cover the silicone implant. Consequently, the relevance of fat grafting may be investigated as an associated technique for improvement of the results of gluteal augmentation. In addition, it is reasonable to emphasize that if autologous fat grafting and implant-based buttock augmentation are equally reproducible and involve similar risk, the authors believe it is possible to combine both techniques in 1 surgical procedure.

The objective of this article is to provide an overview of the intramuscular approach to primary and secondary gluteal augmentation with implants associated with autologous fat grafting. Although gluteal augmentation is a well-studied procedure, previous reports concerning the intramuscular technique have been limited and are related, in particular, to the most recent generations of silicone implants.[8–13] Additionally, there are no detailed clinical reports that specifically address operative planning, outcomes, and complications after simultaneous autologous fat grafting. Gluteoplasty, combining liposuction and gluteal implants, has been previously described by Cárdenas-Camarena and Paillet[11] as an effective procedure for improving the gluteal profile. Unlike these investigators, the authors believe that associating fat injection in the subcutaneous plane provides a more natural outcome. The implant is protected by the intramuscular plane, yielding firm and even projection, and its superior portion is disguised by the grafted fat, which is provided by the fat.

This article provides a detailed description of the authors' method, including preoperative evaluation and intraoperative care for patients undergoing primary and secondary buttock augmentation associated with lipofilling. The surgical technique, advantages, and limitations are also discussed. When combined with clinical expertise, this approach will help plastic surgeons provide their patients with predictable and safer aesthetic outcomes.

THE EVOLUTION OF THE IMPLANT POCKET AND THE INTRAMUSCULAR APPROACH

Gluteal silicone implants may be inserted in 1 of 4 anatomic pockets relative to the gluteus maximus muscle: subcutaneous, subfascial, submuscular, or intramuscular. In the past 10 years, this procedure has been improved by changing the pocket location and type of incision used.[2]

In the 1960s, Bartels and colleagues[5] were among the first to recommend implant placement above the gluteus maximus, using a subgluteal incision. Because of pocket instability and the quality of soft tissue coverage, the subcutaneous technique presented poor long-term outcomes, with some reports of dislocations, implant palpability, asymmetries, and capsular contractures.[2] In the 1980s, Robles and colleagues[7] introduced a new procedure for buttock augmentation by inserting submuscular implants through an incision in the midline of the sacral region. The submuscular pocket located between the gluteus maximus and medius is limited, however, in terms of space and volume. In this technique, the pyramidal muscle cannot be dissected in a caudal direction to avoid compression of the sciatic nerve. Because of this technical limitation, the implant can sometimes be placed too high, with unsatisfactory projection and volume of the lower poles.[8–10] To improve results, Vergara and Marcos[8] described a procedure for gluteal augmentation involving an intramuscular implant pocket. It has been the authors' experience that the intramuscular technique provides adequate coverage of the silicone implant and the ability to place the implant lower because the pocket dissection is not limited by the pyramidal muscle. Furthermore, larger implants can be used with this technique than with the intramuscular pocket. Despite the importance of the initial intramuscular reports,[8] these investigators did not describe the limits of the pocket or details of the intramuscular dissection. Consequently, Gonzalez[9] established surgical parameters for the intramuscular incision to avoid implant visibility. This last technique described the evaluation of 3 reference points (X, Y, and Z) and a line (G) as a guide for placement inside the gluteus maximus.[9,10]

The subfascial approach, which was introduced in the 2000s by de la Peña and colleagues,[16] is interesting for surgeons who have been seeking alternative planes with lower morbidity. Placing the silicone implant inside the muscle may sometimes result in unsatisfactory outcomes, especially in patients who are very physically active. Additionally, some investigators have observed that the intramuscular pocket can present some technical difficulties in terms of muscular detachment in the ideal plane, which can result in palpable implants and pain in the postoperative period.[16]

Despite the controversy concerning the suboptimal soft tissue coverage provided by the subfascial approach and the limitations involved with the intramuscular pocket, some studies have demonstrated satisfactory outcomes in selected patients.[9–13,17,18] There is no consensus, however, on the positioning and coverage of gluteal implants with regard to the intramuscular or the subfascial pocket. Mofid and colleagues[1] stated that intramuscular implant placement is useful in patients with thin subcutaneous tissue, where palpability is a concern. Otherwise, a subfascial pocket may provide better augmentation of the lower pole of the buttock, especially in patients with long buttocks.

In a recent survey, Mofid and colleagues[1] evaluated a 10-question survey that was sent to 83 plastic surgeon members of the American Society of Plastic Surgeons. Data concerning the number of cases performed, implant placement plane and incisional access, and number of complications were recorded. In this sample, 19 respondents (25% response rate) provided data on 2226 patients and a majority of respondents (68.4%) favored intramuscular placement of buttock implants.

Based on the authors' clinical experience and that of other investigators using the intramuscular approach,[17–19] the authors emphasize the importance of the pocket plane in the dynamics between the implant and soft tissues. It has been the authors' impression that besides the positive aspects of the supplementary soft tissue coverage, the intramuscular technique provides more satisfactory postoperative recovery than the total submuscular pocket and avoids implant visibility in patients with poor soft tissue coverage.

Despite these findings, the authors believe that advances in operative techniques are still necessary to improve aesthetic outcomes with lower complication rates. In addition, further studies are needed to compare complication rates between the intramuscular and subfascial techniques.

AUTOLOGOUS FAT GRAFTING

Fat grafting is extensively used in reconstructive and aesthetic surgery to treat contour defects with technical variations in fat harvesting, preparation, and reinjection.[20,21] According to the International Society of Aesthetic Plastic Surgery, in 2009 fat grafting accounted for almost 6% of nonsurgical procedures in the field of aesthetic surgery, with more than 514,000 procedures performed worldwide.[20]

The past 10 years have seen a reintroduction of autologous fat grafting for breast surgery.[21–23] Fat grafting presented advantages in terms of natural and long-term results, even when secondary and tertiary surgical sessions are necessary. In 2008, the American Society of Plastic Surgeons established a committee (Fat Grafting Task Force), which concluded that fat grafting may be considered for breast augmentation and correction of defects associated with oncological conditions.[14] In its report, this task force emphasized that fat grafting can be considered a surgical tool for breast shaping because of its relative ease of use and low morbidity.

Although various surgical procedures have been described to improve survival of fat grafts, including washing, centrifugation, and decantation, there is still controversy about their aesthetic outcomes, complications, and long-term results.[20,21] Coleman and Saboeiro[23] introduced the "structural fat grafting" procedure and pointed out the importance of removing nonviable aspirate components by centrifugation. They also emphasized a nontraumatic method of fat harvesting, centrifugation, and, in particular, small volumes of fat injection to provide maximum contact between the fat and recipient tissue. This technique has gained clinical application and become essential for many procedures described in several further studies.[20,21] The authors' experience in breast and gluteal surgery has confirmed Coleman and Saboeiro's recommendation about minimal fat volumes grafted during injection, maximizing the surface area for contact between the fat and recipient tissue.[24]

In contrast with the centrifugation technique, Khater and colleagues[25] noted that more active preadipocytes were maintained in noncentrifuged adipose tissue and could possibly result in a higher survival for the fat graft. Similarly, Rohrich and colleagues[26] observed that the rate of fat survival after centrifugation was no better than after filtration.

Despite the benefits and satisfactory results described, there is a lack of controlled, prospective clinical studies that evaluate the technical aspects related to autologous fat grafting, such as fat harvesting and processing methods, injection techniques, donor site areas, and outcomes of fat survival.[20,21] Similarly, there is no consensus concerning the viability of cell types between the various fat harvesting and preparation techniques.[20,21]

From the authors' point of view, and despite the good results observed in the authors' sample, the long-term complications of fat grafting in aesthetic gluteal surgery have not yet been reported and determined in a large series. Existing data concerning fat grafting for buttock augmentation are limited to case series and retrospective reviews.[8–13,16–19] Some studies have observed that lipofilling may result in varying degrees of nodule formation and calcifications, which could potentially affect postoperative recovery. Recent clinical data have shown, however, better results for fat grafting, with a lower incidence of complications, less fat necrosis, and fewer unsatisfactory results.[27]

Lipofilling of the buttocks for contouring and gluteal augmentation was popularized by Mendieta[27,28] in the United States. In terms of morbidity, fat grafting provides better versatility and a short recovery time compared with placement of silicone implants. Despite the benefits of each technique, in selected patients the combined technique can improve the gluteal area, with more satisfactory outcomes in terms of implant visibility.

From the authors' point of view, in a group of candidates for gluteal augmentation who have adequate soft tissue coverage and favorable anatomy, there is no need for additional fat grafting, and the intramuscular implant is sufficient to achieve a favorable outcome. But for other patients, combining fat grafting and intramuscular implants represents an alternative when there is not enough soft tissue to cover the selected implant volume. This association can offer the core volume projection of implants and the natural appearance and feel of fat and may be a useful technical alternative in aesthetic gluteal surgery.

SURGICAL PLANNING/TECHNIQUE

Patient Selection

Primary augmentation

In general, most candidates for gluteal augmentation with an adequate donor site can be successfully treated with intramuscular implants associated with lipofilling. Ideal candidates are slim and have poor soft tissue coverage in the gluteal area (for example, pinch test result <2 cm). In the authors' sample, most of the patients were thin, with a body mass index below 20. Despite this limitation in terms of fat volume, adequate volumes of fat could be found in the hip and flank areas. The authors have found that associated lipofilling has not been necessary in patients with a pinch test result greater than 2 cm to 3 cm; this amount of fat is considered a relative contraindication to the present technique and an indication for conventional intramuscular gluteal augmentation (**Box 2**).

Box 2
Intramuscular implants and autologous fat grafting

Patient selection: primary gluteal augmentation

- Gluteal hypoplasia
- Thin patients (body mass index <20)
- Less upper-pole coverage

Patient selection: secondary gluteal augmentation

- Partial or total soft tissue deficiency
- Thin patients (body mass index <20)
- Visible implant contours
- Rippling
- Implant contour palpability

Secondary augmentation

Most candidates for secondary gluteal augmentation can be successfully treated with the technique discussed in this article. These patients frequently present with partial or total soft tissue deficiency with visible implant contours, palpability, and rippling. In patients with thinned or stretched tissue, distortion and irregularities of the implant surface become noticeable. It has been the authors' impression that this aspect is frequently present in thin patients, and consequently implant replacement, pocket change, and fat grafting where needed provide additional soft tissue and camouflages surface irregularities. In the authors' experience with revision, surgery using intramuscular implants associated with fat grafting was indicated for 1 or more of the following primary indications: (1) local soft tissue deficiency/irregularities; (2) implant contour palpability; (3) implant contour visibility; and (4) rippling. Some patients had multiple indications for the use of the technique during their revision procedure. Additionally, the same primary augmentation principles were used (See **Box 2**).

Preoperative Evaluation/Planning

Fat harvesting and fat grafting areas are marked preoperatively with a patient standing. Only 1 point in the gluteal area, the superior edge of the intergluteal fold, is marked with the patient standing position; this marking is paramount for the surgical planning, because once a patient lays down, this point could be displaced (**Fig. 1**).

With the patient in prone position, the ischial tuberosity can easily be identified as a large posterior swelling on the superior ramus of the ischium. It is the most projected bone part that can be found during palpation of the gluteal region. One

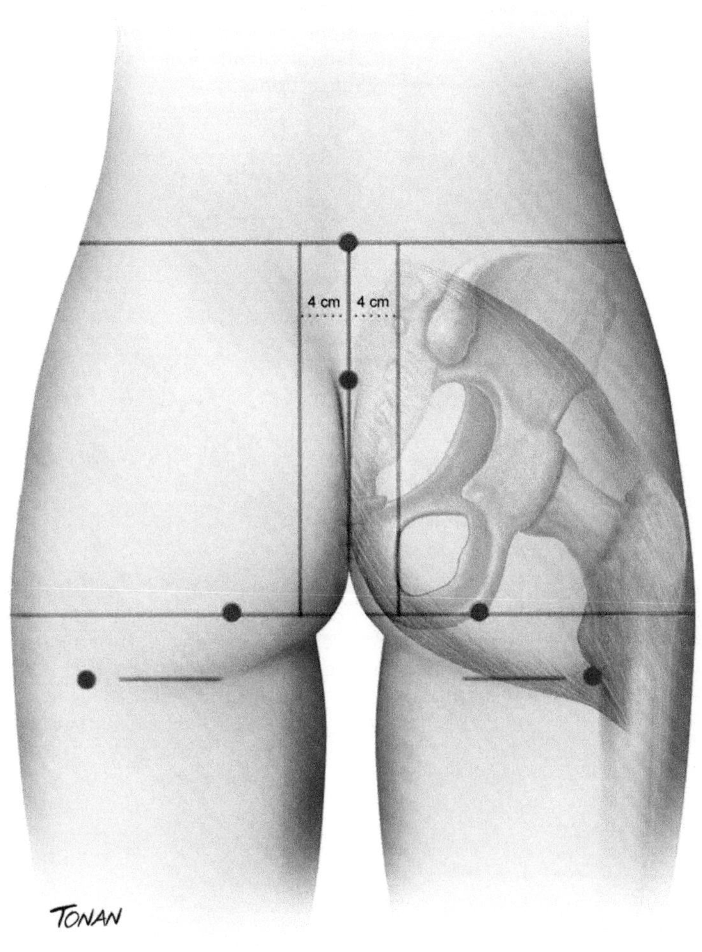

Fig. 1. Medial line drawn on the intergluteal cleft. Two parallel lines, 1 from each side, are 4 cm from the medial line. Another horizontal line is drawn from 1 ischial tuberosity to the other, on the contralateral side.

medial line is drawn on the intergluteal cleft (line A). Next, 2 parallel lines, 1 from each side, are 4 cm from the medial line (line B). Another horizontal line is drawn from 1 ischial tuberosity to the other, on the contralateral side (line C). The identification of the correct location of the ischial tuberosity is critical, because this is the inferior limit of the pocket plane dissection. The superior and lateral limits of the pocket plane dissection are established by imprinting the implant on the gluteal skin: an anatomic implant is placed with its widest part touching the horizontal line (line C) and the medial part of the implant touching line B (**Fig. 2**). The superior limit of the dissection is determined by the superior edge of the implant, and the lateral limit is similarly determined by the lateral portion of the implant. Using the implant dimensions to determine the limits of pocket design permits safe and precise plane dissection and avoids over-undermining of the plane. This maneuver is meant to obtain a tight pocket that keeps the implant definitively positioned, preventing rotation or malpositioning.

Surgical Technique

All patients undergo general anesthesia, and a projection cushion is placed under the hips to project the buttocks and facilitate undermining of the pocket plane. Preparation for gluteal implant surgery begins with either an alcohol-based body wash or a chlorhexidine wash to decrease the bacterial load on the skin. A transparent film dressing is placed over the anus, and a surgical compress is sutured 1 cm above the superior border of the anal area and on the surrounding skin to avoid any possible contact between the implants/instruments with this region.

Intramuscular dissection

A 6-cm skin incision is made on the intergluteal cleft. Unlike other investigators, the authors do

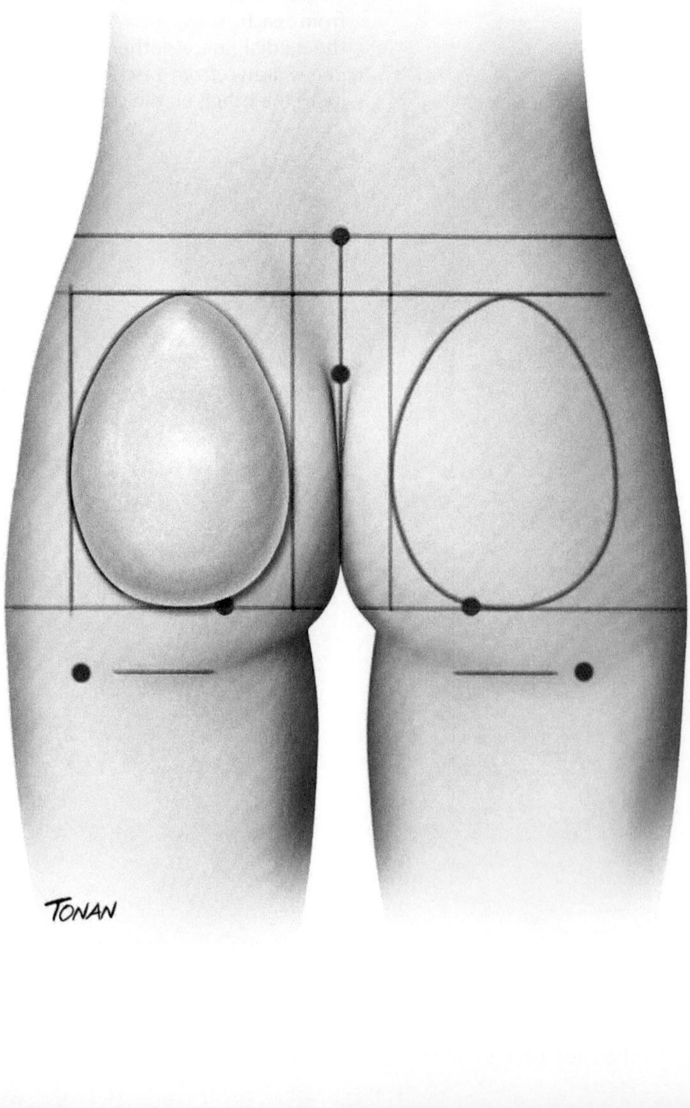

Fig. 2. Imprinting the implant on the gluteal skin: the implant dimensions provide the superior and lateral limits of the pocket dissection.

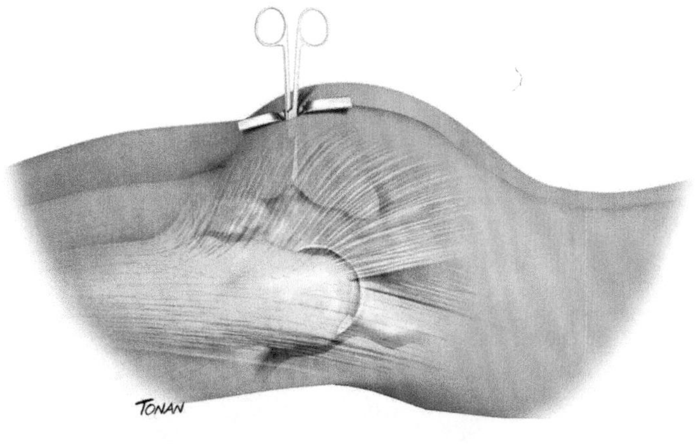

Fig. 3. A 45° dissection in the subcutaneous layer is performed toward the trochanter.

not preserve a skin island on the intergluteal cleft, believing that once the implants are placed, the tension on the incision may increase; if the skin island is resected, the tension on the scar tends to be higher, leading to dehiscence. The authors begin the dissection at 45°, however, to preserve the sacrocutaneous ligament until the identification of the fascia of the gluteus maximus (**Fig. 3**). Undermining above the fascia progresses up to line B. The dissection from the intergluteal cleft to line B should not extend excessively in width, and the previous recommendation is to maintain a 2-cm tunnel (**Fig. 4**). The pocket in the intramuscular plane is created using a blunt dissector and is meant to separate the gluteus maximus muscle into two 3-cm flaps (**Fig. 5**). The limits of the dissections are determined by the implant size, which was marked on the gluteal skin prior to the procedure. To prevent excessive bleeding inside the pocket, a sterile surgical compress immersed with adrenaline solution is placed inside while the contralateral dissection is performed. To avoid rotation/displacement and to ensure implant stability, it is crucial to evaluate the exact dimensions of the implant's height and width, which helps create an adequate pocket and avoid implant rotation (**Box 3**). If an implant has insufficient volume compared with the dimension of the available pocket, rotation/displacement occurs more frequently (**Box 4**).

Implant insertion/closure

The implant is soaked in an antibiotic solution and inserted with the help of sterile plastic funnel devices. Suction drains are placed into the pocket plane and exteriorized in the suprasacral area. The gluteal fascia is closed with interrupted 3-0 nylon sutures and the subcutaneous layer is added to the fascia with 4-0 nylon sutures to avoid accumulation of fluid. The subcutaneous layer of the incision is approximated with inverted, interrupted 3-0 nylon sutures. Skin glues are a good option as scar dressings, because they keep the edges of the incision tighter and act as an impermeable seal to prevent fluid contamination.

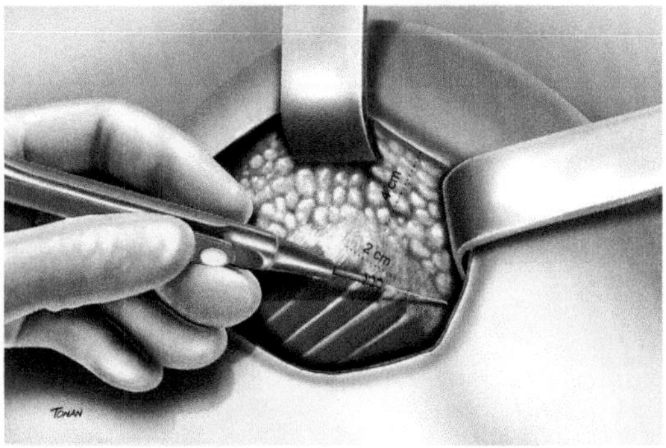

Fig. 4. A subcutaneous tunnel of 2-cm width by 4-cm length is sufficient to initiate the approach on the intramuscular pocket plane.

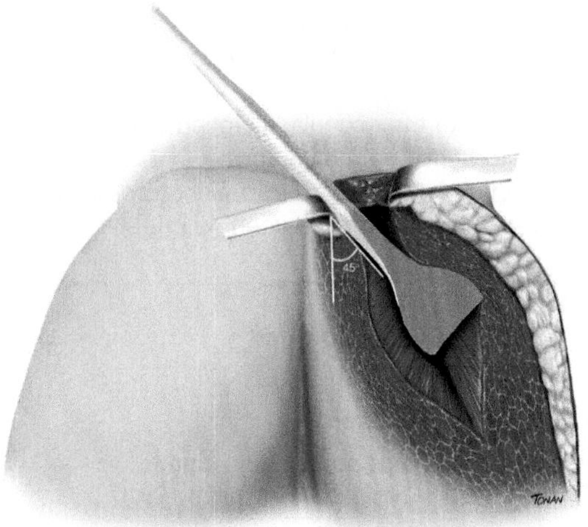

Fig. 5. Blunt dissection of the mayor gluteal muscle and the manufacture of the intramuscular plane.

Box 3
Implants complications: rotation/displacement causes

- Large surgical pocket
- Lateral and superior muscular mobilization
- Seroma, hematoma
- Double capsule
- Postoperative massage

Fat grafting

After the implant is inserted, lipofilling is performed in the areas where extra volume is needed. The authors usually use a modified Coleman and Saboeiro technique for fat graft harvesting.[23] After injection of local anesthesia (40–100 mL/area of 1% lidocaine and 1:100,000 epinephrine), fat is harvested using a blunt 2-mm cannula (Byron Medical, Inc., Tucson, Arizona) with several 0.8-mm holes. The fat is washed and condensed in its own vacuum system; the aspiration is a closed system until the fat is collected and injected into the syringes. The purified fat is transferred into 60-mL syringes with 3-mm cannulas and openings at the tips and injected into the areas marked preoperatively. The cannulas are positioned in the subcutaneous planes through small incisions on the hips and flanks. The technique for injecting fat grafts relies on preoperative topographic markings, where small amounts of fat are infiltrated by means of multiple passes along several planes. The fat is placed in multiple planes from deep subcutaneous to superficial subcutaneous tissue. At this point, care must be taken to avoid penetrating the implant capsule or damaging the silicone implant. Depending on each case, the fat is injected into the trochanteric and subgluteal areas (**Fig. 6**). The injections in the upper pole of the gluteus allow a smooth transition from the hip to the buttock, producing a more natural contour (**Fig. 7**). Fat is injected with retrograde movement of the cannula, injecting approximately 20 mL to 30 mL with each movement. Volumes of fat injections may vary from patient to patient, but in the authors' series, between 40 mL and 120 mL

Box 4
Surgical technique to avoid implant rotation/displacement

- Intramuscular plane
- Precise implant pocket adjustment
- Vacuum drain and postoperative immobilization
- No physical activities and massage

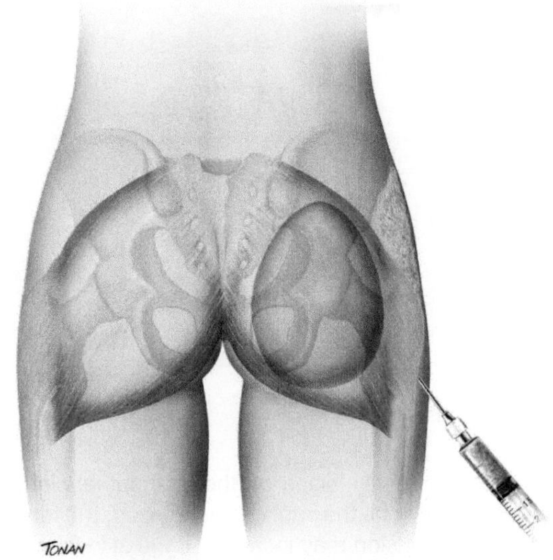

Fig. 6. Fat grafting in the trochanteric areas.

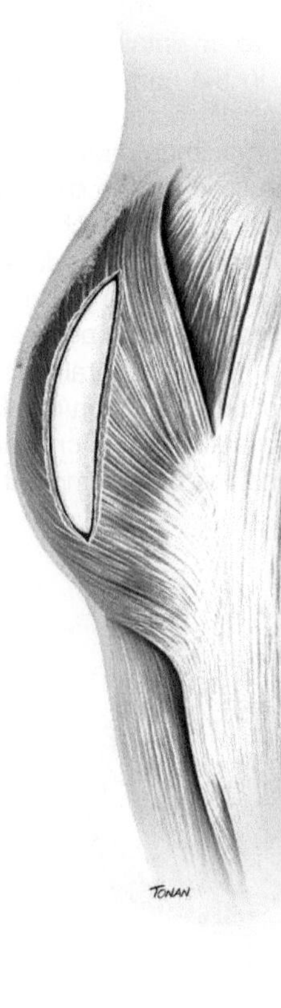

Fig. 7. The injection of fat on the upper pole of the gluteus provides a smooth transition from the dorsal to the buttocks, producing a more natural contour.

was injected on each side. After the injection, the injected area is carefully reshaped to adapt the outline of the desired surface. Elastic bandages and compression are used on the superior portion of the gluteal area to provide flexible strong support, and patients wear a girdle for 2 months (Video 1).

Postoperative Care

All patients receive intravenous antibiotics, and oral antibiotics are continued for 7 days. Immobilization with an occlusive dressing should be used for 3 days to improve scarring. The patients in the authors' series were discharged on the day of surgery or 1 day postprocedure. Early ambulation is encouraged to reduce the risk of venous thrombosis. Muscle relaxants and oral antibiotics are routinely used for 7 days after surgery. Drains are removed at approximately 4 days postprocedure or when drainage is less than 25 mL.

All patients are encouraged to sit on a cushion positioned under the back of the thigh area, allowing the buttocks to hang free. The back should remain straight and the feet on the floor, promoting good posture and relieving pressure on the gluteus.

It is essential for patients to avoid physical activities after implantation to minimize the risk of implant rotation, displacement, seroma, and other complications. As the edema diminishes, the compression band tension requires some adjustment, and patients are seen at appropriate intervals to supervise implant position and band tension. A low waist compression girdle, mid-thigh, is worn immediately after surgery for the first 2 weeks to 3 weeks. This compression garment minimizes swelling after the procedure, providing support to surgical areas for more

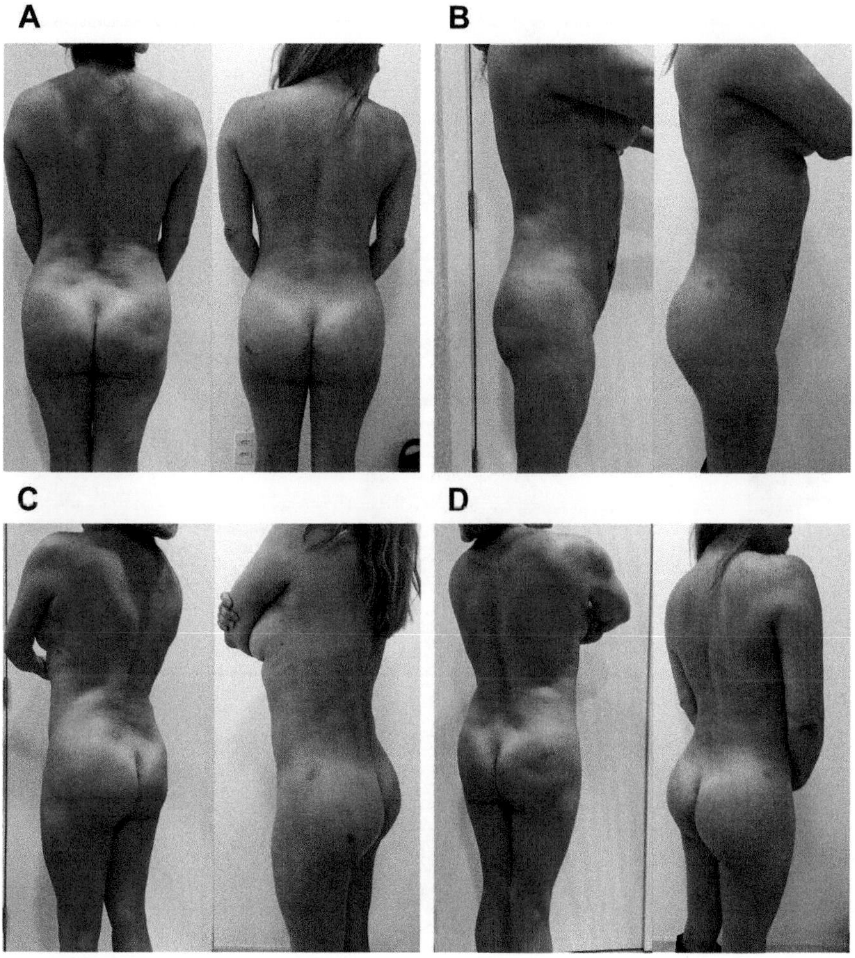

Fig. 8. (*A–D*) Case 1: preoperative posterior view, left oblique view, and left view of a 57-year-old patient with hypoplastic breasts (see **Fig. 2***A, C*). Postoperative (5 d) frontal view, left oblique view, and left view after bilateral anatomic silicone implant (325 mL) and fat grafting (*B, D*).

comfort and allows patients to return to daily routine sooner. Above this garment, a 3-in wide band of soft, elastic fabric is used to provide gentle compression or pressure on intramuscular implants. Fabric hook-and-loop fastener strips at each end allow adjustments as the edema decreases overtime.

RESULTS

Results after gluteal augmentation using the technique described previously have been very satisfactory in the authors' patients. Complications and surgical revisions have been rare. The authors' results verified that most complications occur in the initial postoperative period, and all were minor and predictable and did not affect the final aesthetic result. The level of satisfaction was assessed at least 6 months postprocedure; satisfactory aesthetic results were obtained, with maintenance of a natural gluteal shape. At this time, a majority of the patients were either very satisfied or satisfied with their results. The final result was generally good, and a soft transition between the subcutaneous tissue and implant edge was observed in all cases. One of 31 patients (3.22%) underwent a breast augmentation procedure at the same time as the gluteal surgery. One of 31 patients (3.22%) had fat injected into a reconstructed

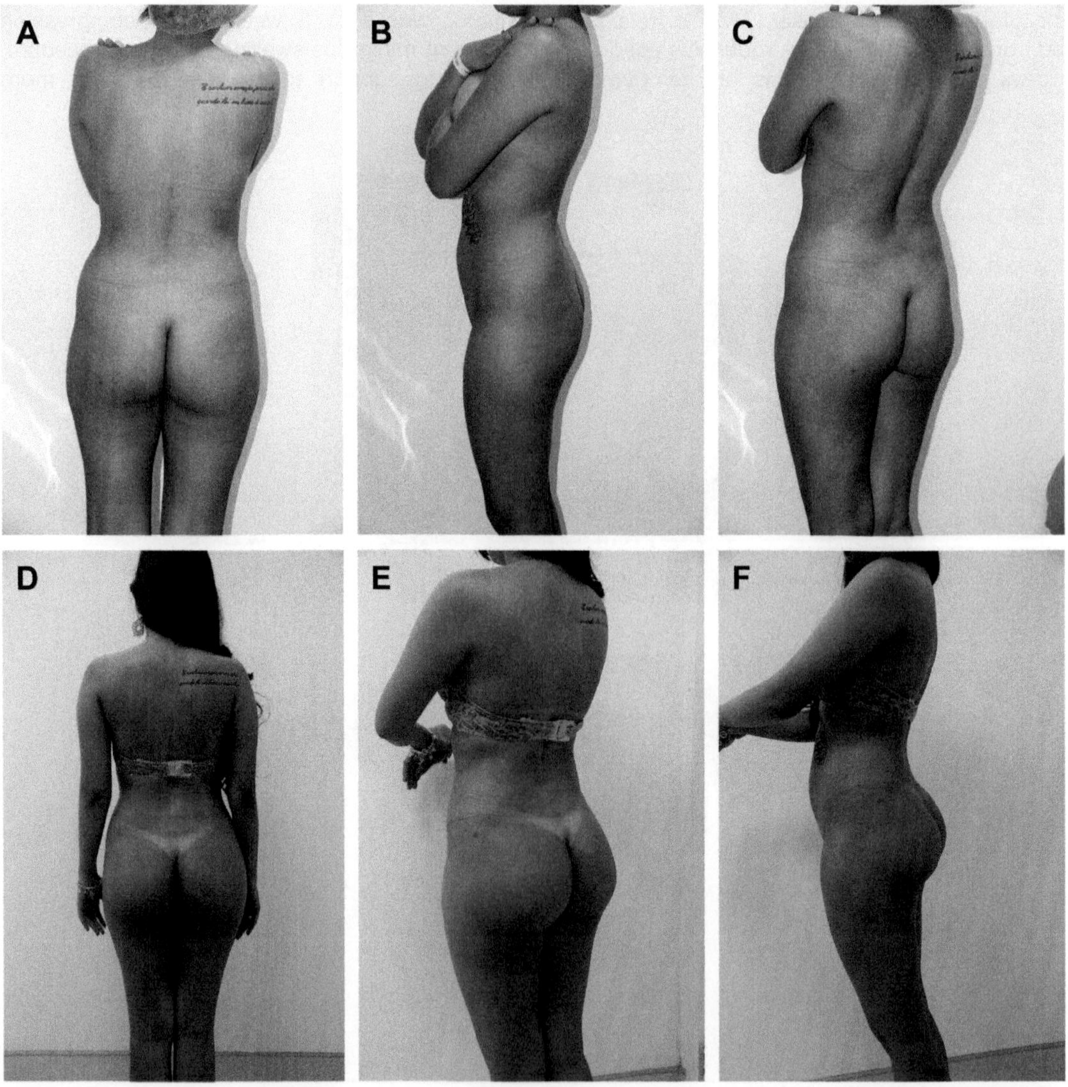

Fig. 9. (*A–F*) Case 2: preoperative posterior view, right oblique view, and right view of a 23-year-old patient with hypoplastic buttocks (see **Fig. 3***A*, *C*, and *E*). Postoperative (1 y) posterior view, right oblique view, and right view after bilateral anatomic silicone implant, 375 mL, associated with autologous fat grafting (*B*, *D*, and *F*).

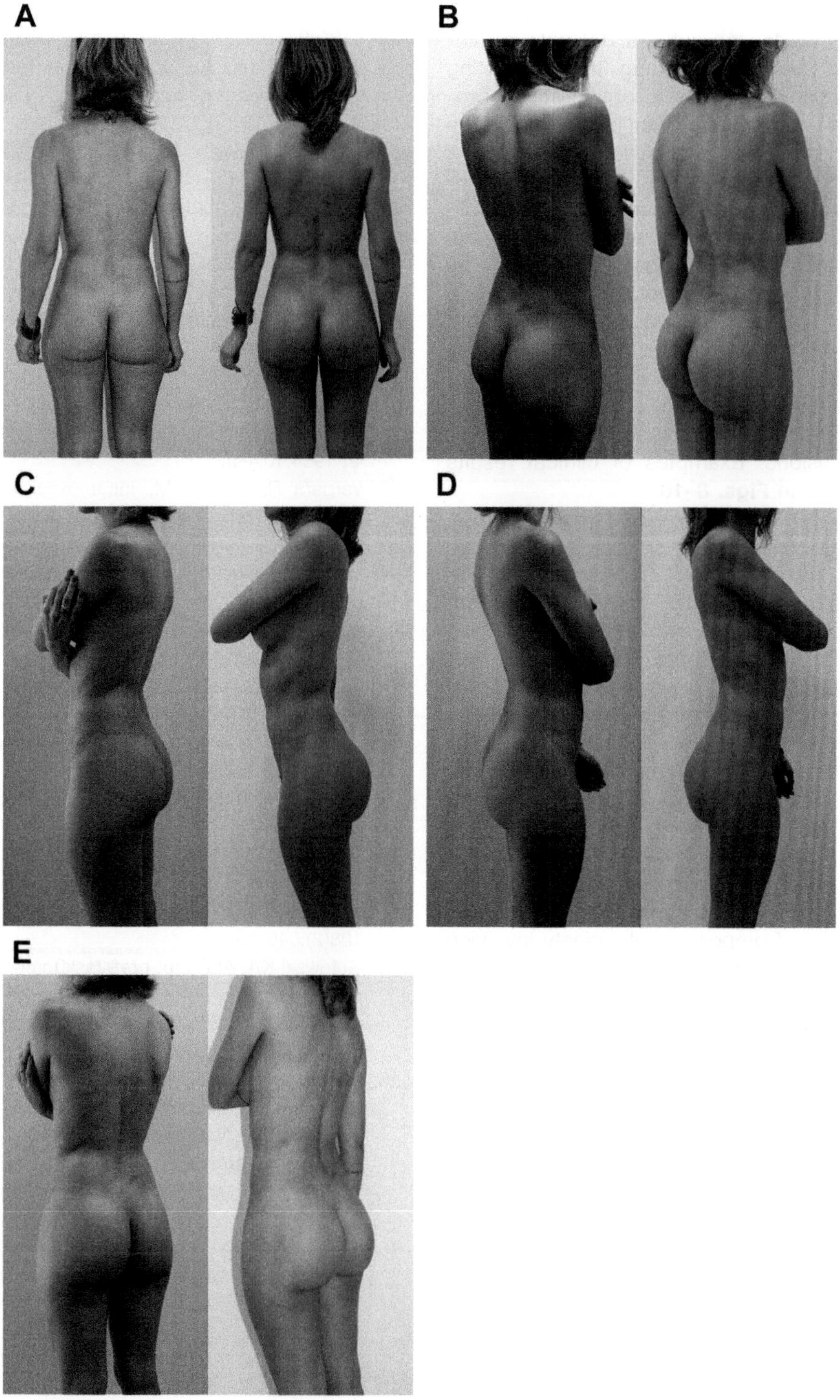

Fig. 10. Case 3: preoperative (*left*) posterior view, right oblique view, and right view of a 29-year-old patient with hypoplastic breasts and hypoplastic buttocks (*A, C,* and *E*). Postoperative (*right*) (1 y) frontal view, right oblique view, and right view after bilateral implant with a 180-mL implant on the breast and a 235-mL on the gluteus associated with autologous fat grafting (*B, D*).

breast at the same time as the gluteal procedure. In this study, the authors did not use implants with volumes exceeding 350 mL, opting for lower-volume implants to obtain stable projection, and the volume was achieved by the use of fat. In the authors' series, there were 2 cases of wound dehiscence (6.44%). The authors attribute the low dehiscence rate to application of the technical changes in the skin closure technique, previously described by Serra and colleagues.[19] No patients in this study developed seroma, hematoma, or implant displacement postprocedure. As of this writing, no capsular contracture has been observed; however, a larger number of patients and longer follow-up period are necessary to draw significant conclusions. Examples of clinical results are illustrated in **Figs. 8–10**.

SUMMARY

Advances in intramuscular dissection and fat grafting techniques have led to improved aesthetic outcomes for the gluteal area. The authors believe that this technique can play a useful role in gluteal aesthetics, and the experience demonstrates that this is a simple and predictable procedure. A majority of complications were minor and did not affect aesthetic outcome. Regardless of the aesthetic benefits, the association of autologous fat grafting and silicone implants presents some limitations; the main drawbacks are the need for previous training and surgical skills and longer operative time. Composite gluteoplasty involving buttocks augmentation simultaneously using implants and fat is a versatile approach to the gluteal region and combines the core volume projection of silicone implants with the natural look and feel of overlying fat. Like in breast surgeries, smaller-volume implants can be used and camouflaged by fat grafting.

SUPPLEMENTARY DATA

Supplementary data related to this article can be found online at https://doi.org/10.1016/j.cps.2017.12.004.

REFERENCES

1. Mofid MM, Gonzalez R, de la Peña JA, et al. Buttock augmentation with silicone implants: a multicenter survey review of 2226 patients. Plast Reconstr Surg 2013;131(4):897–901.
2. Sinno S, Chang JB, Brownstone ND, et al. Determining the safety and efficacy of gluteal augmentation: a systematic review of outcomes and complications. Plast Reconstr Surg 2016;137(4):1151–6.
3. Wong WW, Motakef S, Lin Y, et al. Redefining the ideal buttocks: a population analysis. Plast Reconstr Surg 2016;137(6):1739–47.
4. American Society of Plastic Surgeons. 2016 cosmetic surgery national data bank statistics. Available at: http://www.surgery.org/sites/default/files/Stats2015.pdf. Accessed July 25, 2017.
5. Bartels RJ, O'Malley JE, Douglas WM, et al. An unusual use of the Cronin breast prosthesis. Case Report. Plast Reconstr Surg 1969;44(5):500.
6. González-Ulloa M. Gluteoplasty: a ten-year report. Aesthetic Plast Surg 1991;15(1):85–91.
7. Robles JM, Tagliapietra JC, Grandi M. Gluteoplastia de aumento: implante submuscular. Cir Plast Iberolat 1984;10:4–5.
8. Vergara R, Marcos M. Intramuscular gluteal implants. Aesthetic Plast Surg 1996;20:259–62.
9. Gonzalez R. Augmentation gluteoplasty: the XYZ method. Aesthetic Plast Surg 2004;28(6):417–25.
10. Gonzalez R. Gluteal implants: the "XYZ" intramuscular method. Aesthet Surg J 2010;30(2):256–64.
11. Cárdenas-Camarena L, Paillet JC. Combined gluteoplasty: liposuction and gluteal implants. Plast Reconstr Surg 2007;119(3):1067–74.
12. Cárdenas-Camarena L, Silva-Gavarrete JF, Arenas-Quintana R. Gluteal contour improvement: different surgical alternatives. Aesthetic Plast Surg 2011;35(6):1117–25.
13. Cárdenas-Camarena L, Arenas-Quintana R, Robles-Cervantes JA. Buttocks fat grafting: 14 years of evolution and experience. Plast Reconstr Surg 2011;128(2):545–55.
14. Gutowski KA. ASPS fat graft task force. current applications and safety of autologous fat grafts: a report of the ASPS fat graft task force. Plast Reconstr Surg 2009;124:272–8.
15. American Society of Plastic Surgeons. Fat transfer/fat graft and fat injection: ASPS guiding principles, January, 2009. Available at: http://www.plasticsurgery.org/Documents/medical-professionals/health-policy/guiding-principles/ASPS-Fat-Transfer-Graft-Guiding-Principles.pdf. Accessed July 17, 2013.
16. de la Peña JA. Subfascial technique for gluteal augmentation. Aesthet Surg J 2004;24:265–73.
17. Aboudib JH, Serra F, de Castro CC. Gluteal augmentation: technique, indications, and implant selection. Plast Reconstr Surg 2012;130(4):933–5.
18. Serra F, Aboudib JH, Marques RG. Intramuscular technique for gluteal augmentation: determination and quantification of muscle atrophy and implant position by computed tomographic scan. Plast Reconstr Surg 2013;131(2):253e–9e.
19. Serra F, Aboudib JH, Marques RG. Reducing wound complications in gluteal augmentation surgery. Plast Reconstr Surg 2012;130(5):706e–13e.

20. Largo RD, Tchang LA, Mele V, et al. Efficacy, safety and complications of autologous fat grafting to healthy breast tissue: a systematic review. J Plast Reconstr Aesthet Surg 2014;67:437–48.
21. Gir P, Brown SA, Oni G, et al. Fat grafting: evidence-based review on autologous fat harvesting, processing, reinjection, and storage. Plast Reconstr Surg 2012;130:249–60.
22. Spear SL, Wilson HB, Locjwood MD. Fat injection to correct contour deformities in the reconstructed breast. Plast Reconstr Surg 2005;116:1300–5.
23. Coleman SR, Saboeiro A. Fat grafting to the breast revisited: safety and efficacy. Plast Reconstr Surg 2007;119:775–85.
24. Sampaio Goes JC, Munhoz AM, Gemperli R. The subfascial approach to primary and secondary breast augmentation with autologous fat grafting and form-stable implants. Clin Plast Surg 2015; 42(4):551–64.
25. Khater R, Atanassova P, Anastassov Y, et al. Clinical and experimental study of autologous fat grafting after processing by centrifugation and serum lavage. Aesthetic Plast Surg 2009;33:37–43.
26. Rohrich RJ, Sorokin ES, Brown SA. In search of improved fat transfer viability: a quantitative analysis of the role of centrifugation and harvest site. Plast Reconstr Surg 2004;113:391–5.
27. Mendieta CG. Gluteal reshaping. Aesthet Surg J 2007;27(6):641–55.
28. Mendieta CG. Gluteoplasty. Aesthet Surg J 2003; 23(6):441–55.

Intramuscular Gluteal Augmentation
The XYZ Method

Raul Gonzalez, MD*, Ricardo Gonzalez, MD

KEYWORDS

• Buttocks implants • Gluteoplasty • XYZ method • Intramuscular implants • Complications

KEY POINTS

- Visibility of the gluteal implants is a sequela that is not well accepted by patients as it causes a change in their lifestyle and body image issues.
- Superficial augmentation planes such as the subcutaneous or subfascial plane are more likely to result in implant visibility than the intramuscular plane.
- Pocket dissections with thin segments of muscle covering the implant can lead to implant visibility.
- The intramuscular dissection for buttocks implants should split the muscle entirely at its midthickness, avoiding thin segments of muscle that atrophy over time.
- The sandwich plane as described in the XYZ method splits the muscle at its midthickness and places the implant inside the muscle as a burger in a bun, avoiding thin segments on the muscle.

BUTTOCKS IMPLANTS AS AN OPTION FOR REMODELING BUTTOCKS

Buttocks implantation was one of the first procedures used to remodel buttocks. This technique began to be used in the 1980s, mainly in Latin America before the popularization of fat grafting.[1–6] Nevertheless, from the beginning, buttocks implants have been associated with high complication rates, and surgeons have not been encouraged to recommend this procedure.[7,8] Even so, it is important to note that complications generally result from 2 factors: the anatomic plane used or poor technique. The subcutaneous, subfascial, and submuscular planes may lead to less aesthetic results and to complications inherent to those locations.[9–11] When performed correctly, the intramuscular implant technique can offer outcomes that are not always achieved through other methods. Low complication rates when compared with the other planes, or even with breast implants, are achievable.[12–17]

Roundness and good projection of the buttocks are easily obtained with implants. Even if an implant cannot lift ptotic buttocks, it can provide a lift effect because of the visual improvement of the projection of the upper pole.

RESHAPING IS MORE IMPORTANT THAN AUGMENTATION

When reshaping buttocks, the surgeon has several options including fat grafting and implants. Some physicians who are not familiar with buttocks reshaping may have doubts about recommending 1 procedure over another. In most cases, the correct option is not a question of preference but rather indication, and it is important to understand the patient's wishes clearly.

Unlike fat grafting, implants achieve the desired round shape through a concentrated projection, whereas the volume of fat grafted can spread, thereby reducing focal augmentation. This concentration of the volume is desirable in many

Disclosure Statement: The authors have nothing to disclose.
Clinica Raul Gonzalez, R. Amadeu Amaral, 661 - Vila Seixas, Ribeirão Preto - São Paulo, 14020-050, Brazil
* Corresponding author.
E-mail address: Doctor.raulgonzalez@gmail.com

Clin Plastic Surg 45 (2018) 217–223
https://doi.org/10.1016/j.cps.2017.12.006
0094-1298/18/Published by Elsevier Inc.

cases, because it helps project the buttocks in a posterior direction instead of laterally. This projection results in a perky shape rather than large buttocks. This outcome meets the needs of some patients who do not want large buttocks and prefer medium-sized yet round buttocks with posterior projection.

Patients who request reshaping do not necessarily have flat buttocks, and grafting large amounts of fat is not what every patient is looking for. The authors have observed that most patients have properly sized buttocks and only require filling in specific areas such as the trochanteric depression, the upper pole of the buttocks, or the sciatic depression in order to obtain the roundness and projection desired. These areas can present impressive changes when they are filled with just 200 to 300 cc on each side.

FAT GRAFTING OR IMPLANTS?

A large amount of fat must be harvested for fat grafting on the buttocks. This is not possible in thin people, in whom implants are the only option. In most patients seeking major liposuction, one may easily utilize a procedure that uses the liposuctioned fat to reshape the buttocks.

Consequently, even surgeons with vast experience in buttocks implants often use fat grafting more frequently than buttocks implants. In the authors' practice, more fat grafting is performed than gluteal implants. More than 70% of the authors' cases of buttocks implants occur in conjunction with some amount of fat grafting (a common association of procedures) in selected areas to help reshape the buttocks and improve the outcome.

WHY CHOOSE THE INTRAMUSCULAR PLANE OVER SUPERFICIAL PLANES?

Buttocks implant may be placed in deeply, such as in the submuscular and intramuscular planes, or superficial as in the subcutaneous and subfascial planes. Each of these planes have attributes that can provide different long-term outcomes. The intramuscular plane is least likely to present implant visibility problems and complications of any kind.

The use of superficial planes is contraindicated in thin patients because of the visibility of the implant.[12,14] When used in patients with good adipose coverture, the subfascial plane can look good initially, but after some years the fascia can loosen, and the implant may become visible. The more superficial an implant, the more visible it is. In some cases, the implant can only be seen when the patient is moving, bending forward, or contracting the gluteal muscles. Postoperative pictures of patients showing good recent results standing up may not always represent the actual outcome. Another issue that is frequently associated with the subfascial plane is late seroma formation. Although the rate of late seroma is high, no data have been published about the frequency of this outcome.

One disadvantage of the retromuscular plane is the restricted space available for implant placement. Only the area above the piriformis muscle can be used, because the sciatic nerve below the muscle is unprotected, and contact with the implant can cause nerve pain. When this plane is used, the upper pole is filled more than the caudal pole, and a double-bubble effect can result.

All the problems that stem from use of the subcutaneous, subfascial, and retromuscular planes (such as seromas, visibility, or double-bubble) can be avoided by changing to the intramuscular plane. Consequently this plane is generally preferred for buttocks implants.

THE GLUTEUS MAXIMUS MUSCLE AND PRINCIPLES FOR CREATING THE POCKET

The lower gluteal nerve diverges into several branches entering the gluteus maximus muscle (GM) through the anterior aspect and one through the posterior aspect. Because most of these branches are not encountered during undermining, they are largely preserved with minimal damage to a few branches. Nevertheless, in order to preserve adequate muscular function and obtain good aesthetic results, some principles must be followed when creating an intramuscular space:

1. Undermining should be restricted to the GM.
2. Undermining should split the GM muscle in the middle, leaving the same amount of muscle in front of and behind the implant.

THE SANDWICH PLANE WITHIN THE GLUTEUS MAXIMUS MUSCLE

The authors call this plane created by splitting the GM in the middle the sandwich plane. This plane allows the implant to maintain its position during muscle contraction. When 1 area in the plane is more superficial than another, the balance of the muscular force is broken. The deeper area has more muscle fibers and is stronger than the superficial area. When the muscle contracts, the contraction pushes the implant against the thinner wall of the pocket. Continued pressure on the thin muscular wall eventually causes muscular atrophy.

Furthermore, thin layers of muscle can also lead to muscle fiber atrophy caused by ischemia, or by denervation or inadequate passage of electric stimuli in a muscle with little volume. Any undermining close to the posterior surface of the muscle and its fascia results in a thin muscle segment that covers the implant posteriorly and poor blood supply leading to muscle atrophy. The thinner the muscle, the poorer the blood flow to that muscle segment. It is also more likely that this thin segment will be denervated. In this situation, the implant may be visible in dynamic conditions such as bending forward, raising the legs, or contracting the muscle.

Most surgeons who create an intramuscular space without adequate training fear injuring deep structures such as the sciatic nerve. Most poor results usually stem from undermining too superficially or creating a pocket that is not entirely in the muscle.

DIFFICULTIES CREATING A SANDWICH PLANE

Creating a space within the gluteal muscles is not an easy procedure. Most of the dissection, which is the most important part of the surgery, is performed blindly. Even if the muscle fibers can be seen during the procedure, it is difficult to identify the correct plane and depth within the muscle. It is difficult to ascertain whether the muscle is really being separated at the midpoint of its thickness to create an adequate sandwich. There are no surgical planes to be followed, and skin markings are not useful.

THE XYZ METHOD AND THE GEOMETRIC PLANE GUIDED BY ANATOMIC REFERENCES

Lack of a surgical plane for dissection and blind dissection are the main challenges in obtaining a correct sandwich plane. Despite these challenges, anatomic references can be useful for guidance. This is the main purpose of the XYZ method: to perform a geometric dissection within the muscle guided by anatomic references in order to create a proper sandwich plane.

The XYZ points are located within the GM muscle, in the sandwich plane. By joining the first 2 points (X and Y) with a dissector to create a line, one can then move this line toward the third point (Z), thereby creating a geometric plane.

THE SURGERY

Skin Marking

The top of the intergluteal sulcus (line A) is marked with the patient standing. All additional marks are drawn in the operating room, with the patient prone. From line A downward, a 4 to 5 mm wide and 7 cm long spindle shape is marked over the sulcus. An inverted heart-shaped figure is marked, as shown in **Fig. 1**.

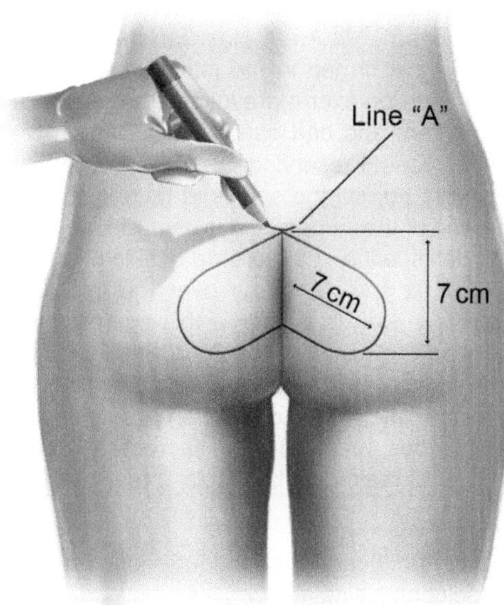

Fig. 1. An inverted heart figure is marked, with line A at its top limit. This drawing will guide subcutaneous undermining to expose the GM. The main axis of each side of the heart is 7 cm long and follows the direction of the muscle fibers, at approximately a 45° angle with the intergluteal sulcus. The spindle marked over the sulcus is also 7 cm in length.

Exposing the Muscle and Preserving the Sacrocutaneous Ligament

The inverted heart is abundantly infiltrated with Klein solution, using a 21G 1 1/4 needle (at an oblique angle), which usually touches the prefascial area in most patients; 40 cc of solution are usually infiltrated on each side and 40 cc over the intergluteal sulcus. If not infiltrated, dissection of this area can be particularly bloody. The 2 parallel lines of the spindle are cut at 90° until the subcutaneous layer is reached, after which dissection proceeds at 45°, preserving the sacrocutaneous ligament, until the muscular fascia is reached. The sacrocutaneous ligament was described by the lead author[3,11–13] and is responsible for the structure and depth of the intergluteal sulcus. When this incision is closed, this ligament will be useful for rebuilding the sulcus at its original depth. Undermining to expose the muscle should preserve the fascia as much as possible and use the inverted heart drawing as a guide.

Preserving the Sacrocutaneous Ligament

The sacrocutaneous ligament is a strong ligamentous structure that joins the medial sacral bone crest and coccyx to the buttocks skin and is responsible for the depth of the intergluteal sulcus.

It was described by the lead author in previous publications.[3,11–13] As the incision to expose the muscle is performed in the intergluteal sulcus, a straight incision over it provokes a detachment of this ligament and can cause late ablation of the natural crease. Preserving this ligament helps the surgeon to rebuild the sulcus at its original depth at the end of the surgery and is useful in preventing major dehiscence. A small strip of skin (7 cm × 4–5 mm) in a spindle shape over the intergluteal crease is 1 way to preserve this ligament when accessing the muscle. The 2 parallel lines of the spindle are cut at 90° until the subcutaneous layer is reached, after which dissection proceeds at 45° on both sides, preserving the sacrocutaneous ligament, until the muscular fascia is reached.

Exposing the muscle

The inverted heart is abundantly infiltrated with Klein solution, using a 21G 1 1/4 needle (at an oblique angle) usually touching the prefascial area in most patients. Approximately 40 cc of solution are usually infiltrated on each side and 40 cc over the intergluteal sulcus. If not infiltrated, dissection of this area can be particularly bloody. Undermining to expose the muscle should preserve the fascia as much as possible, and the inverted heart drawing should be used as a guide.

Point X

In order to split the muscle at the sandwich plane, the surgeon should be able to identify the midpoint of the muscle thickness at 2 points: at the opening incision adjacent to the sacrum, called here point X, and at the lateral edge close to the iliac crest, called here point Y.

Once the muscle is exposed, an incision is made along the muscle fibers by cutting the fascia and opening the muscle, creating a cleft 5 to 6 cm long and 3 cm deep. Point X is a spot 2.5 to 3 cm deep inside this cleft.

Close to the sacrum, the muscle thickness varies from 4 to 5.5 cm. During surgery, this thickness can be easily confirmed by introducing the index finger through the muscle incision in the caudal direction, pressing deeply until the sacrotuberous ligament can be felt. This ligament is easily identified, because it feels as firm as a human finger. Because this ligament is the anterior limit of the muscle at that particular spot, the distance between the posterior surface of the muscle and this ligament indicates the muscle thickness. To calculate the midpoint of the thickness (the location of point X), this thickness is divided by 2, but in practice the minimal thickness that should be left, as muscle cover is 2.5 cm in thinner muscles, and 3 cm when muscle thickness exceeds 5 cm (**Fig. 2**).

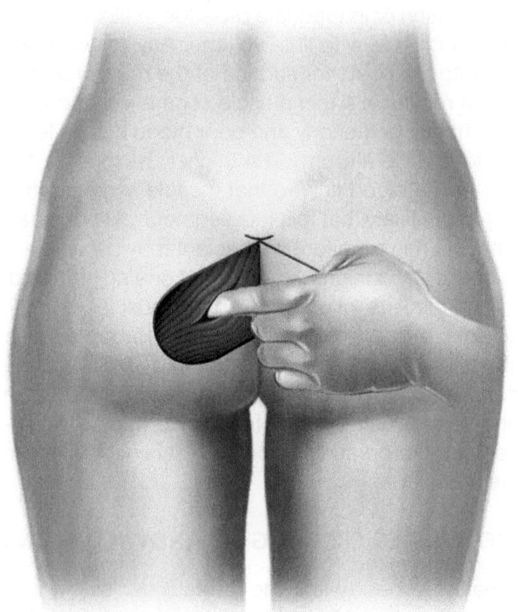

Fig. 2. After the muscle is exposed (with fascia preserved), a cleft 6 cm long and 3 cm deep is created along the muscular fibers. This incision is initially made with a scalpel and subsequently enlarged with the fingertip. The X point is located 2.5 or 3 cm deep inside this cleft, according the thickness of the muscle.

Line G

This line indicates the lateral edge of the GM, located 5 cm lateral to the upper-posterior iliac spine, over the iliac crest. First, the iliac crest is palpated and marked. Next, the authors start at the posterior-superior iliac spine and measure 5 cm laterally, marking a line on the iliac crest that demarcates the lateral limit of the gluteus maximus at its origin over this crest. The authors palpate and find the trochanter, marking its projection. A line is then drawn from the lateral edge of the muscle on the iliac crest up to posterior-lateral aspect of the trochanter, as seen in **Fig. 3**.

The Point Y

At its most cephalic portion, the lateral limit of the GM is approximately 2 cm thick. At this spot, the GM is adhered to both the iliac crest and the iliac bone; more specifically, half the muscle adheres to the iliac crest (roughly 1 cm at this point), and the other half, which is also approximately 1 cm, adheres to the iliac bone. If, during the procedure, the authors can identify the point where the crest and the bone are connected, they can identify the midpoint of muscle thickness at this spot. In practice, the lateral limit is identified by drawing

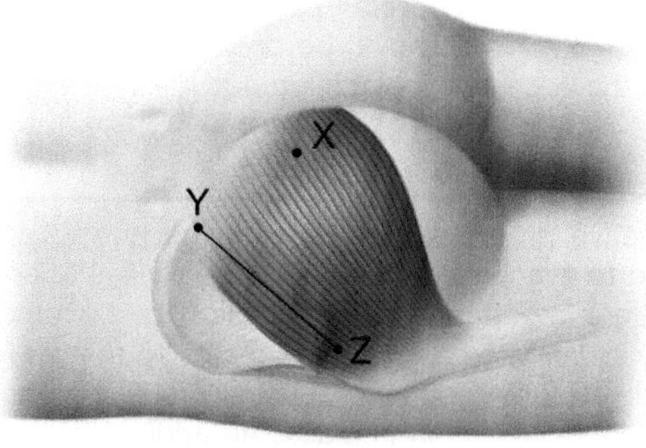

Fig. 3. Line G indicates the lateral limit of the GM, based on the surface anatomy. From the posterior-superior iliac spine, a spot is marked 4 to 5 cm laterally over the iliac crest. Line G connects this spot and the farthest projection of the trochanter. Point Y is defined over this line, showing where the intramuscular dissection must stop.

line G, as described previously. The midthickness of the muscle can then be pointed out at this line by sliding the finger downwards from the crest, always pressing the muscle until the fingertip can be felt to be 1 cm deep within the muscle mass. This maneuver will bring the fingertip close to the point where the iliac crest is joined to the iliac bone, which in turn is the midpoint of this muscle's thickness. This point, which called here Y, is extremely useful; along point X described previously, it creates a line within the GM muscle making the midpoint of its thickness. Joining these 2 points is the first step in bisecting the muscle properly.

Creating a line joining X and Z

Once line G and points X and Y are determined, the next step in bisecting the muscle in the ideal plane is to join these 2 points together with a detacher. This is a bimanual maneuver in which 1 hand holds the detacher at point X, and the fingertip of the other hand indicates point Y, as shown in **Fig. 4**.

Creating a plane using line X-Y

Line X-Y will help create a geometric plane. By definition, a geometric a plane is a figure resulting from the movement of a line toward a known point. Following this idea, when line X-Y is rotated (represented here by the dissector), one can obtain a plane inside the muscle. This rotation proceeds until it approaches the trochanter, creating a triangular dissection, as seen in **Fig. 5**.

Enlarging the Triangular Pocket

When the previously described procedure is complete, the upper part of the pocket is almost complete. The pocket is exposed using a 12 cm

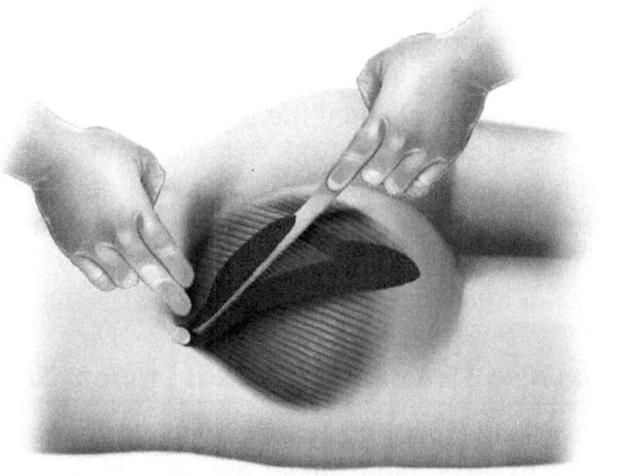

Fig. 4. In a bimanual maneuver, the GM is bisected linearly at the midpoint of its thickness. One hand indicates point Y over line G, pressing the fingertip until it reaches 1 cm inside the muscle mass. As the muscle at this area is 2 cm thick, a spot 1 cm inside the muscle is more or less at the midthickness. Using the other hand, a strong dissector (30 cm long and 2.5 cm wide) is placed at the first spot of the dissection (point X) and proceeds close to the bones of the area, first abutting the sacral bone and then the iliac bone, always guided by the tip of the finger on the other hand (point Y).

retractor with a right blade and without teeth on the uppermost part and a 10 cm retractor on the lower portion. A fiber optic light can be introduced to identify any remaining septa; these should be

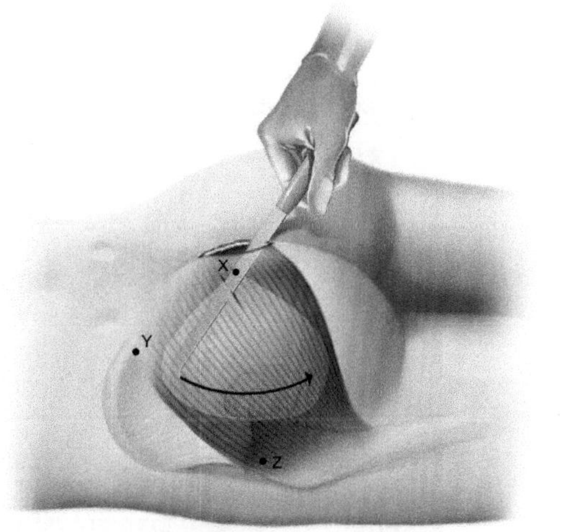

Fig. 5. By placing the detacher on the strong muscle fibers in the sacral area and using these fibers as support, the instrument easily rotates from point X to the contralateral aspect of the trochanter, point Z. This rotation creates a small triangular pocket containing some remaining strong muscular septa, which should be disrupted using the index finger as a dissector. Next, retractors can be introduced inside the pocket created to continue the procedure, enlarging it according to the size and shape of the implant.

cut with a dissector slightly wider than the instrument used initially. Next, the caudal aspect of the pocket is enlarged. The instrument the authors devised to complement the undermining procedure is a large forceps with flat, diamond-shaped tips here called a duck's bill. This tool completes the separation of muscle fibers, breaks many of the interfascicular septa, and can practically finish the undermining.

Obtaining Symmetry in Pockets on Both Sides

When inadequate technique without reference points to guide detachment are used for buttock augmentation, one of the most frequent complications is the asymmetry. With the XYZ technique, the upper undermining split in the muscle is guided by the iliac bone. The detacher follows the same upper limit of the bone on both sides. From an aesthetic viewpoint, the implant should be placed as high as possible in the intramuscular pocket, which helps produce a nice projection in the upper pole of the buttocks. The pocket should be enlarged according to the shape and size of the implant, and should not be too large or too tight; as a result, the pocket should be enlarged using sizers and feeling if the pocket corresponds well to the implant. After both implants are placed within the pockets, they must be compared and adjusted. In some cases, some complementary enlargement using fingers may be required to obtain asymmetry. The oval implant should be positioned vertically, with the larger section at the top.

Closing the Incisions

Negative pressure drains inside the pocket are used to evacuate some blood (usually 50–80 cc), and are important to avoid sciatic-type pain that may occur when this fluid migrates to the nerve area. A 2-day period is usually sufficient for the drains to be left in place. An additional drain in the area that was detached to expose the muscle is useful for avoiding small seromas in this region. To close the muscle, the authors prefer a running 2-0 absorbable suture, followed by another running suture using the same absorbable suture that approximates the roof and floor (subcutaneous and muscle layers) of the inverted-heart-shaped detached area, performing a quilting suture. This suture continues beyond the muscle and proceeds until it includes some of the subcutaneous tissue previously cut at 45° on the sacrocutaneous ligament.

The strip of skin left to preserve the sacrocutaneous ligament at the beginning of the procedure is de-epithelialized; there is a suture joining the deep dermis on 1 side, the sacrocutaneous ligament, and the deep dermis on the other side is created to reconstruct the intergluteal sulcus.

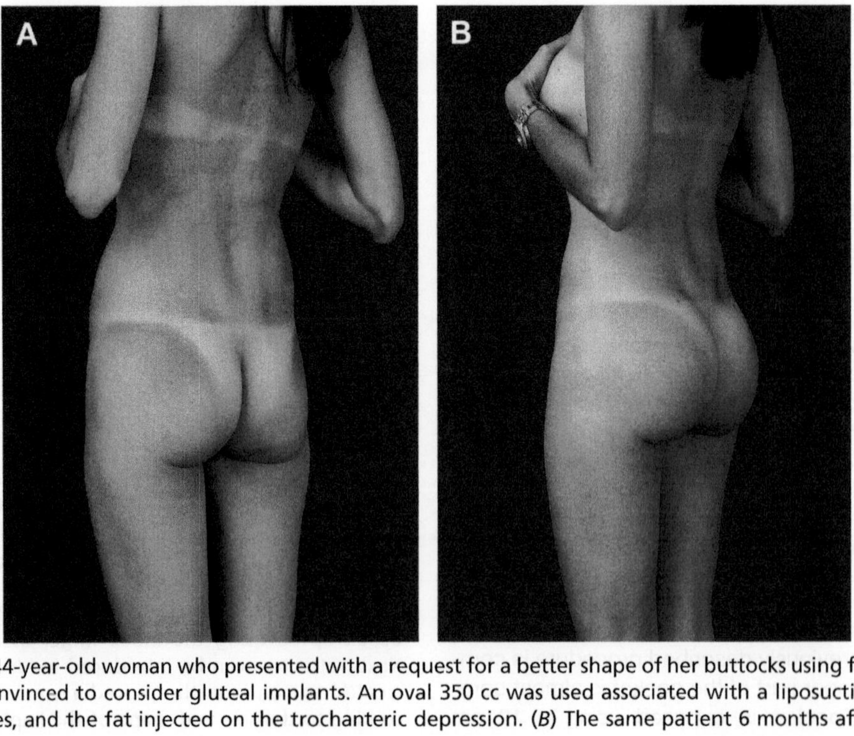

Fig. 6. (*A*) 44-year-old woman who presented with a request for a better shape of her buttocks using fat grafting. She was convinced to consider gluteal implants. An oval 350 cc was used associated with a liposuction on hips, love handles, and the fat injected on the trochanteric depression. (*B*) The same patient 6 months after surgery.

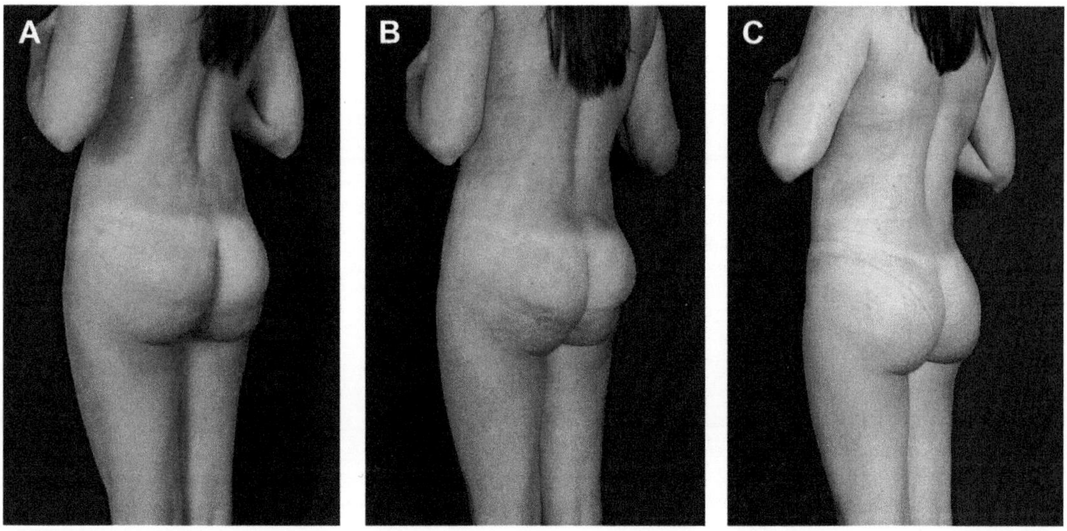

Fig. 7. (*A*) This 36-year-old patient presented with complaints of visibility of her implants mainly in the upper pole. On computed tomography the implants were inside the muscle just on the lower aspect of the implant, explaining the reason of the visibility. (*B*) When contracting the muscle, is possible to see the implant popping up and out. The lower aspect of the muscle contracts due this dynamic effect. (*C*) The implants were removed, the pocket was hermetically closed using 2-0 Vicryl suture, and a drain was left in the neo-pocket to avoid seroma. This is a frequent complication with removal and replacement of implants. After 4 months, the implants were replaced using the XYZ technique. The picture shows the patient 6 months after the second procedure.

Postoperative Care

This procedure can be particularly painful, and maintenance of an epidural catheter is useful for controlling pain. Ropivacaine 0.15%, 20 cc every 6 hours, prevents pain effectively. The patient is usually maintained in the prone position the hospital for 48 hours during this treatment. After discharge, the patient is encouraged to walk and sit normally. During the first week, the patient must avoid remaining in a prone position too long in order to prevent migration of the edema to the sciatic nerve area. After a week, driving is permitted (**Figs. 6** and **7**).

REFERENCES

1. Gonzalez-Ulloa M. Gluteoplasty – a ten years report. Aesthetic Plast Surg 1991;15:85–7.
2. Robles JM, Tagliapietra JC, Grandi M. Gluteoplastia de aumento: implante submuscular. Cir Plast Iberolat 1984;X:4–9.
3. Gonzalez R. Gluteoplasty: personal modifications of the Robles technique. In: Toledo S, editor. Recent Advances in Plastic Surgery 90. Sao Paulo, Brazil: Editora Grafica do Estadao; 1992. p. 166–71.
4. Gonzalez R. Prótese para a região glútea (Prostheses for gluteal área). In: Tournieux AAB, editor. Atualização em Cirurgia Plástica. São Paulo (Brazil): Robe Editorial; 1992. p. 555–70.
5. Vergara R, Marcos M. Intramuscular gluteal implants. Aesthetic Plast Surg 1996;20:259–62.
6. De la Peña JA. Subfascial technique for gluteal augmentation. Aesthet Surg J 2004;24(3):265–7.
7. Cocke WM, Ricktenson G. Gluteal augmentation. Plast Reconstr Surg 1973;52:93.
8. Bruner TW, Roberts LT III, Nguyen K. Complications of buttocks augmentation: diagnosis, management and prevention. Clin Plast Surg 2006;33(3):449–66.
9. Gonzalez R. Late intracapsular seroma in subfascial buttock augmentation: a case report. Aesthetic Plast Surg 2006;30(5):599–604.
10. Flores-Lima G. Cutaneous fistulas and acute seroma after subfascial gluteal implants. Aesthetic Plast Surg 2008;32(5):810–2.
11. Gonzalez R. Augmentation gluteoplasty: the XYZ method. Aesthetic Plast Surg 2004;28:417–25.
12. Gonzalez R. Gluteal implants: the "XYZ" intramuscular method. Aesthet Surg J 2010;30(2):256–64.
13. Gonzalez R. Buttocks reshaping – posterior contour surgery: a step-by-step approach. Rio de Janeiro (Brazil): Editora Indexa; 2006. p. 109–60.
14. Flores-Lima G. Surgical pocket location for gluteal implants: a systematic review. Aesthetic Plast Surg 2013;37:240–5.
15. Flores-Lima G, Eppley BL. Body Contouring with solid silicone implants. Aesthetic Plast Surg 2009;33:140–6.
16. Gonzalez R. Remodelagem glutea. In: Pitanguy I, editor. Cirurgia Plastica – uma visão de sua amplitude. Sao Paulo, Brazil: Editora Atheneu; 2016. p. 553–62.
17. Gonzalez R, Mauad F. Intraoperative ultrasonography to guide intramuscular buttock implants. Aesthet Surg J 2012;32(1):125–6.

Subfascial Gluteal Implant Augmentation

Jose Abel de la Peña Salcedo, MD, FACS*, Guillermo J. Gallardo, MD, Guillermo Ernesto Alvarenga, MD

KEYWORDS

• Buttock augmentation • Gluteal implants • Gluteal augmentation • Subfascial gluteal implants

KEY POINTS

- Preoperative planning and use of templates are crucial for determining implant volume and position.
- Preoperative markings are crucial in guiding the surgical procedure and should be performed with the patient in a standing position.
- The gluteal point of maximal projection should lie at the pubic bone level on a lateral view.
- Buttock implants should always be placed vertically, and orientation is aided with a white line across the implant equator.
- Buttock augmentation is major surgery; therefore, adequate precautions should be taken to avoid significant complications.

INTRODUCTION

The attractiveness of the buttocks is judged in proportion to the waist.[1] According to Singh,[2] there is 1 female body shape that men universally find most attractive (full buttocks, narrow waist). The ideal female proportions can be condensed into a waist-to-hip ratio of nearly 0.7 (measuring the waist at its narrowest and the buttock at the level of maximum circumference).

In addition to this overall proportional relationship, there are various characteristics associated with attractive youthful buttocks. These include (1) a marked lumbosacral lordosis with a downward pelvic tilt, (2) a very feminine cleavage as the buttocks separate superiorly, (3) inferior buttock separation creates a diamond shape together with the internal upper thighs, (4) maximum projection where the buttock equator joins an imaginary vertical line between the medial and central one-third of the buttocks, (5) minimal infra-gluteal crease, and (6) no ptosis.[3,4]

THE SUBFASCIAL PLANE

Because the subcutaneous, submuscular, and intramuscular techniques have inherent problems associated with the dissection plane, the subfascial plane can ideally accommodate a gluteal implant and overcome the shortcomings of other approaches (**Fig. 1**).[1,5] This technique is based on extensive cadaver dissections and study of each distinct anatomic layer. The gluteal fascia is very strong at the origins and insertions. It covers the gluteus maximus muscle, the largest and most superficial muscle in the region, and is a significant contributor to the projection of the

Disclosure: The authors have nothing to disclose.

Plastic Surgery Institute, Hospital Ángeles Lomas, Vialidad de la Barranca s/no consultorio 490 Col. Valle de las Palmas Huixquilucan, Mexico City 52763, Mexico
* Corresponding author.
E-mail address: doc@institutodecirugiaplastica.mx

Clin Plastic Surg 45 (2018) 225–236
https://doi.org/10.1016/j.cps.2017.12.012

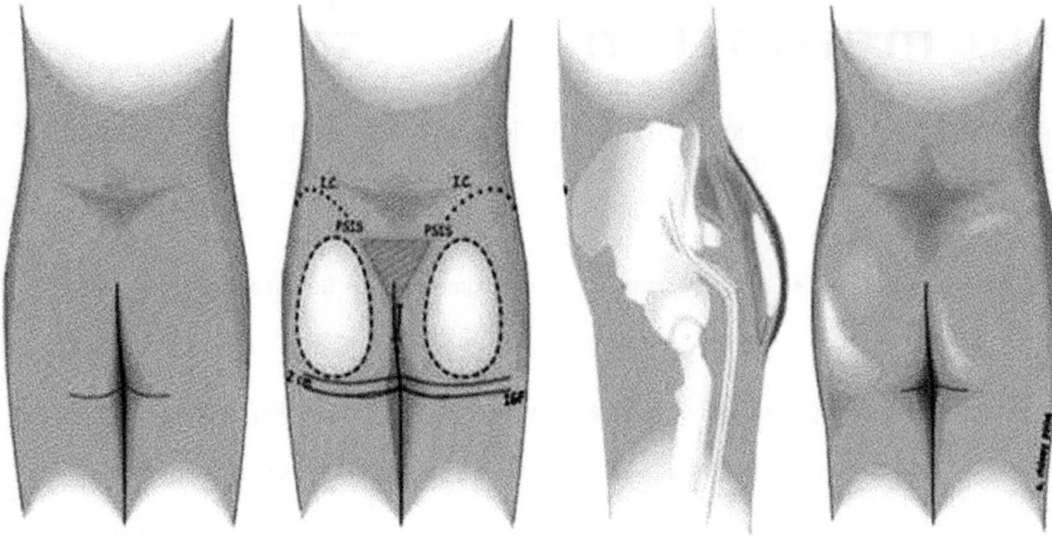

Fig. 1. Relevant anatomy and position of a subfascial implant, which must be centered in the buttock and completely covered by the fasciocutaneous flap. The sciatic nerve, visible on the lateral view, is a safe distance away from the implant pocket. (*From* de la Peña JA. Subfascial technique for gluteal augmentation. Aesthet Surg J 2004;24:265–73; with permission.)

buttocks. The anterior two-thirds of the gluteus medius muscle, also covered by the gluteal aponeurosis, provide bulk to the upper one-third of the buttocks. The gluteal aponeurosis' origin is on the posterior iliac bone, the sacrum, and the coccyx; laterally, it inserts on and envelops the greater trochanter and extends to the iliotibial line. This aponeurosis covers the entire gluteal region and is capable of holding gluteal implants in an adequate position because the fascia is stronger at the origin and insertion sites, and is compliant in the middle.[6] Consequently, when an implant is placed in this space, an anatomic contour is created naturally.

The gluteal aponeurosis sends expansions to the skin, which insert into the deep dermis. They work as a system to adhere the skin and subcutaneous tissues in the gluteal region. Aponeurotic expansions are distributed in a transverse direction (**Fig. 2**), along the axis of the muscle fibers throughout the gluteal region.[7] This system of fascial attachments should be maintained in any gluteal implant surgery. The aponeurotic expansions to the skin are preserved, and the subaponeurotic space allows proper positioning of an implant without risking injury to the deep neurovascular structures (**Fig. 3**).

TREATMENT GOALS

Patient treatment is focused on enhancing size, contour, and projection of the gluteal region because of hypoplasia, hypotrophy, or aging. In other cases, where patients present with a mild lumbosacral lordosis, the volume gained by the implant creates the illusion of a more noticeable angle. To help create an adequate gluteal cleavage, liposuction of the waist is needed in some cases. The inferior buttock–inner thigh diamond can be created by liposuction of the inferior inner quadrant of the gluteus and the inner thigh. For most patients seeking gluteal augmentation,

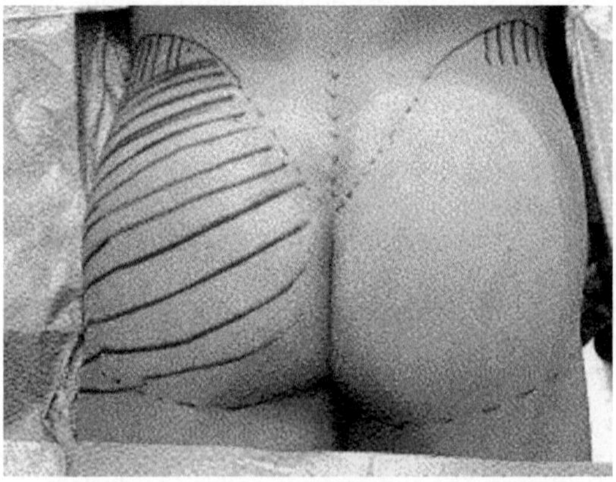

Fig. 2. The aponeurotic expansions run from the gluteal aponeurosis to the dermis in the direction of the *red lines* drawn on the skin. (*From* de la Peña JA, Rubio OV, Cano JP, et al. Subfascial gluteal augmentation. Clin Plast Surg 2006;33:408; with permission.)

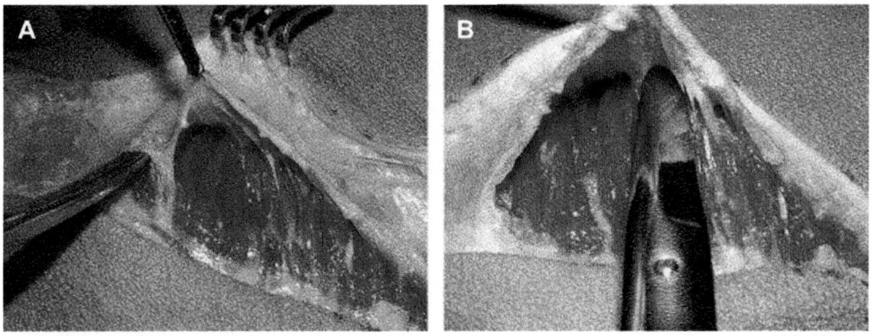

Fig. 3. (*A*) Aponeurotic expansions traverse the superior layer of the gluteus maximus muscle. (*B*) Dissection between the aponeurotic expansions is essential for creation of the implant pocket. (*From* de la Peña JA, Rubio OV, Cano JP, et al. Subfascial gluteal augmentation. Clin Plast Surg 2006;33:409; with permission.)

ancillary procedures, such as liposuction of adjacent areas, are often required to achieve optimal results.

PATIENT SELECTION

Thin patients with an athletic build and little or no ptosis are the ideal candidates for subfascial augmentation. When significant buttock ptosis exists, the skin typically has poor elasticity and weak underlying support structures. Overweight and even moderately obese patients may also benefit from this technique, but often require more extensive liposculpture. If large volume liposuction is needed, staging the procedures is probably wise. Massive weight loss patients are good candidates if they undergo excisional procedures to correct the back and gluteal regions. Patients with skin laxity may also require skin excisions.[1]

Subfascial gluteal augmentation can be successfully done in most patients who lack projection of the buttocks, who desire gluteal shape improvement, and who are properly selected for cosmetic surgery. The procedure may be performed with small anatomic implants used for gluteal-pexy or large implants to increase projection and volume. Small implants around 175 mL and 250 mL can be placed to lift the buttocks, that is, gluteal-pexy, resulting in an improved gluteal shape without an evident increase in volume. Because implants are placed below the gluteal aponeurosis and on top of the gluteus maximus muscle, anatomically shaped implants are the best suited.

The anatomic system we designed for subfascial augmentation consists of templates for preoperative skin markings, sizers, and either elastomer or highly cohesive silicone gel-filled implants.[8] The best elastomer implants are those with the maximum softness available.

PREOPERATIVE PLANNING AND PREPARATION

Patient preparation begins at the time of the initial consultation when postoperative instructions are carefully explained so appropriate patient expectations are established. The patient is also instructed to refrain from taking any aspirin, vitamin E, omega fatty acids, and homeopathic supplements (except for *Arnica montana*) because of the risk for increased bleeding during surgery.[1] They are admitted to the hospital the night before surgery to mark the skin and administer an enema.

With the patient in a standing position, markings are made using custom-designed templates (**Fig. 4**). The template must be centered over the gluteal region

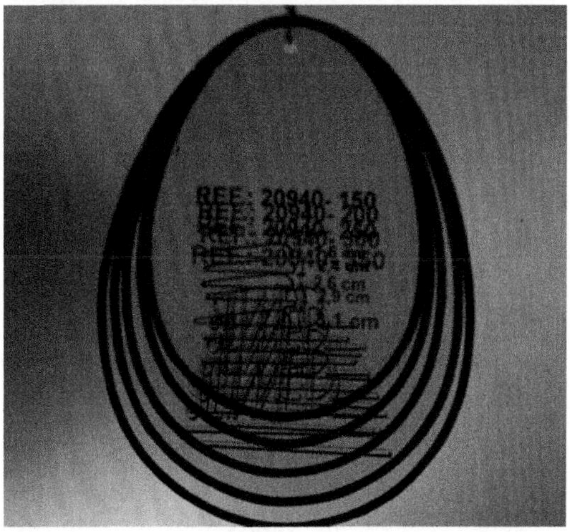

Fig. 4. Set of templates used for preoperative evaluation of implant size. (*From* de la Peña JA, Rubio OV, Cano JP, et al. Subfascial gluteal augmentation. Clin Plast Surg 2006;33:410; with permission.)

leaving at least 5 cm between the template and the infragluteal fold and 2 cm lateral to the sacrum (**Fig. 5**).

Determining the implant size is simplified by knowing the exact measurements of the template that best accommodates the buttocks (**Fig. 6**), and patient expectations. The most appropriate size can be selected before surgery and confirmed with implant sizers during surgery (**Fig. 7**). Anatomically designed implants with varying projections are now available.[1]

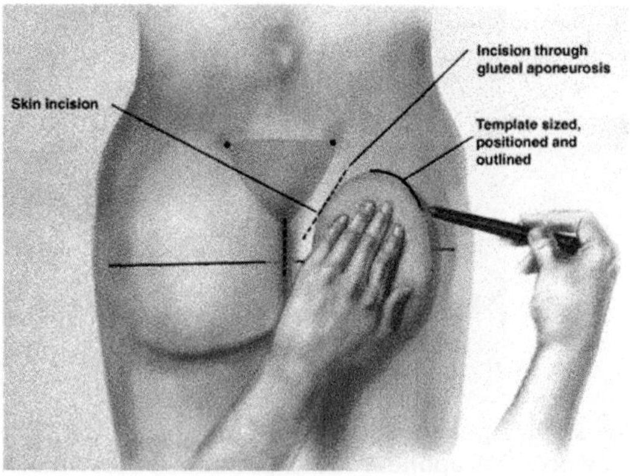

Fig. 6. Bilateral paramedian presacral incisions are used and a beveled dissection is carried out up to the border of the sacrum, the gluteal fascia in incised, and a subfascial pocket is created over the gluteus maximus muscle. (*From* de la Peña JA, Rubio OV, Cano JP, et al. Subfascial gluteal augmentation. Clin Plast Surg 2006;33:411; with permission.)

PATIENT POSITIONING

The procedure can be performed under general or spinal anesthesia, but we favor general anesthesia because spinal anesthesia causes vasodilation in the operating field. The patient is placed in a prone position with a unitary catheter in place, antiembolism and circumferential compression stockings are fitted, and pressure relief gel pads are set on the elbows, shoulders, iliac bones, and knees. A pressure relief face mask is used in a neutral position. The gluteal area is prepped from the popliteal fossa to the upper back. An iodopovidone-soaked gauze is placed over the anus, a sterile lap sponge is secured with 2-0 silk over the gauze to cover the anus and the inner gluteal zone to avoid contamination.[9] Finally, an antimicrobial plastic film (3M Ioban Antimicrobial Incise Drapes, 3M, Maplewood, MN) is placed on the caudal portion of the buttocks below the planned incision.

PROCEDURAL APPROACH

The skin is injected with a mixture of 2% lidocaine with epinephrine and 7.5% ropivacaine. The skin is incised using 6 cm bilateral paramedian incisions 5 cm above the anus, a beveled dissection is carried up to the muscular aponeurosis at the lateral border of the sacrum, an 8- to 10-cm incision into the aponeurosis is made parallel to the sacral border entering the subfascial dissecting plane (**Fig. 8**). Tumescent solution, 100 to 150 mL, is instilled with a cannula. This step enables the identification of the avascular plane deep to the fascia and facilitates sharp dissection of the septa in the subfascial plane, permitting the elevation of an intact fasciocutaneous flap (**Fig. 9**). The septa parallel the direction of the muscle fibers and, therefore, radiate out in a fanlike pattern.[10]

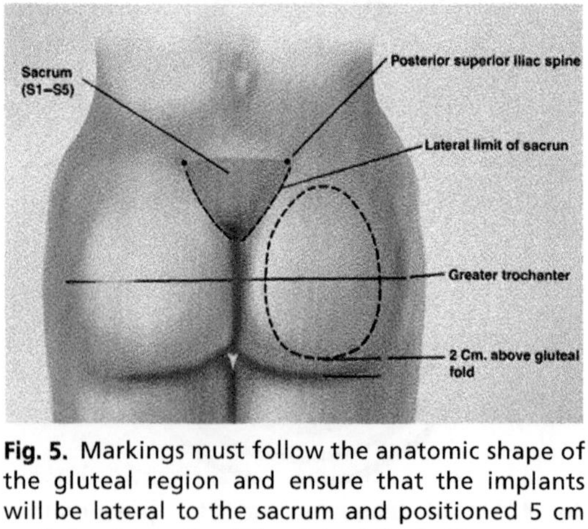

Fig. 5. Markings must follow the anatomic shape of the gluteal region and ensure that the implants will be lateral to the sacrum and positioned 5 cm or 2 in above the infragluteal fold. (*From* de la Peña JA, Rubio OV, Cano JP, et al. Subfascial gluteal augmentation. Clin Plast Surg 2006;33:410; with permission.)

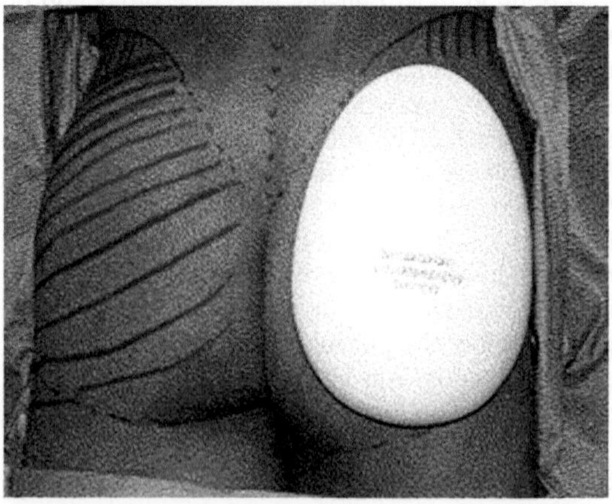

Fig. 7. The sizer must be adequate for the gluteal region. (*From* de la Peña JA. Subfascial technique for gluteal augmentation. Aesthet Surg J 2004;24:268; with permission.)

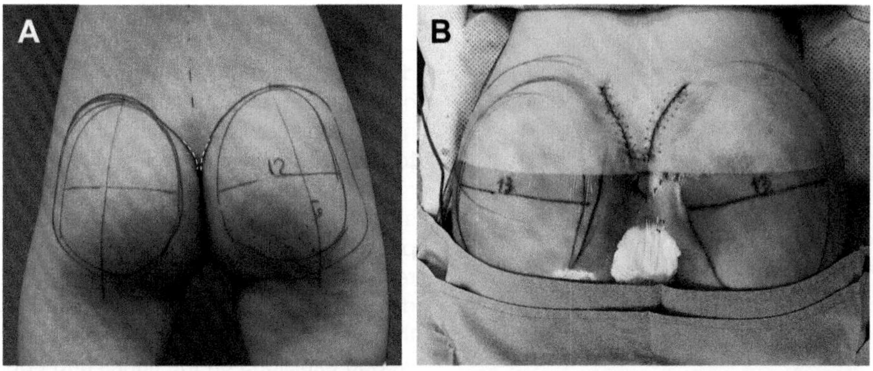

Fig. 8. (*A*) The operation is planned using templates that fit the buttock area of the patient and 6 cm bilateral paramedian presacral skin incisions at least 5 cm superior to the anus. (*B*) This is a patient with a buttock localized adjuvant disease and a previous ultrasonic liposuction of this area, where the incisions were placed higher on the buttocks to avoid any complications.

Double-ended, blunt, round dissectors are used initially to separate the avascular plane and preserve the septa and the aponeurosis. Undermining is facilitated if dissection is carried out from medial to lateral, and from cephalic to caudal using a fiberoptic retractor (**Fig. 10**). A long cautery tip is used to dissect the septa, as well as a pair of long cauterizing scissors (**Fig. 11**). Branches of the superior and inferior gluteal arteries are coagulated and a few vessels that run through the gluteal aponeurosis septa. Both pockets should be dissected before placement of any implant to ease dissection of the contralateral pocket (**Figs. 12** and **13**). Once the pockets are dissected, a sizer is used to evaluate the volume and shape of the pocket and to confirm the correct implant size for the patient (**Fig. 14**).

Before the introduction of microtextured implants, we placed drains exiting superiorly and laterally on the buttocks. Today, we no longer use drains routinely. It was initially thought that both macrotextured implants and polyurethane-covered implants would avoid seroma formation because of the high adhesion they have to the surrounding tissues. As the breast implant literature has shown, this is not the case, and seromas rarely occur, if at all, with smooth implants. Microtextured implants behave similarly to smooth implants. As such, and because of the high mobility of the buttock compared with the breast, we have preferred microtextured implants over any other shell type; we have not had any seromas in our series to the time of writing. The implant is then inserted, making sure that it is perfectly aligned on its axis and fitting loosely inside the pocket (**Fig. 15**).[1] We insist that all gluteal

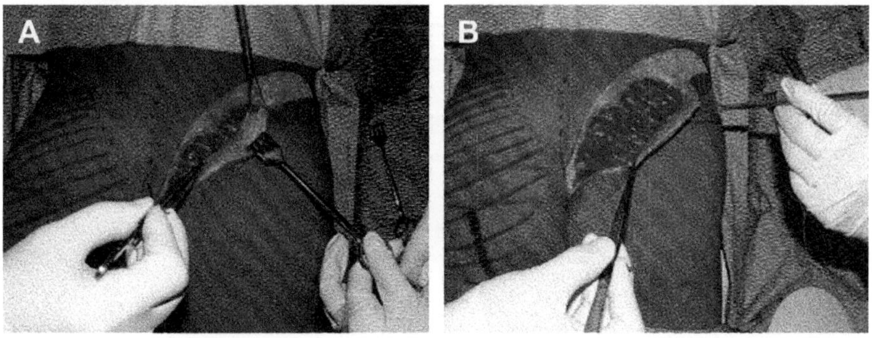

Fig. 9. Markings of important anatomic landmarks. (*A*) Incision of the gluteal aponeurosis begins at the lateral border of the sacrum. (*B*) Subfascial undermining starts from the incision in the gluteal aponeurosis. (*From* de la Peña JA, Rubio OV, Cano JP, et al. Subfascial gluteal augmentation. Clin Plast Surg 2006;33:411; with permission.)

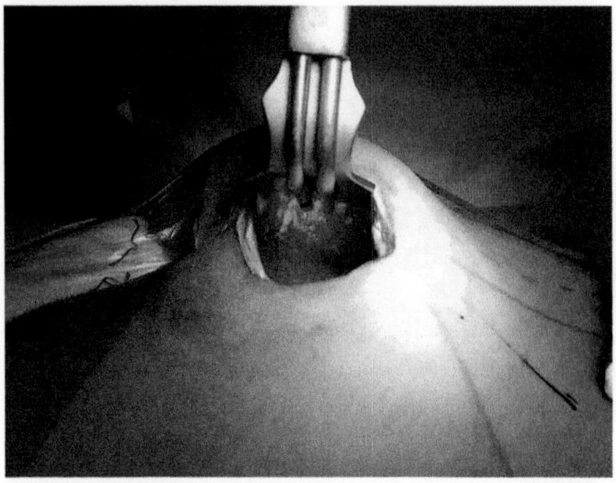

Fig. 10. Fiberoptic retractors with a smoke extraction port are helpful during undermining and elevation of the fasciocutaneous flap.

implants must have a white line through their horizontal axis to facilitate and ensure proper vertical alignment inside the pocket (**Fig. 16**). Implants should never be placed in an oblique manner because this placement causes a double bubble contour inferolaterally (**Fig. 17**).

Once the implants have been inserted, closure begins by suturing the gluteal aponeurosis with both an interrupted 2-0 cutting needle nylon suture and a running 2-0 round needle polyglactin 910 suture ensuring a watertight closure, making sure that no tension is placed on the suture line. Then, the deep and superficial subcutaneous layers are closed separately over the sacrum with a cutting needle 2-0 polydioxanone. The dermis is then closed up using a watertight suture with a 3-0 polydioxanone on a cutting needle and a 4-0 running nonabsorbable monofilament suture, for example, nylon, is placed on the skin and reinforced with a topical skin adhesive.

Skin resection in patients requiring skin excisions should always be done superiorly, on the cephalic part of the buttocks. The incision and resection should be planned in such a way that dissection of the subfascial plane is carried out through it. The surgery is planned with bilateral wedge excisions on the flanks and upper buttock area of both skin and subcutaneous tissue. Dissection is carried out as described after tumescent solution is instilled to create a subfascial pocket through the superior incision. The rest of the procedure is carried out in the same fashion as described, and closure is executed verbatim.

POTENTIAL COMPLICATIONS AND THEIR MANAGEMENT

The most common complication reported is wound dehiscence. Bilateral paramedian sacral incisions have decreased wound dehiscence from 30% in midsacral incisions to 5.0% to 7.9%. Wound management to facilitate healing by secondary intention is used to avoid implant exposure, which only occurs in approximately 2% of cases. This approach includes meticulous local wound care and serial dressing changes. Wound care is initially carried out daily

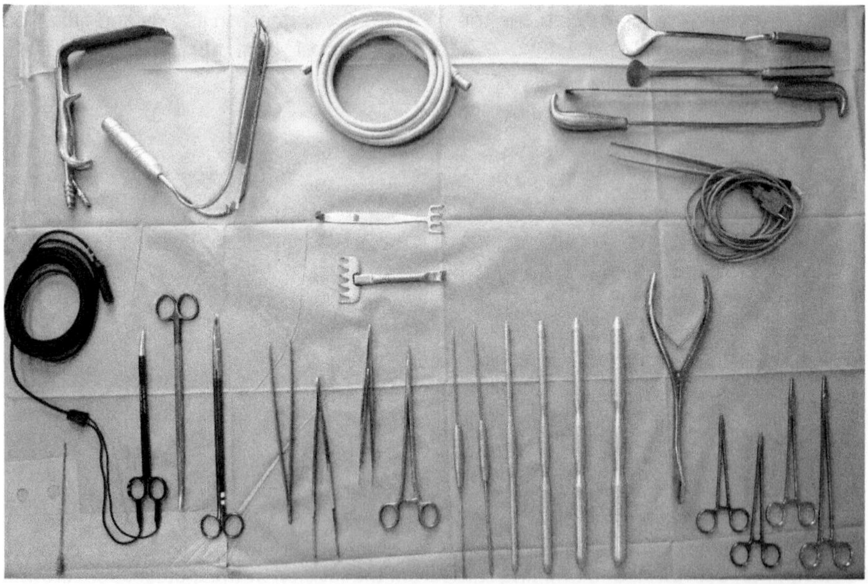

Fig. 11. Surgical instruments typically used for subfascial gluteal augmentation implant placement.

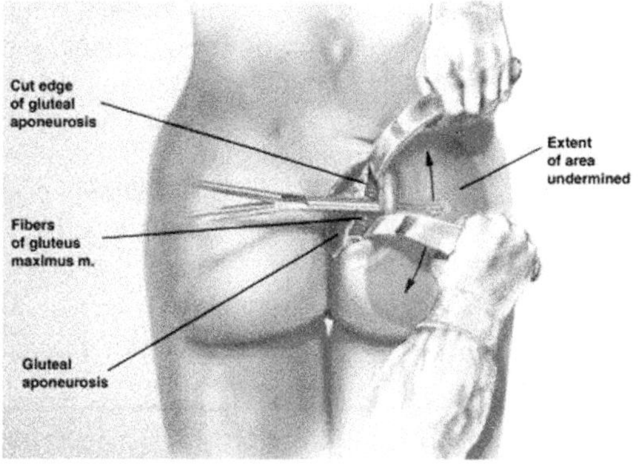

Fig. 12. Subfascial pocket dissection is carried out before placing the sizer to ensure adequate contour correction. (*From* de la Peña JA, Rubio OV, Cano JP, et al. Subfascial gluteal augmentation. Clin Plast Surg 2006;33:412; with permission.)

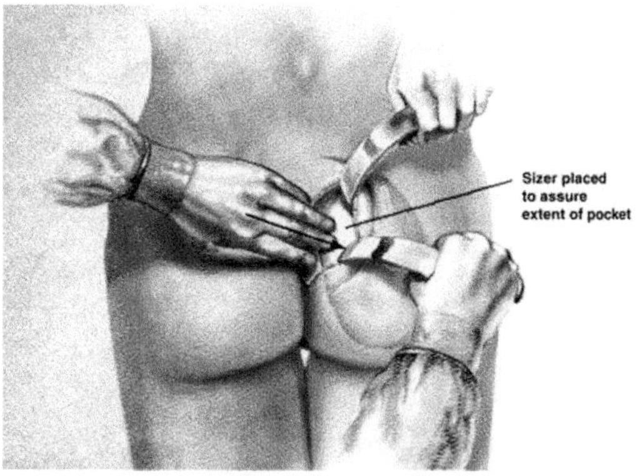

Fig. 14. Once the pocket is completed, insert a sizer, evaluate the pocket, and assess implant size. The implant should fit snugly in the space. (*From* de la Peña JA, Rubio OV, Cano JP, et al. Subfascial gluteal augmentation. Clin Plast Surg 2006; 33:414; with permission.)

after showering with an antiseptic chlorine and hydrogen peroxide based solution (Microdacyn 60, Oculus Innovative Sciences, Petaluma, CA). After irrigation with this solution, the wound is treated with either a silver-containing gel or a silver alginate dressing, and then covered with a *Triticum vulgare*–containing dressing (Italldermol) and a dry nonadherent antimicrobial impregnated dressing (Telfa by Medtronic, Minneapolis, MN). The wound is then isolated with a plastic skin dressing (3M Tegaderm Transparent Film Dressing) to keep it out of contact with the contralateral incision or any external contamination. The wound is always cultured and the antibiotic regime is modified appropriately. Any scar revision can be performed 3 to 6 months after the wound is healed.[10]

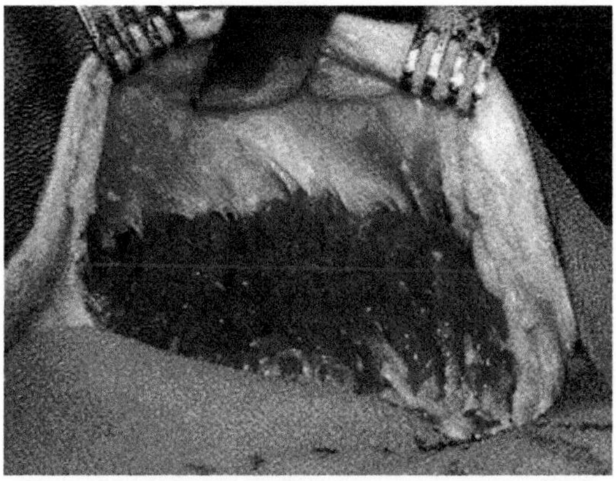

Fig. 13. Cadaver dissection demonstrates the fasciocutaneous flap that is raised during pocket dissection. A large incision has been made only for demonstration purposes. A normal incision is 6 to 7 cm in length and 1 cm lateral to the intergluteal crease. (*From* de la Peña JA. Subfascial technique for gluteal augmentation. Aesthet Surg J 2004;24:268; with permission.)

Seroma can lead to implant displacement, asymmetry, and infection, and must, therefore, be evacuated. Late seroma occurs mainly with textured implants 3 to 6 months postoperatively and has an incidence of 3.0% to 3.7%. Successful resolution of late seromas, in our experience, requires implant exchange (substitution for smooth implants), partial capsulectomy, and drainage.[10,11]

The incidence of infection is less than 1% and treatment usually requires temporary removal of the implant. Gluteal sensitivity is lost during the first 6 weeks after surgery, and full recovery may take up to 4 months.

Other uncommon complications include capsular contracture, implant rotation, and skin ulceration, which have an incidence of less than 1% each and require surgical explantation for their resolution.[12]

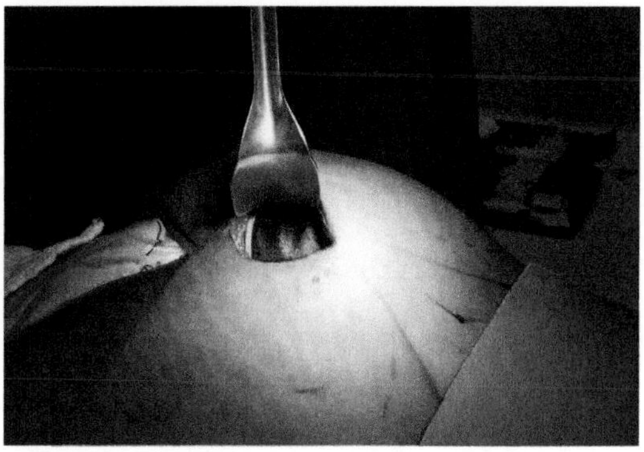

Fig. 15. The buttock equator must coincide with the white line equator mark on the implant to help guarantee a correct implant position.

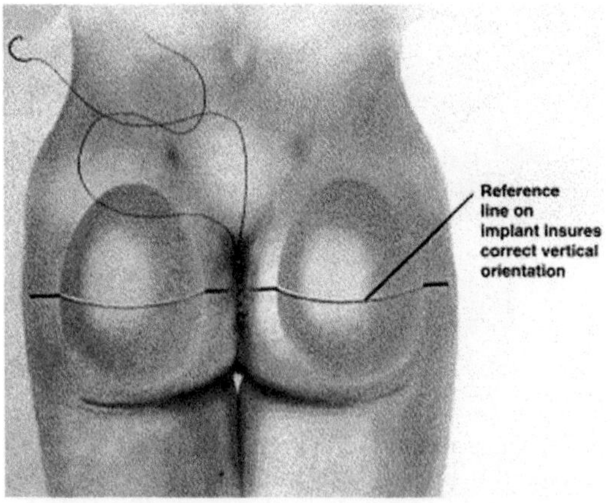

Fig. 16. This posterior view shows an implant in its correct position in relation to the sacrum, intergluteal sulcus, and lateral limits. The midline incision depicted in the drawing has been abandoned in favor of 2 paramedian incisions. (*From* de la Peña JA. Subfascial technique for gluteal augmentation. Aesthet Surg J 2004;24:269. with permission.)

POSTOPERATIVE CARE

Because wound dehiscence typically occurs between days 12 and 16 in our series, patients are instructed to stop activities that cause wound pressure, stretching, or friction. After 2 weeks, the patient may return to normal activities, but physical exercise and sitting down is withheld for a whole month; it is only permitted when voiding.[10] To use the toilet, the patient is advised to use a raised toilet seat to reduce tension on the suture line. If the patient desires to sleep in a supine position, a pillow should be placed under the lumbar region and below the upper thighs for at least 3 weeks.

Garments

Compressive garments are worn for 6 weeks to place light pressure on the upper part of the buttock. A compression girdle is fitted to decrease tension on the incision. A 3-panel abdominal binder is used on top of the girdle to keep the buttocks together.

Wound Care

Once wound dressings are taken off, the patient continues with irrigation of the area with an antiseptic solution daily and after voiding. A shower is allowed 24 hours after surgery. An antibiotic (moxifloxacin) is used preoperatively and continued postoperatively for 10 days. During the patient's weekly visits, the wound is covered with additional topical skin adhesive to ensure wound impermeability.

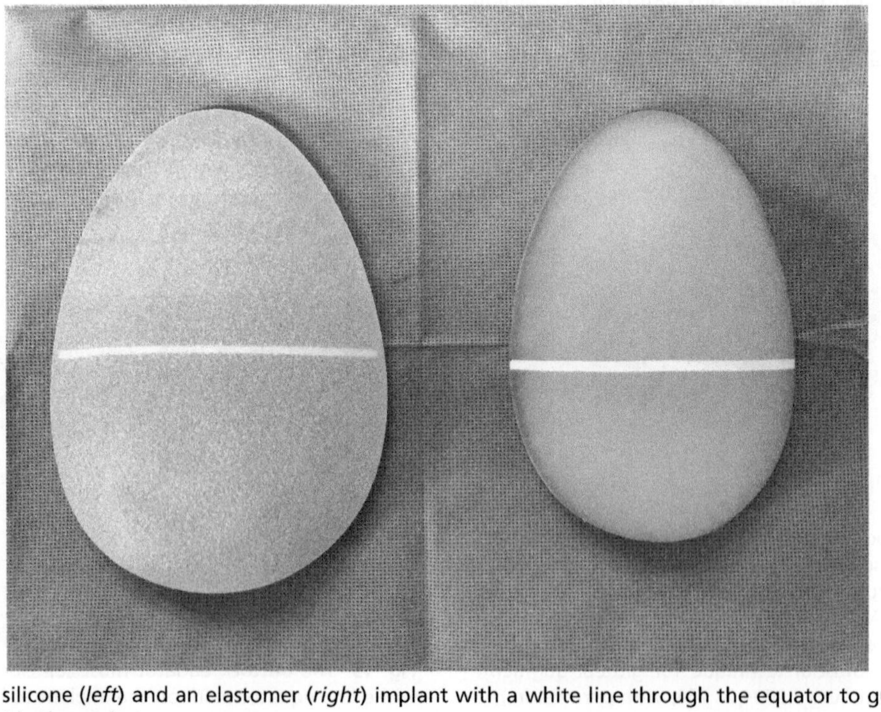

Fig. 17. A silicone (*left*) and an elastomer (*right*) implant with a white line through the equator to guide positioning inside the pocket.

Pain Management

Most patients experience either little or no discomfort at all. A course of nonsteroidal antiinflammatory drugs are always prescribed, together with ice packs for at least 10 days.

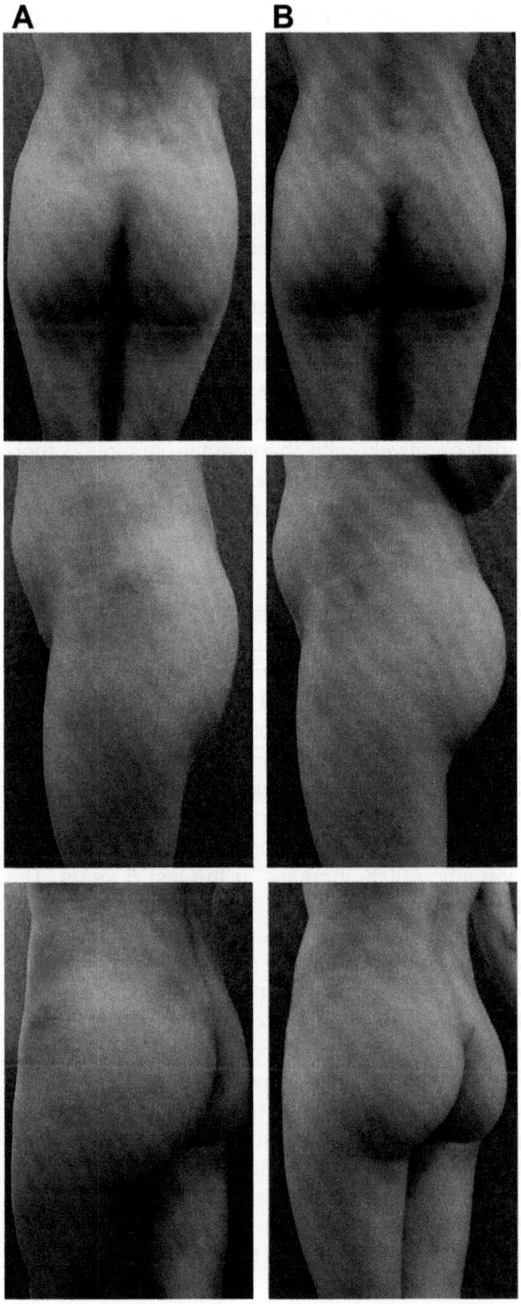

Fig. 18. (*A*) Preoperative and (*B*) postoperative photographs of an ideal patient with gluteal augmentation with a 225-mL subfascial implant.

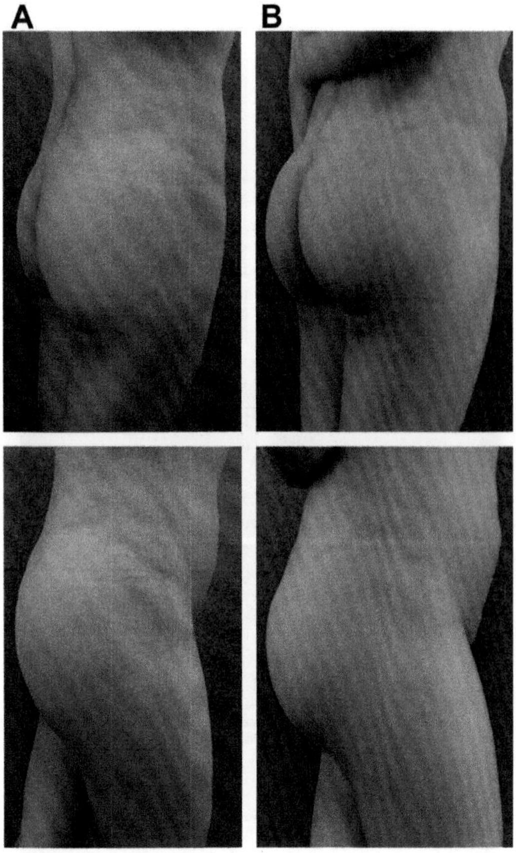

Fig. 18. Continued

RECOVERY

Patients usually return to work after 3 weeks. Physical exercise can be resumed after 8 weeks. If wound dehiscence occurs, an additional 6 weeks of restricted activity may be required. A patient who experiences a dehiscence typically may resume unrestricted activity at 12 weeks postoperatively. The implants will initially feel very firm and it will take 3 months for them to soften.

OUTCOMES

A healthy 31-year-old patient, an ideal candidate for gluteal augmentation with implants as described, presented with insufficient buttock volume for gluteal augmentation. Two 225-mL polyurethane anatomic gel implants were placed in the subfascial plane. There were no complications during her recovery and her incisions healed adequately (**Fig. 18**).

A 52-year-old patient presented with severe laxity owing to aging of the buttocks and a desire to increase their volume. A 330-mL anatomic polyurethane silicone implant was placed bilaterally in the subfascial plane. She had an unremarkable postoperative recovery (**Fig. 19**).

A 30-year-old patient presented with an interest in buttock augmentation surgery, even though she had a good volume to begin with. After evaluation it was decided that she would obtain the desired result with waist liposuction and buttock augmentation with implants. Two 330-mL microtextured implants were placed bilaterally. The patient presented postoperatively with a partial, less than 2 cm bilateral and superficial wound dehiscence that was treated conservatively with secondary closure, antiseptic solution, and local and systemic antibiotics as described in our treatment plan (**Fig. 20**).

Finally, a 48-year-old patient with a history of liposculpture and an obtuse lumbosacral angle desired buttock augmentation. A pair of 300-mL microtextured silicone implants were placed in a subfascial pocket bilaterally. She was cared for postoperatively with therapeutic ultrasound therapy in an attempt to decrease inflammation. No complications were seen postoperatively (**Fig. 21**).

SUMMARY

Gluteal augmentation with silicone implants is a safe and effective procedure with high patient satisfaction and a low complication rate if performed appropriately and care is taken throughout the entire process. Despite gluteal augmentation with implants being practiced for more than 30 years, significant patient awareness and demand for buttock contouring began approximately 10 years ago. Buttock augmentation has shown a dramatic 600% increase in the last 5 years. The first treatment option for these patients is gluteal fat grafting,[13] but not every patient is a good candidate for this type of surgical treatment. Planning and refinement of the described technique has had a long learning curve because of a high initial incidence of wound infection. This reason is why a double incision was favored over a single incision, one per side to isolate each implant pocket, and why the incisions are now placed further away from the anus.

The use of implants, sizers, and templates, and initiating the dissection laterally to the sacral border, have contributed to a significant decrease

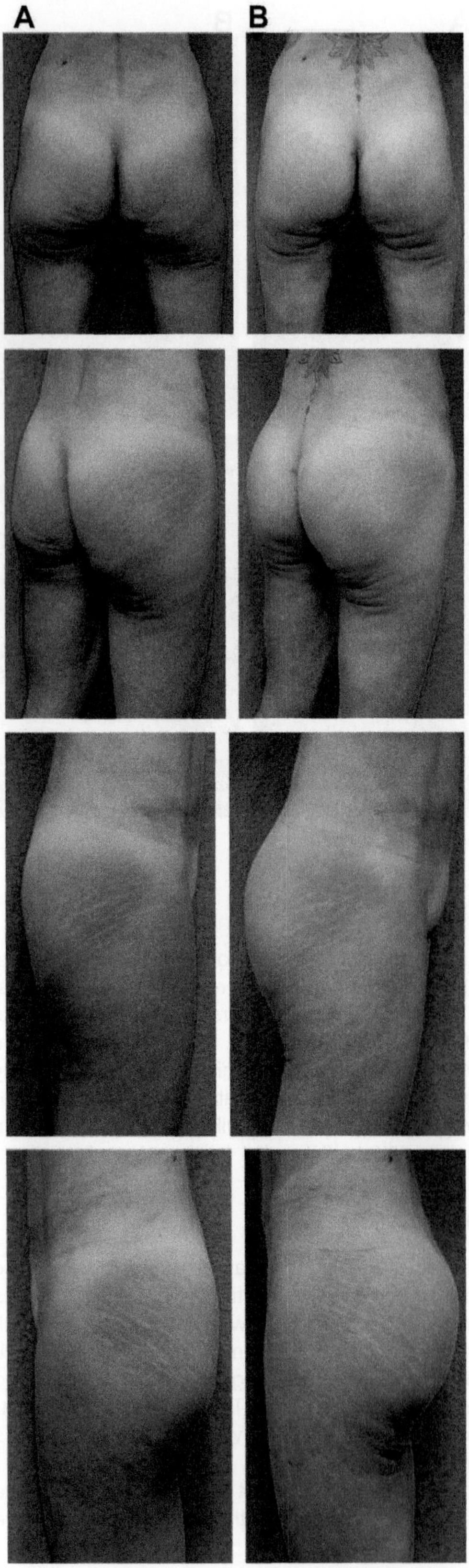

Fig. 19. (*A*) Preoperative and (*B*) postoperative photographs of a patient with severe skin laxity treated with gluteal augmentation with 330-mL subfascial implants.

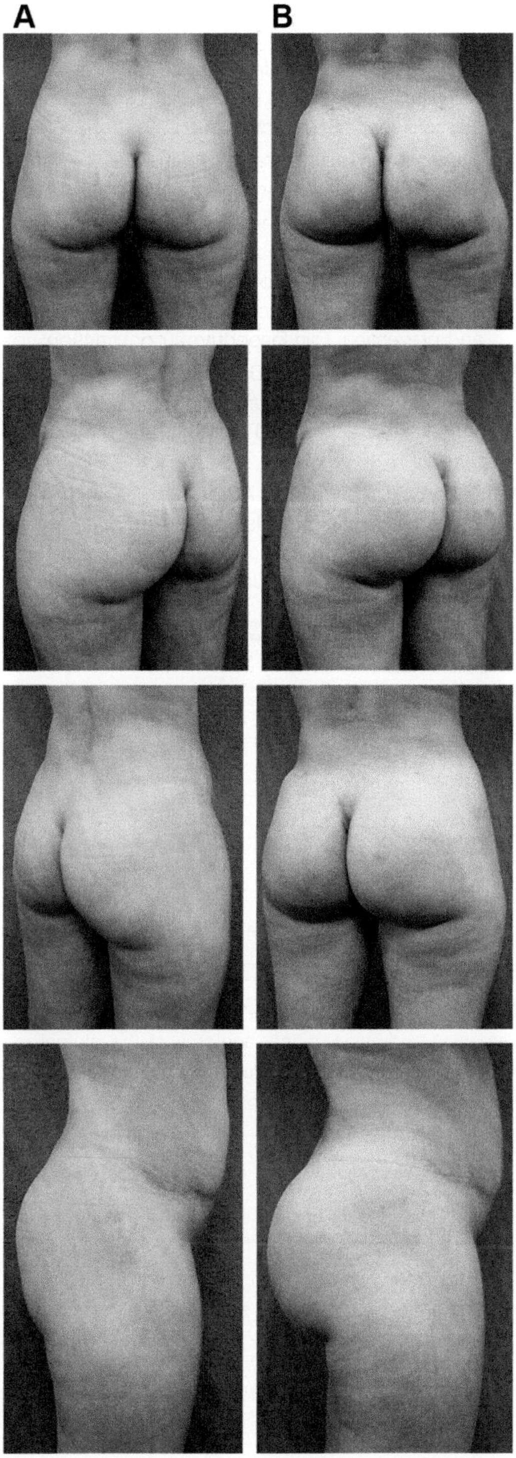

Fig. 20. (*A*) Preoperative and (*B*) postoperative photographs of a patient with an adequate preexisting buttock volume who desired gluteal augmentation. The 330-mL subfascial implants were placed bilaterally.

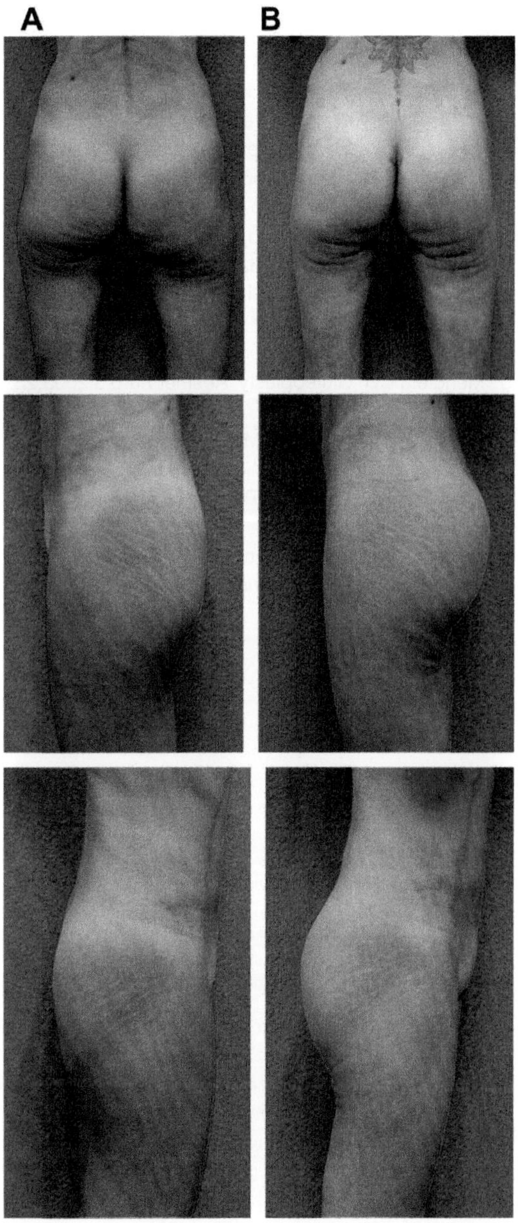

Fig. 21. (*A*) Preoperative and (*B*) postoperative photographs of a patient with a flattened lumbosacral lordosis who desired gluteal augmentation. The 300-mL subfascial implants were placed bilaterally.

in the frequency of complications. Once the sizer is in place, it is very important to check that the aponeurosis can be closed without tension. Finally, the use of specialized surgical instruments has contributed to an easier dissection overall, which has decreased morbidity and operative time.

REFERENCES

1. De la Peña JA, Rubio OV, Cano JP, et al. Subfascial gluteal augmentation. Clin Plast Surg 2006;33:405–22.
2. Singh D. Universal allure of the hourglass figure: an evolutionary theory of female physical attractiveness. Clin Plast Surg 2006;33:359–70.
3. Cuenca-Guerra R, Lugo-Beltran I. Beautiful buttocks: characteristics and surgical techniques. Clin Plast Surg 2006;33:321–32.
4. Centeno RF, Young VL. Clinical anatomy in aesthetic gluteal body contouring surgery. Clin Plast Surg 2006;33:347–58.
5. Mendieta CG. Gluteoplasty. Aesthet Surg J 2003;23:441–55.
6. De la Peña JA, López HM, Gamboa LF. Augmentation gluteoplasty: anatomical and clinical considerations. Key Issues in Plastic Cosmetic Surgery 2000;17:1–12.
7. De la Peña JA. Subfascial technique for gluteal augmentation. Aesthet Surg J 2004;24:265–73.
8. De la Peña JA, Rubio OV, Cano JP, et al. History of gluteal augmentation. Clin Plast Surg 2006;33:307–19.
9. Tardif M, De la Peña JA. Gluteal augmentation. In: Aston SJ, Steinbrech DS, Walden JL, editors. Aesthetic plastic surgery. Saunders Elsevier; 2009. p. 837–44.
10. Bruner TW, De la Peña JA, Mendieta CG, et al. Gluteal augmentation. In: Neligan PC, editor. Plastic surgery. 3rd edition. Saunders Elsevier; 2012. p. 599–615.
11. Bruner TW, Roberts TL III, Nguyen K. Complications of buttocks augmentation: diagnosis, management, and prevention. Clin Plast Surg 2006;33:449–66.
12. Mofid MM, Gonzalez R, De la Peña JA, et al. Buttock augmentation with silicone implants: a multicenter survey review of 2226 patients. Plast Reconstr Surg 2013;131:897–901.
13. Roberts TL III, Weinfeld AB, Bruner TW, et al. "Universal" and ethnic ideals of beautiful buttocks are best obtained by autologous micro fat grafting and liposuction. Clin Plast Surg 2006;33:371–94.

Improvement of the Gluteal Contour

Modern Concepts with Systematized Lipoinjection

Lázaro Cárdenas-Camarena, MD[a,b,c,d,*], Héctor Durán, MD[a,b,c,d]

KEYWORDS

• Fat grafting • Buttock fat grafting • Brazilian butt lift • Gluteal augmentation • Technique

KEY POINTS

- Properly evaluating the patient and identifying the areas that require treatment with subtraction or addition of volume are keys to being able to achieve an adequate result.
- This report describes the steps and technique that allow us to remove fat properly and infiltrate it correctly without contaminating it, along with the technique for infiltrating it.
- Identifying and planning important points for patients are keys for achieving more adequate results.
- A beautiful buttock is characterized not only by the increase in its volume, but also by the adequate proportions of the areas that surround it.
- Proper postoperative management will yield better long-term results by minimizing reabsorption.

INTRODUCTION

Delivering a beautiful buttock contouring result is not just a matter of adding fat and giving more volume. Advances in morphology, psychology, and anatomy have shown that giving shape to the buttock is much more complex than just increasing its volume. Achieving good results requires an understanding of the complex anatomy that gives us aesthetically pleasing and reliable outcomes. It is important that we understand that the relationships between the areas surrounding the buttock may be more important than the volume itself. Shape has more relevance than volume. Shape is subject to the relationships between the waist, the hips, and the legs. A large buttock is no better than a well-formed small buttock. Patients are demanding more and more volume in this area, and as a result we are also facing aesthetic deficiencies when we focus exclusively on this goal without taking into account gluteal contour. As with breasts, an appropriate volume with a beautiful shape is the main objective. To think that a very large buttock will satisfy the expectations of all patients is to ignore aesthetics and set an incorrect goal. Similarly, we cannot achieve an aesthetic buttock without considering the 3 anatomic regions that give harmony: the lumbar region, waist, and legs.

This knowledge is derived from important studies on Brazilian butt lifting[1]; the first use of the term has been attributed to Brazilian authors. The shape in relation to the type of gluteal frame, mainly in the form of a round “A” or a square “V”

The authors have nothing to disclose.

[a] International Society of Aesthetic Plastic Surgery (ISAPS); [b] Iberolatinoamerican Plastic Surgery Federation (FILACP); [c] Mexican Association of Plastic Esthetic and Reconstructive Surgery (AMCPER); [d] American Society of Plastic Surgeons (ASPS)
* Corresponding author. Innovare Specialized Plastic Surgery, Avenue Verona 7412, Col Villa Verona, Zapopan, Jalisco 45019, México.
E-mail address: drlazaro@drlazarocardenas.comu

Clin Plastic Surg 45 (2018) 237–247
https://doi.org/10.1016/j.cps.2017.12.005
0094-1298/18

are concepts that we must understand to create a beautiful buttock.[2]

TREATMENT GOALS AND PLANNED OUTCOMES

As with other surgeries, proper planning is a part of success. We must know the expectations of the patient to know their aesthetic desire. We must also consider the characteristics of the buttock that may benefit them, not only aesthetically, but also in relation to their anatomy and race. In Asian or Caucasian patients or those patients with a body mass index of less than 25 kg/m^2, a small, short, aesthetic buttock with a concentrated volume in the buttock maximus area, with a waist-to-hip ratio of 0.70 to 0.65, may be achieved. However, in Latin patients, African Americans, or those with a body mass index of greater than 25 kg/m^2, a ratio of less than 0.65 will be favored by structuring a buttock that forms a same unit with the hip, being voluminous, very round, and very marked in the supragluteal region. However, some athletic patients who request a buttock with more definition will not favor very full projection with less lateral projection that highlights a gluteal frame in a round shape and may even mark the origin of the fascia lata (**Figs. 1–3**).[3]

PREOPERATIVE PLANNING AND PREPARATION

All patients should be checked preoperatively for hemoglobin, coagulation times, bleeding time, prothrombin times, and thromboplastin times. Glucose assessment and other studies may be required, along with evaluations of internal medicine, endocrinology, or cardiology. All indications should be discussed with the patient, and smoking, aspirin, and any dietary supplement that is not indicated should be discontinued for at least 2 to 3 weeks preoperatively. Consideration should also be given to the use of preoperative iron and vitamin K supplementation, and the patient and family should be informed about the risks of the procedure; it is also very important that informed consent be signed. To achieve an excellent gluteal contour, patient analysis requires not only observing the anatomic characteristics, but also the patient's desires and the real possibilities. This process can be achieved by analyzing the preexisting fat volume and observing the proper contour of the adjacent structures. In this way, based on analysis and systematization, we can perform procedures with consistent results. If we perform liposuction and infiltration in a systematic way, using the same order, positions, approach, and equipment, we can achieve better standardization of our procedures and improve our results (**Fig. 4**).

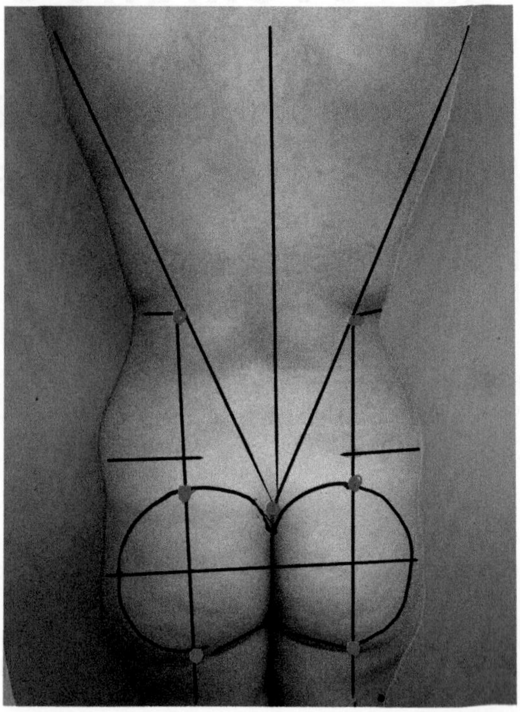

Fig. 1. Latin 30-year-old woman, in its preoperative photograph and planning. (1) Abdomen: Excellent donor fat, no scars, and good skin quality. (2) Symmetry: The left side was fuller than her right side. In her left buttock, it was less projected and also wider. (3) Irregularities: Just a few in her inferior buttocks quadrants at 6 o'clock. (4) Incisions: Planned as the technique in the intersections. (5) Hip-waist ratio: 0.75 actual ratio. Needs reduction at her waist and some fat infiltration at her hips at the transverse midgluteal line (a) back of the 12th rib or elbows. Needs liposuction and reduce fat toward the posterior axillary line. (b) Gluteal frame and point of greatest projection. Square frame, point of great transversal projection needs fat grafting to enhance hip-waist ratio. (6) Leg and lower gluteal fold: It extends beyond the midvertical gluteal line, needs fat grafting to enhance buttock support and erase the line. (7) Anatomic points to emphasize and thickness of the flaps: Thickness is okay, risk for irregularities low. (8) Transitions: Soft to enhance roundness.

MARKING

The design is created with the patient standing with their back facing the physician. The midline is marked, and then 2 lines that extend from the posterior axillary fold to the upper intergluteal line on both sides. This line delimits the lateral areas to which liposuction can be extended. We then draw a horizontal line that joins both elbows and

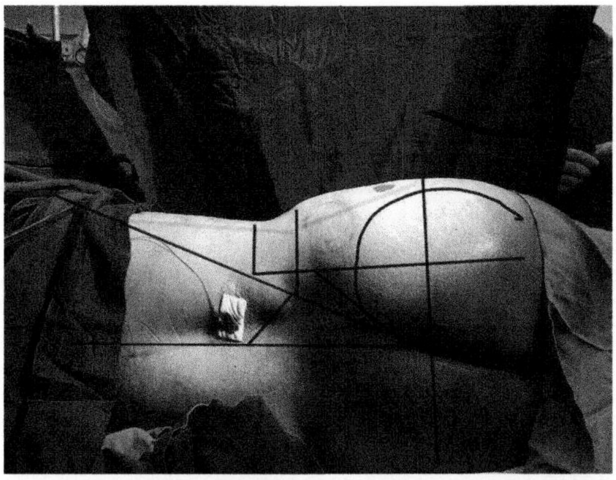

Fig. 2. Intraoperative photograph of a 30-year-old female patient lying on her side. The markings show areas with fat deposits that require suctioning to achieve aesthetic improvement.

that generally corresponds with the 12th rib. This line indicates the area to be improved with liposuction, that is, the waist, which must begin to increase in thickness as you proceed downward to the point of greatest projection, taking care not to leave a step at the level of the iliac spines; doing so converts the gluteal frame into an A frame. The posterior iliac spines are also marked, and a vertical line is added dividing the buttock right in the middle that goes superiorly until it meets the union of the axillary lines and those of the rib. Finally, the circumference of the buttock is delimited, emphasizing any asymmetry or difference between the heights. When marking the buttock, we must include 2 lines: the first a circle that corresponds with the base of the original buttock, and a second line that will be seen once we press on the most central portion of the buttock that corresponds with the zone where we want to expand the base of the buttock. We should also check if there are areas where fat should be added. We must also verify that the area from the buttock that is most projected corresponds with the height of the mons pubis. It is also important to verify that the infragluteal fold does not extend beyond the midline of the buttock or ischial tuberosity. If so, we must mark the line projected outside the midline and ischial tuberosity, and infiltrate it with fat to prevent it from extending beyond what is considered aesthetic. We mark the incisions in another color. If there are asymmetries, irregularities, or other characteristics to be highlighted, they are also marked.[4]

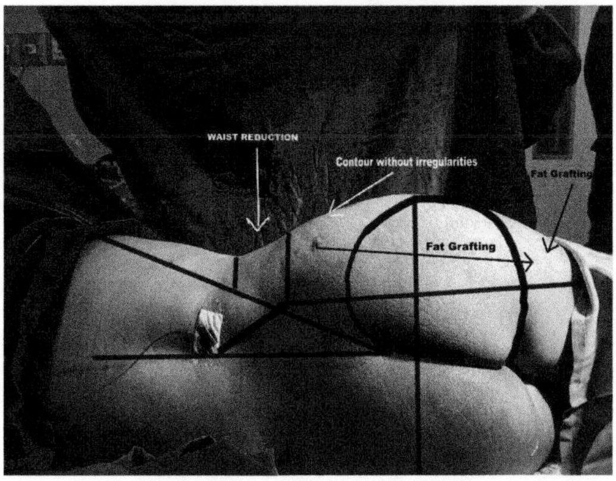

Fig. 3. Patient lying on the side with the liposuction already finished. Smaller waist with wider hip. Lipoinjection was also performed in the external quadrant of the gluteus and the external infragluteal portion.

PATIENT PREPARATION

Before surgery, the patient is prepped in the standing position. This position allows adequate preparation of all areas to be treated. The patient is placed on the surgical table, which has been previously prepared with sterile sheets so that the patient's position can be changed. The anesthesiologist can perform general anesthesia or an epidural block, and a Foley catheter is then placed. We must always take note of the patient's temperature. There are devices that work very well for this purpose; however, for body contouring, the use of forced air is not very practical because the sheets generally do not cover most of the body, they are bulky, and they do not work adequately with extensive exposure of the body. For this purpose, preheating the patient for 1 hour before beginning surgery and using warm solutions or a circulating hot water mattress have proven to be very useful to avoid hypothermia.

SURGICAL PROCEDURE

We begin with abdominal liposuction because that allows us to obtain enough volume of fat to infiltrate. Two incisions are used in the inguinal region and in the umbilicus. Incisions may also be needed below the breast to access the upper abdominal region. Infiltration is performed using a super wet or tumescent technique, usually using 3 L-size bags with isotonic saline solution, with 3 ampules of adrenaline per bag. We do not use lidocaine, because it is not required when using general anesthesia or the epidural block technique. Liposuction is performed with 3- and 4-mm atraumatic cannulas and 60-mL syringes. The thickness of the flap is determined by the pinch maneuver and by observing the regularity of the flap by lifting the cannula. Fat is collected in a closed container. Subsequently, the patient is placed in the left

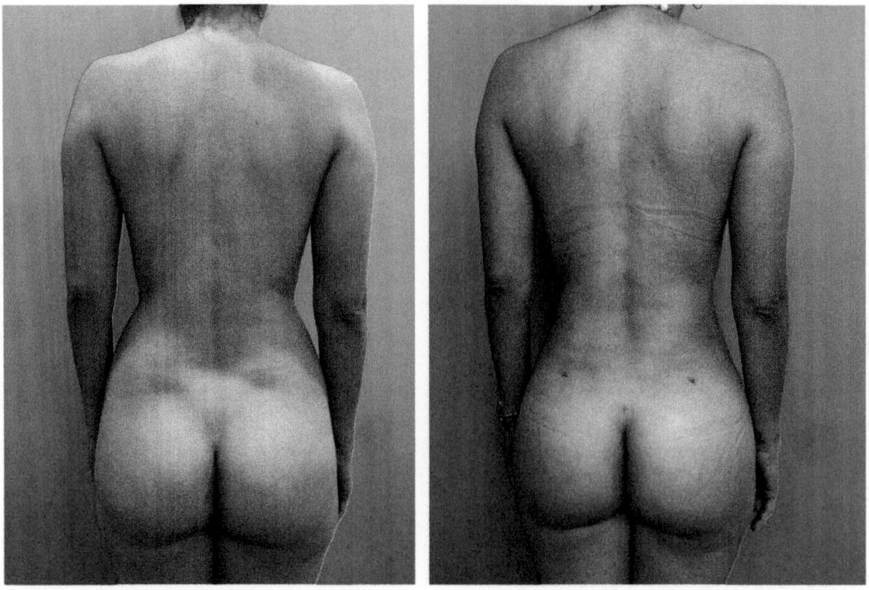

Fig. 4. Preoperative and postoperative photographs of a 28-year-old female, who desired a narrow waist with a fuller buttock, but no hip enhancement at 3 months after surgery. Because her upper back did not have problems, we did not perform liposuction in that area.

and right lateral decubitus positions to perform liposuction of the gluteal frame, and later in the ventral decubitus position to perform liposuction of the lumbar area and to infiltrate the buttocks. For the preparation of the fat to be injected, decanting and manual cleaning are performed, eliminating any connective tissue. Clindamycin (300 mg) is added to the prepared fat, infiltrating it in multiple paths and in different planes as described elsewhere in this article, avoiding the deep intramuscular planes. We currently infiltrate the fat with movements similar to those made during liposuction. After confirming symmetry, silicone drains 3 to 5 mm in length are placed in the wounds to allow fluid to drain for 5 to 7 days (**Figs. 5–11**).

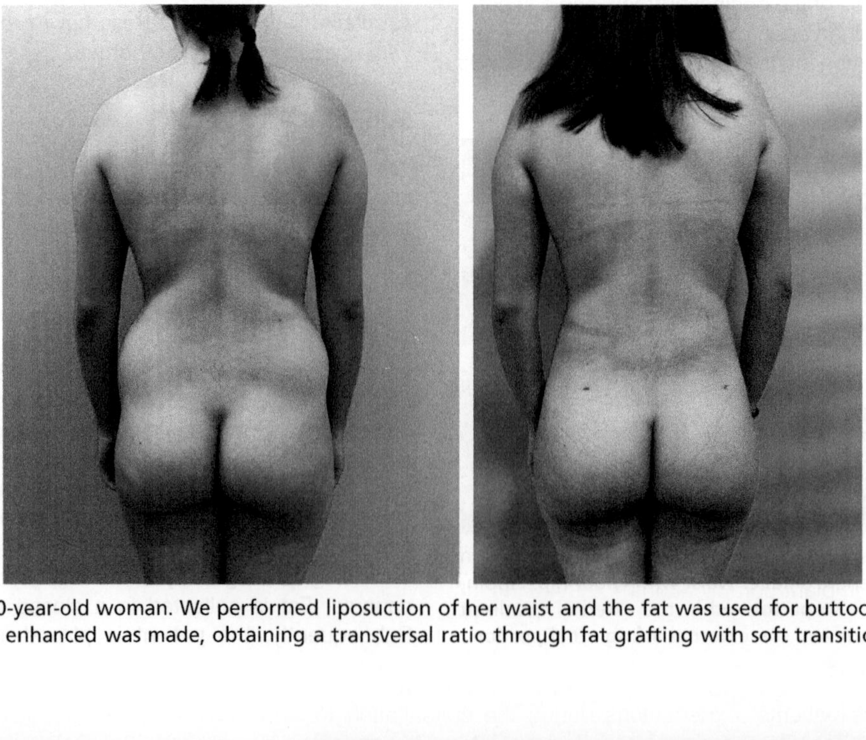

Fig. 5. A 20-year-old woman. We performed liposuction of her waist and the fat was used for buttock augmentation. Hip enhanced was made, obtaining a transversal ratio through fat grafting with soft transitions.

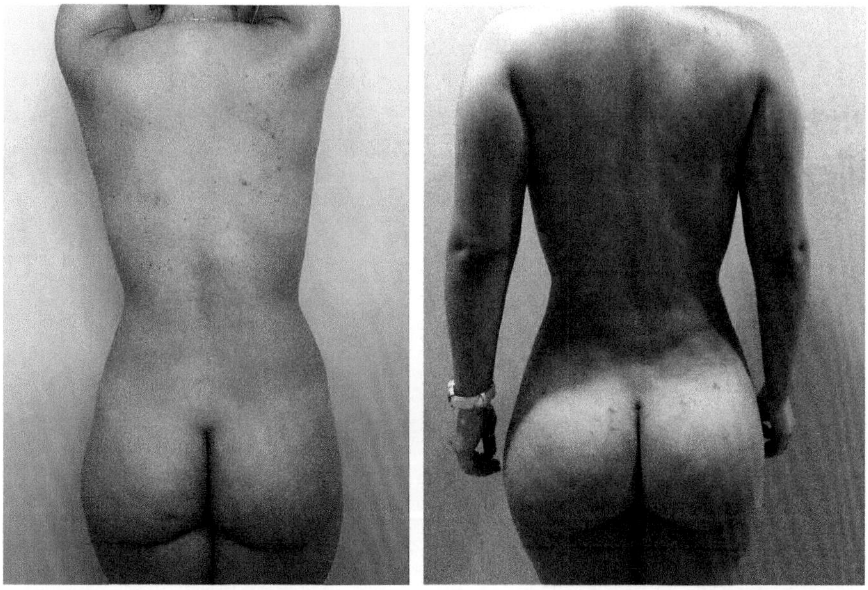

Fig. 6. A 28-year-old with 2 previous pregnancies. She had an excellent skin quality and wanted full surgery. Three months postprocedure. Waist was narrowed and 1000 mL of lipoinjection was made per side. Asymmetry also was corrected with soft transition.

SURGICAL PLAN

To perform a procedure, according to the analysis of the surgical plan, we use a protocol called the systemized liposuction system. There are 8 points in the systemized liposuction system, which allow us to take into account all of the key elements before and during surgery to obtain a good result. Having photos before surgery and using them during surgery, highlighting the key points and surgical plan, will prevent us from overlooking areas to be treated. These 8 points are as follows:

1. Abdomen
2. Symmetry
3. Irregularities

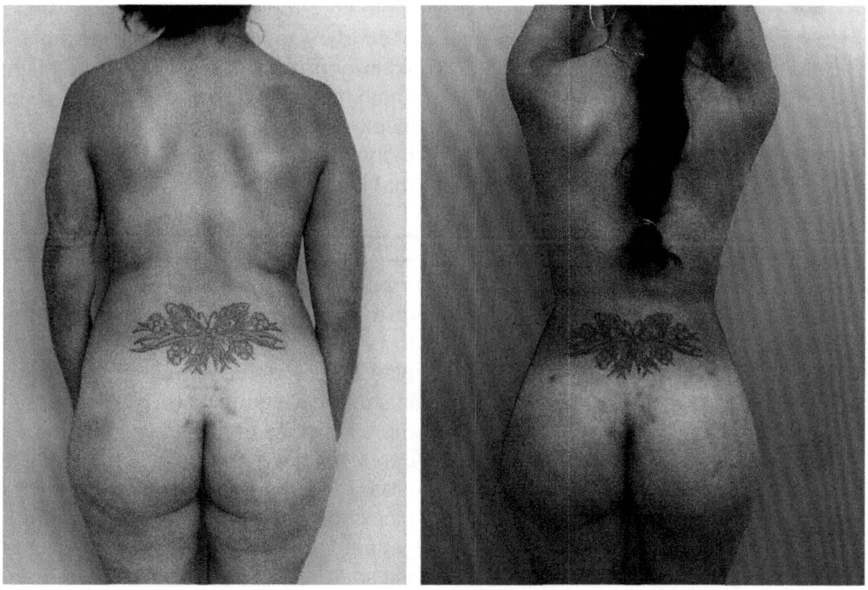

Fig. 7. A 34-year-old woman who wanted a full surgery performed. Suction of upper back was not made. Narrowing the waist, and fuller buttock fat grafting, with a better contour was achieved.

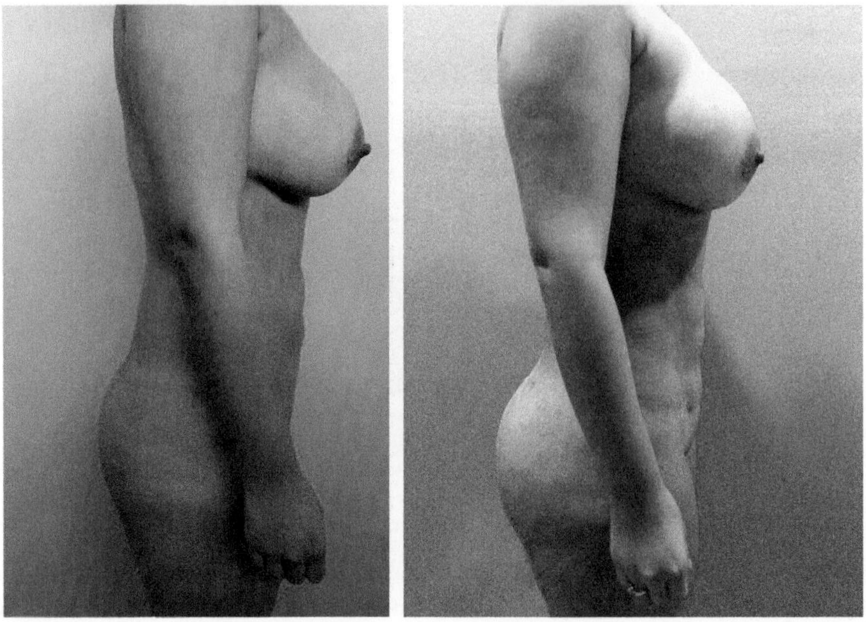

Fig. 8. A 28-year-old woman. Better buttock projection is achieved with lipoinjection of the buttocks.

4. Incisions
5. Hip-to-waist ratio
   a. Posterior area at the level of the 12th rib or elbows
   b. Gluteal frame and point of greatest projection
6. Leg and lower gluteal fold
7. Anatomic points to emphasize and thickness of the flaps
8. Transitions

Abdomen

The abdomen is important during because it is generally where the best quality and the greatest volume of fat can be obtained. If the abdomen is virgin, we will know the quality and volume of the fat that we can count on to infiltrate the buttocks.

Symmetry

Several studies have shown that asymmetry in the buttock is very frequent among patients.[5] It is important to highlight these aspects and to point them out to the patient, planning the procedures to reduce these asymmetries. The most frequent irregularity is a scoliosis or difference in hip height owing to shortness of one leg. During the examination, the surgeon will be able to observe a difference in the height of the shoulders, impacting the height of the iliac spines and, therefore, in the buttocks. The gluteal frame may have an important asymmetry, which can also be properly observed in the size of the gluteal maximus muscle up to the infragluteal fold. Asymmetries are frequently observed in width, height, and projection, which generates differences in volume between the buttocks. These differences should be considered at the time of surgery because it is difficult to achieve symmetry.

Irregularities

If asymmetry is frequent, irregularities are even more so. Problems such as scars, and retractions secondary to intramuscular injections and infections generate visible alterations of the contour. Often, the method for handling these irregularities involves releasing them with cannulas or specific techniques,[6] and later filling with fat the space that is created.

Incisions

Proper planning of incisions for lipoinjection allows us to not only discuss potential outcomes, but also to plan the best approach with the patient. This plan should also allow a safe approach to gluteal infiltration. Depending on the height of the patient, more incisions may be required on the back if the cannulae do not allow us to reach the desired areas. The most frequent incisions for gluteal lipoinjection are as follows. Midline above the intergluteal fold allows us to approach the region of the sacrum, but also to infiltrate the buttock safely. Two lateral incisions are also frequently made in the area of greatest gluteal height because we

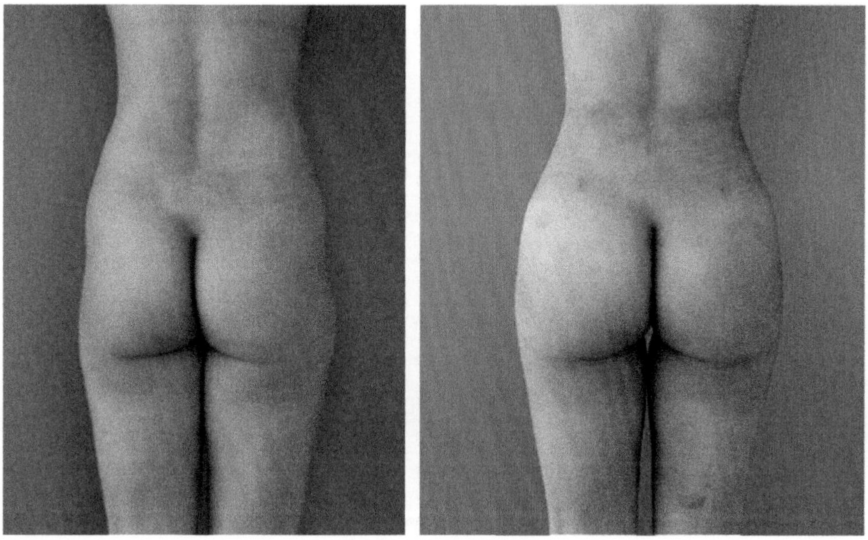

Fig. 9. A 22-year-old woman: 1250 mL of fat obtained through liposuction. There were 300 mL infiltrated on each buttock. The patient did not want any hip infiltration.

can approach upper areas easily. A lateral incision below the iliac crest will also allow for good access to other zones.[7] Another potential incision is in the infragluteal fold, but it is not recommended that this incision be placed further than the midline of the buttock. This incision will allow us to perform infiltration of the point of greatest projection, but also to infiltrate the buttocks and the transition zones. However, the infragluteal incision should never be used to infiltrate fat deep into the midline. It is imperative that you avoid the deep intramuscular area because of the risk of injury to large vessels and gross fat embolization. Thus, this incision should always be used upward and outward in a plane parallel to the surgical table or the patient.

Hip-to-Waist Ratio

Psychologist Davendra Singh taught us that, in terms of physical attractiveness, the relationship between the waist and hip is important.[8] We must always strive to maintain this relationship, taking different cultural and racial preferences into account. The wishes of the patient and what can realistically achieved should both influence any decisions. The objective is to maintain a

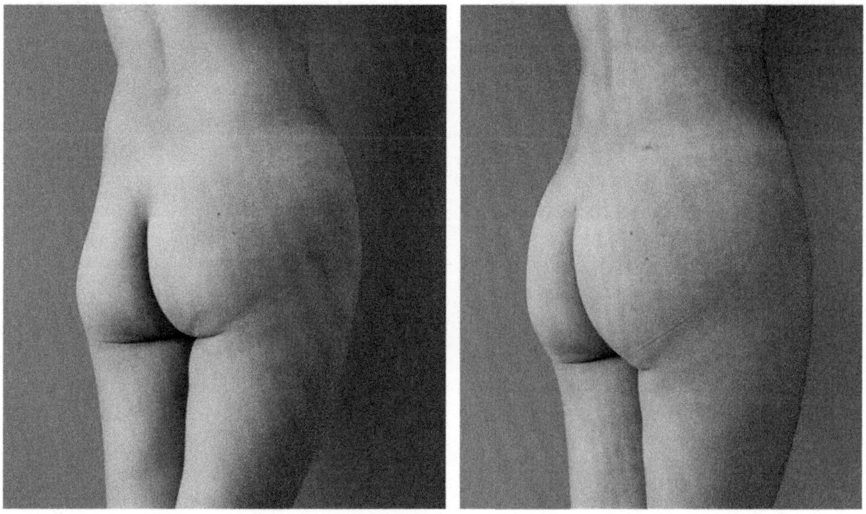

Fig. 10. A 36-year-old woman. There were 350 mL infiltrated on each buttock and 150 mL on each hip.

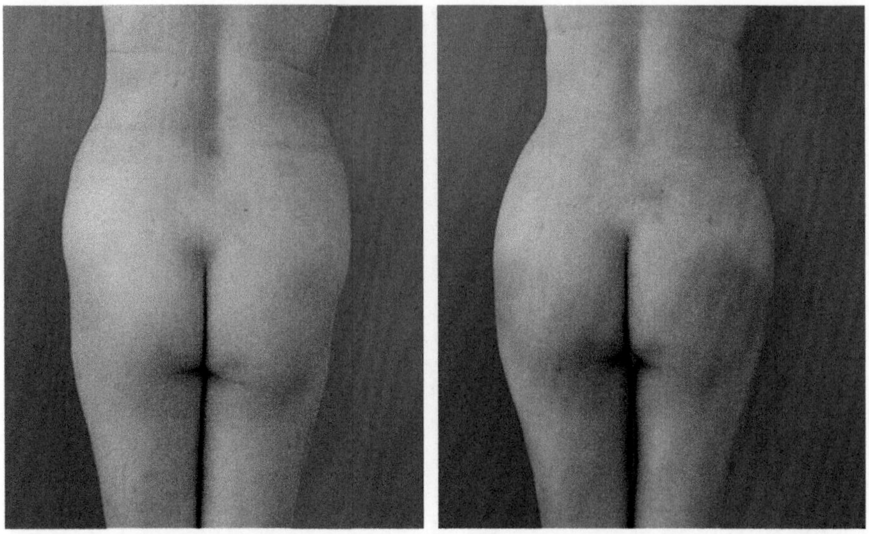

Fig. 11. A 26-year-old woman, with important asymmetry and hip atrophy, making a "V" shape. There were 3250 ml of fat obtained through liposuction. It was infiltrated as 425 mL on each buttock and 275 mL and 375 mL on the right and left hips, respectively.

relationship between the hips and waist between 0.70 in the most conservative patients and up to 0.65 in those requesting greater volume.[9] Therefore, during surgery, we must monitor this relationship by analyzing measurements, knowing that the proportion in the buttock will decrease once the fat is reabsorbed. In contrast, the waist is fairly stable because the thoracic bony structures will not allow a greater decrease that what is present intraoperatively after liposuction.

Posterior area at the level of the 12th rib or elbows

The posterior area is one of the most important elements that surround and participate in the aesthetics of the buttock. We can decrease the fat in the upper back, but the most important thing is to achieve the smallest side-to-side diameter at the waist level. There are 3 ways to determine where the waist level is located. The first is the height of the 12th rib, the second is a crease in the back that generally corresponds with this level, and finally another simple guide is that when the patient is facedown, with their arms at their sides, the height of the elbows will correspond with this zone. If we want to approach this area with inconspicuous incisions, they can be placed in the axilla at the level of the posterior axillary line. A more comfortable incision is in the back on the brassiere line. This area usually has a more compact fat that is difficult to remove and tends to bleed easily. Despite these difficulties, because of the thickness of the skin, irregularities are an uncommon occurrence.

We must also not forget the area that corresponds with the sacrum and the lumbar region above the buttock. This area is important to demarcate because it defines the buttock, and achieves an aesthetically pleasing lordosis. This area can usually be treated through an intergluteal incision and liposuction is very safe. It is important is to be careful to avoid irregularities in an attempt to remove too much fat. We must also consider that this area tends to bleed in the immediate postoperative period and to accumulate fluid in the form of seroma. It is recommended that either the wound is left open or a small drain is placed to facilitate drainage.

Gluteal frame and the point of maximum projection

The gluteal frame is one of the most important features in gluteal aesthetics.[10] The gluteal border, which consists of the muscles and lateral bone structures (the ilium and greater trochanter) with the underlying fat, form a figure that is usually grouped in A or V circular or square shapes,[2] depending on all these structures. Knowing how to mold this area is important to obtain a harmonious figure and to achieve the correct waist-to-hip ratio. Generally, the most appropriate and simple way to mold it is with the patient in the lateral decubitus position. In the ventral decubitus position, it is more difficult to do it because the pressure exerted by the tissues on these structures changes the shape. The approach can usually be made from an incision in the highest region of each buttock or from that of the infragluteal fold.

The point of greatest projection is a key structure. It is an anatomic point that, in and of itself, greatly influences the aesthetics of the gluteal frame. Unlike the frame that is usually molded by means of liposuction, a suitable projection point is achieved by fat infiltration. This structure is the area between the ilium and the greater trochanter, and is generally deficient in volume.[11] The appropriate way to mold it is with the patient in the lateral decubitus position and prone, because we must manage the transition between the muscle and the gluteal frame.

Lower Gluteal Leg and Fold

The region of the infragluteal fold has been generally ignored or inadequately treated. For many years, it was thought that this area should be suctioned aggressively, and it was never taken into account that buttock support and projection depend on it. The aesthetic line of the infragluteal fold should generally be short, no longer than the midline of the buttock, and should descend from the midline to the side. A long line that extends beyond the midline will result in an unpleasant appearance, forming a square buttock or a V-shaped deformity.

Correcting this area is quite a challenge, and generally, fat infiltration directed from the center of the buttock toward the thigh is required. This anatomically based approach is helpful because the gluteus maxims muscle descends to insert itself into the trochanter. In patients with a very voluminous or ptotic inferomedial aspect of the buttock, liposuction or even resection of this area may be required. The only indication for liposuction below the buttock is the banana-roll deformity. This area should be treated conservatively with superficial liposuction to correct it. However, a volume deficiency of the external gluteal zone, which requires volume, is much more common.

Anatomic Points to Highlight and the Thickness of the Flaps

Determining the thickness of the regions in which liposuction is to be performed is important when our patients ask us for high-definition liposuction. The sacral area should usually have a thickness of no more than 1 cm to the pinch test. In the more lateral areas, where the skin is thicker, flaps with a thickness of 1.5 to 2.0 cm can be left. Trying to leave flaps thinner than 1 cm usually generates irregularities or changes of color (marble skin) that are difficult to correct. The area where a significantly thicker flap must be maintained is in the area of the buttock proper or where we want to achieve a build-up of fat that normally exists.

Transitions

An important aspect of high-definition liposuction in the buttock is knowing where to remove volume and where to increase volume. Although there are areas that should be left thin, there are also areas that should not be thinned because thinness in these areas generally will not look good. An example is the region of the supragluteal external lower back. Although the sacral or medial, supragluteal region should be left very demarcated, the external region should keep a smoother transition.[12] This is the last point where we a hope to achieve a refined aspect to our contouring. It is important to pay attention to areas that require subtraction or addition of volume, but also with areas of transition between these zones. We should always try to deliver a smooth transition, except in rare high-definition liposuction cases, where an abrupt transition zone is desired. However, preoperatively defining which areas should be smooth and which should be abrupt will allow us to deliver fineness and aesthetically pleasing results. In general, transitions are defined by the underlying anatomic structures; therefore, in a muscular zone with a lot of movement, the transition must be smooth. However, if we have an insertion zone or muscle raphes, our transitions may be more marked.

SYSTEMIZED FAT GRATING

Systematization in gluteal fat infiltration is recommended from the bottom to the upper part of the buttock and from deep to superficial. This approach will generate the shape the buttock and will lift the tissues. We suggest this order when performing fat infiltration: infragluteal crease, point of greatest projection and gluteal frame, transition of the buttock, buttock base, and buttock projection and definition.

Infragluteal Crease

Performing the infiltration of this area helps not only to create a broader base from which the buttock will rest, but also to push it upward by a purely mechanical effect. Additionally, treating it adequately and infiltrating sufficiently will allow the gluteal crease to be shortened and oriented more vertically.

Point of Greatest Projection and Gluteal Frame

The point of greatest projection is important because it will provide the curvature of the gluteal frame. Treating it properly is the basis for being able to change the shape from a V or square shape to an A shape. Defining it is important because it helps us to generate a larger or more harmonious shape. The definition of the point of greatest projection can be affected depending on the planned aesthetic objectives. For example, a more athletic buttock should have more fat in the upper gluteal region to achieve a smooth transition and not too much fat at the point of greatest projection. A more bulky, Latin or African American buttock will require more fat to be placed in the middle to lower third or in the lower third.[13]

Transition of the Buttock

Treating the transition between the gluteal frame and the gluteal volume will help us to achieve a smoother appearance. This treatment allows the curves to unite in a single, natural curve.

Buttock Base

Fat is placed in deeper areas of the buttock corresponding with the superficial muscular planes. It is imperative to avoid deep medial infiltration to avoid the gluteal vessels and macroscopic fat embolization.[14] It is in this step where we can shape the width and thickness of the buttock and where we can also extend the buttock upward, if making it longer is desired.

Buttock Projection and Definition

The last area to infiltrate is the most superficial area of the buttock, with the goal of achieving definition and projection. We must identify which area is best to project and concentrate the fat there, which usually corresponds horizontally with the middle third or to the height of the pubis or point of greatest projection.

POSTPROCEDURAL CARE, POTENTIAL COMPLICATIONS, AND THEIR MANAGEMENT

At the end of the surgery, a cotton bandage is applied, placing more volume and compression in the thinner sacral region. Patients are taken to the recovery room and are then admitted to the hospital while keeping them in the ventral decubitus position. They are discharged the next day with a compression garment and cotton in the treated areas. They are prescribed analgesics and broad-spectrum antibiotics for 5 days. The patient is asked to start with early ambulation on the first day to reduce the risk of venous thromboembolism. It is also necessary to verify that the patients are well-hydrated so that the risk of fat embolism syndrome is minimized. They should also bathe daily; after bathing, they should apply an antiseptic on the wounds, followed by sterile gauze cotton and bandages for 1 week. The implementation of preventive pharmacologic chemoprophylaxis is determined based on the Caprini score.[15]

At 1 week postoperatively, we recommend that the postoperative compression garment be placed. We do not place the garment immediately postoperative because excess inflammation and edema can generate necrosis of compressed zones. We do not recommend massages in the first postoperative month. Immediate complications (0–3 days) can be bleeding, fulminant fat embolism, or visceral perforation. Delayed complications (3–21 days) may include bleeding, fat embolism syndrome, deep venous thrombosis, pulmonary thromboembolism, infection, edema, seromas, and fat necrosis. Late complications (21 days onward) include irregularities, asymmetry, loss of sensation, seroma, and fat necrosis. In our series, we have performed more than 1000 surgeries, and we had early complications that occurred during the first 3 days, as bleeding in 2% of the operated patients. We had 2 patients with fat embolism syndrome, which began 48 hours after surgery and were resolved in the intensive care unit without major problems. Intermediate complications that appeared between 3 and 21 days after surgery were bleeding in 0.5%, deep vein thrombosis in 0.1%, and seromas in 2% in the area of lumbar liposuction. Alterations that occurred after 21 days were irregularities (3%), asymmetries (2%), fat necrosis (1%), and seromas (1%).

REHABILITATION AND RECOVERY

In the first 7 days, early ambulation is recommended at home. Starting in the second week, rehabilitation with therapeutic ultrasound treatments 3 times a week should be performed. This treatment is indicated on the liposuctioned areas and avoided in the infiltrated areas. Return to normal activities should occur between the second and third weeks, and aerobic exercise is recommended beginning in the fourth week.

OUTCOMES

Generally, results can be observed within the first few weeks postoperatively. Final results can be appreciated after 3 months and are permanent if the patient maintains proper dietary habits.

SUMMARY

Gluteal lipoinjection performed in a systematized manner, following protocols designed for fat harvesting and infiltration, will provide predictable and standardized results. This approach will help to ensure a high degree of satisfaction for both surgeon and patient alike.

REFERENCES

1. Toledo LS. Gluteal augmentation with fat grafting the Brazilian buttock technique: 30 years' experience. Clin Plast Surg 2015;42(2):253–61.
2. Mendieta CG. Gluteal reshaping. Aesthet Surg J 2007;27(6):641–55.
3. Lee EI, Roberts TL, Bruner TW. Ethnic considerations in buttock aesthetics. Semin Plast Surg 2009;23(3):232–43.
4. Morley-Forster PK. Unintentional hypothermia in the operating room. Can Anaesth Soc J 1986;33(4): 515–27.
5. Centeno RF, Young VL. Clinical anatomy in aesthetic gluteal body contouring surgery. Clin Plast Surg 2006;33(3):347–58.
6. Wall SH, Lee MR. Separation, aspiration, and fat equalization. Plast Reconstr Surg 2016;138(6): 1192–201.
7. Mendieta CG. Gluteoplasty. Aesthet Surg J 2003; 23(6):441–55.
8. Roberts TL, Weinfeld AB, Bruner TW, et al. "Universal" and ethnic ideals of beautiful buttocks are best obtained by autologous micro fat grafting and liposuction. Clin Plast Surg 2006;33(3):371–94.
9. Wong WW, Motakef S, Lin Y, et al. Redefining the ideal buttocks: a population analysis. Plast Reconstr Surg 2016;137(6):1739–47.
10. Singh D. Universal allure of the hourglass figure: an evolutionary theory of female physical attractiveness. Clin Plast Surg 2006;33(3):359–70.
11. Kirwan L. Three-dimensional liposculpture of the iliac crest and lateral thigh. Aesthet Surg J 1997; 17(5):334–6.
12. Hoyos AE, Prendergast PM. High definition body sculpting. 2014. https://doi.org/10.1007/978-3-642-54891-8.
13. Singh D, Dixson BJ, Jessop TS, et al. Cross-cultural consensus for waist-hip ratio and women's attractiveness. Evol Hum Behav 2010;31(3):176–81.
14. Cárdenas-Camarena L, Bayter JE, Aguirre-Serrano H, et al. Deaths caused by gluteal lipoinjection: what are we doing wrong? Plast Reconstr Surg 2015;136(1): 58–66.
15. Pannucci CJ. Evidence-based recipes for venous thromboembolism prophylaxis. Plast Reconstr Surg 2017;139(2):520e–32e.

Gluteal Augmentation and Contouring with Autologous Fat Transfer: Part I

Ashkan Ghavami, MD[a,b,*], Nathaniel L. Villanueva, MD[c]

KEYWORDS

• Gluteal augmentation • Fat grafting • Gluteal contouring • Fat transfer • S-curve butt lift
• Brazilian butt lift • Buttock fat transfer • Buttock augmentation

KEY POINTS

- Appropriate patient selection, preoperative marking, and planning are keys to achieving aesthetically pleasing buttock contour and desired volume.
- Gluteal fat transfer must be performed using small aliquots with constant cannula motion in the subcutaneous layers and superficial to intermediate gluteal musculature depth.
- Avoiding overcorrection is important, because increased pressure within the buttock may decrease fat graft viability and create potential soft tissue buttock ptosis.
- Patients should avoid placing pressure on the buttocks for 2 weeks and take conscious care to avoid excess sitting for another 4 to 8 weeks postoperatively.

Video content accompanies this article at http://www.plasticsurgery.theclinics.com/.

INTRODUCTION

As the number of gluteal augmentation procedures performed annually in the United States steadily increases, the demand for augmentation with fat transfer has also seen a dramatic increase in recent years.[1] There are several advantages associated with the use of fat transfer for gluteal augmentation.[2–10] The key advantages are precise contouring and reshaping of the gluteal region, improvement of overall body aesthetics in a 360° fashion, and the use of autologous tissues. Fat transfer permits focused augmentation of the buttock and thigh region as well as reduction of adjacent body regions. The combination of augmentation adjacent to reduction achieves the patients' contouring goals in ways that cannot be accomplished with implants alone or autoaugmentation flaps. Fat harvesting through liposuction allows for improvement of regional and global body contour aesthetics. Specifically, liposuctioning of fat in the lower back, flanks, thighs, and more distant sites are powerful adjuncts to overall body contouring as well as sources of fat for gluteal augmentation. The removal of fat from the lower back and torso with simultaneous augmentation of the buttocks superiorly and medially enhances the gluteal silhouette with 360° "S-shaped" curves (**Fig. 1**). The combination of liposuction and gluteal fat transfer allows for the creation of concavities that transition to convexities forming the "S" curvilinear body contour, leading to aesthetically pleasing results. Furthermore, the use of autologous tissues avoids the complications associated with use of gluteal implants, which include seroma, capsular contracture, implant migration, wound-healing complications, thinning of native tissues, and implant-related infections and exposures.[11–14] However, the gluteal fat transfer procedure has

Disclosure Statement: The authors have nothing to disclose.

[a] Division of Plastic and Reconstructive Surgery, Department of Surgery, David Geffen School of Medicine at UCLA, 200 UCLA Medical Plaza, Suite 465, Los Angeles, CA 90095, USA; [b] Private Practice, Ghavami Plastic Surgery, 433 North Camden Drive, Suite 780, Beverly Hills, CA 90210, USA; [c] Department of Plastic Surgery, University of Texas Southwestern Medical Center, 1801 Inwood Road, Dallas, TX 75390, USA
* Corresponding author. 433 North Camden Drive, Suite 780, Beverly Hills, CA 90210.
E-mail address: ashghavami@yahoo.com

Clin Plastic Surg 45 (2018) 249–259
https://doi.org/10.1016/j.cps.2017.12.009

plasticsurgery.theclinics.com

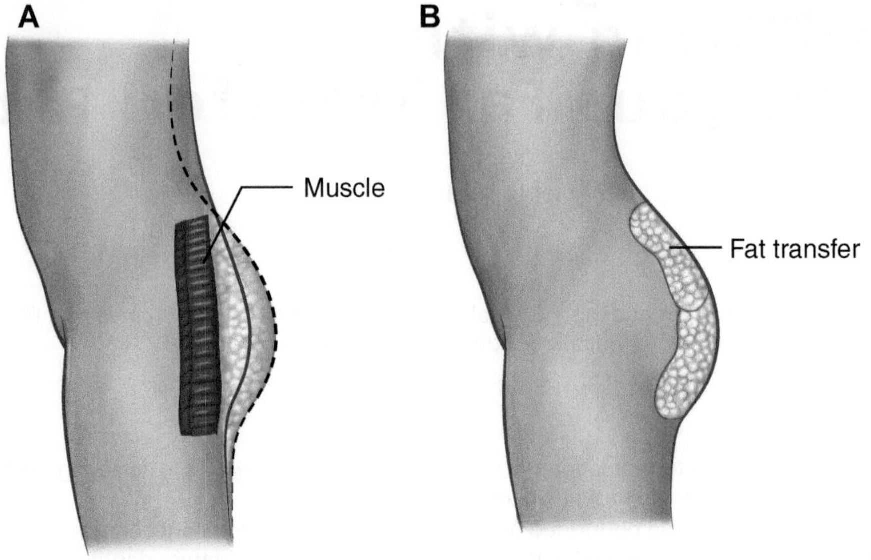

Fig. 1. The principle of subtraction of lipodystrophy regions adjacent to the buttock where addition of fat grafts will create a more curvaceous "S-curve" silhouette in which newly created concavities are next to convexities. (*A*) Location of fat reduction next to augmentation. (*B*) Regions of fat augmentation in superficial, deep subcutaneous, and superficial fascial locations.

also been associated with several complications, including fat necrosis, infection, abscess formation, contour irregularities, sciatic nerve injury, fat embolism, thromboembolism, and death.[15–21] Despite these known complications, improvements in patient selection, surgical technique, and perioperative management can lead to an improved safety profile, with excellent short- and long-term results. The procedure has evolved to produce more consistent and predictable results with a dramatic reduction in complications when precise technique is used. In the authors' opinion, it is arguably superior to other modalities of gluteal augmentation. Herein, the authors describe their technique for patient selection, harvesting, processing, and fat injection, which has been safely and effectively performed by the senior author (A.G.) over the past decade.

PREOPERATIVE PLANNING AND PREPARATION

The ideal patient for gluteal augmentation with fat transfer should have sufficient donor fat to allow for an appreciable augmentation. However, a dramatic transformation of the torso and buttocks can be achieved in thin patients with modest liposuction and fat transfer to specific gluteal zones. Patients who have very low body fat composition are generally considered poor candidates for this procedure, but in some cases, they can be instructed to gain weight in order to optimize lipoaspirate yield.

During the patient selection process, it is important to identify the patient's goals and have a thorough discussion about the degree of augmentation possible and to set realistic contouring expectations based on the patient's anatomic morphology. Expectation management is critical to the success of the procedure and patient satisfaction. The patient should be asked to prioritize areas of importance, such as the upper buttock fullness, projection, posterior lateral fullness, or lateral hip to trochanteric fullness. This is particularly important in thin patients who may not have enough fat to augment all areas. It is also important to review the patient's medical comorbidities and current medications. This allows the surgeon to appropriately risk stratify the patient and hold medications, which increase the risk of perioperative complications like fish oils, aspirin, nonsteroidal anti-inflammatories, and so forth. Tobacco use must cease at least 4 weeks before surgery and preferably for at least 3 to 6 months postoperatively because it may decrease fat graft survival rates. Thromboembolic risk factors should be evaluated and discussed with the patient, which includes possible use of thromboembolism prophylaxis in the postoperative period.[22]

TREATMENT GOALS AND PLANNED OUTCOMES

Surgical Planning

Once the surgical goals have been defined with the patient, successful execution of the procedure depends on gluteal shaping rather than simply the volume of fat transfer. Using the gluteal frame classification system as described by Mendieta[23] can help define the aesthetic goals. There are 4 general frame shapes, which are the A, V, H, and round frames. Identifying and appropriately evaluating the patient's frame allows for proper identification of surgical goals. Understanding how V and H frames can be altered to achieve the more desirable A frame are important for achieving aesthetic goals. Avoiding excessive fat transfer to the midlateral and inferior lateral areas is important because they are notorious for having decreased fat graft survival. In general terms, 2 aspects of shape preferences, projection and lateral fullness, should be discussed with patients. Some patients desire a more athletic frame with less lateral fullness and therefore a waist:hip ratio greater than 0.7. Other patients may desire an exaggerated hourglass or S-curve shape with more lateral fullness (with or without marked projection) and less than a 0.7 waist:hip ratio.

Marking

The patient should be marked in the standing position. The areas of liposuction should be marked in the standard fashion with an understanding how zones adjacent to the buttock will affect gluteal shape. For example, the flank region is almost always markedly reduced and can be one of the best donor sites. Areas that require release of ligamentous attachments (fascial zones of adherence) and have different capacities for accepting fat should be identified. The markings are based on several factors, including skin laxity, fat and muscle distribution, and bony structure. Identification and assessment of the lateral trochanteric region and the need for augmentation at this location are important during this evaluation because they significantly contribute to the lateral contour of the gluteal profile and the waist:hip ratio. As with all plastic surgery, the inherent bony, muscular, and soft tissue morphology will determine prioritization of available donor fat. The iliac crest should also be identified because it is a transition zone that serves as the deepest and most inferior point of liposuction and the upper edge of the gluteal region. Laterally, the iliac crest height, width, shape, and distance from the lowest rib will determine the potential for waist definition in the flanks (**Fig. 2**). Areas of dimpling throughout the gluteal region should be identified for selective release/augmentation during the case.

PATIENT POSITIONING

The patient is prepared and draped for surgery in the supine position. Foley insertion is mandatory to assess fluid resuscitation. Sequential compression devices are used. There are multiple approaches to patient positioning during surgery; however, the authors prefer to begin the operation with the patient in supine position and turn the patient prone to complete the procedure. When the patient is placed prone and prepared/draped,

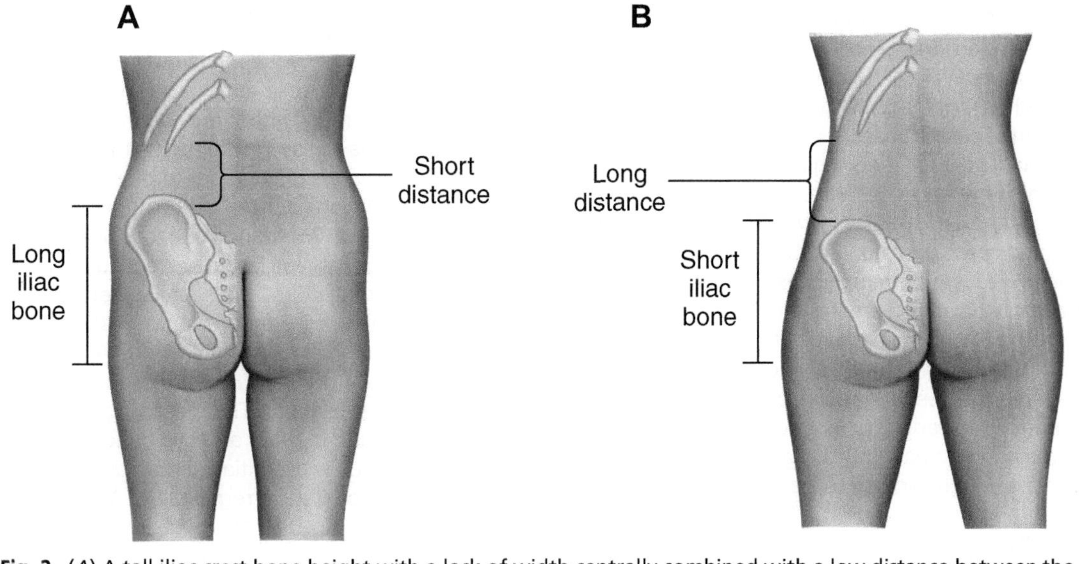

Fig. 2. (*A*) A tall iliac crest bone height with a lack of width centrally combined with a low distance between the iliac and lowest rib. This is the most complex morphology to enhance and requires aggressive flank liposuction along with substantial augmentation in the midlateral buttocks in most patients when an hourglass waist:hip ratio is desired. (*B*) Most favorable morphology in which iliac height is proportionate and further caudal from the lowest rib. A flared or wider iliac bone is present.

infiltration should be performed first to take advantage of the adrenaline vasoconstriction as fat is injected into the buttocks. Another variation of positioning is performed with the patient alternating from lateral decubitus positions, but the authors do not think this allows for good visualization of gluteal symmetry and can create abnormal buttock contours and deformation of the tissues. This approach has a higher learning curve.

PROCEDURAL APPROACH

Fat Harvest

Fat harvesting is performed using standard liposuction techniques with the surgeon's preference of tumescence and cannulas. The patient should also be given a dose of preoperative antibiotics according to the Surgical Care Improvement Project recommendations.[24] The authors use high-oscillation, power-assisted lipoaspiration. Using 4- and 5-mm flared Mercedes tip cannulas, the subscarpal fat is released and then removed. This allows adequate removal, contouring, and redraping of the tissues postoperatively. Aspiration is largely done with blunt tip Mercedes tip cannulas of 4 and 5 mm diameter. The larger cannula diameters minimize trauma to the fat lobules, which improves viability.[25,26] Smaller cannulas may be used for more precise excision of superficial fat deposits in thinner patients. The power-assisted oscillation of the cannula without suction is occasionally used to release superficial and deeper bands before performing liposuction. Pretunneling with the cannula off suction and post-aspiration tunneling with the cannula off suction are effective methods of mobilization of the fat to be aspirated and evenly distributes the remaining fat, respectively. Multiple access incisions are placed at various points to allow a cross-hatched pattern of cannula passes at various depths in order to avoid contour irregularities. During liposuction, key areas of fat removal are the lower back, sacral region, and flanks. Fat removal in these areas allows for improved definition of the gluteal region. The sacral area is important because removal of lipodystrophy in this region creates an apparent increase in lower back lordosis and projection of the upper pole gluteal projection. However, excessive liposuction in this area can destroy lymphatics, similar to the mons pubis area, leading to an increased incidence of seromas. Seromas in this region can be managed in office with aspiration as needed.

Fat Preparation

Fat preparation is an essential component to graft survival.[25–27] The authors' preferred method is to drain or aspirate the aqueous component of the lipoaspirate once the fat has decanted in the liposuction canister. The fat is then strained through a commercial strainer, without touching the fat, removing further aqueous components and obtaining a greater content of more purified fat lobules. Revision and secondary liposuctioned zones will contain scar and fibrous tissue, which may be aspirated and require direct removal before placing fat lobules into 60-mL Toomey injection syringes. The fat is mixed with a total of 300 mg clindamycin solution for each strained batch. The fat is then transferred into 60-mL Toomey syringes and prepared for injection to the gluteal region. The strainers are covered with towels or paper to avoid theoretic contamination in this open, exposed part of processing. Although proponents of closed systems claim contamination is an issue, there has been no evidence to suggest that infection rates are increased or viability rates are reduced with this processing technique. In more than 1000 buttock fat transfers using the simple technique described here, the senior author (A.G.) has only seen 4 infections, 2 of which required intravenous antibiotics. One of these patients developed infection in the thighs and not in areas of fat injection. All 4 cases resolved with incision and drainage (one requiring 2 incision and drainage sessions), with no need for further revision or regrafting.

Fat Injection

Fat transfer is the most technically unforgiving component of the procedure. The fat graft survival depends on various aspects of harvesting and transfer; specifically, injury or death from shearing, nutritional depletion, overinjection in one area, and/or excessive pressure are important to avoid.[25–27] The most important technical aspect of fat transfer is to lay multiple small aliquots of fat, which allows the injected fat to be surrounded by healthy, well-vascularized tissue and surrounding native fat cells. Avoidance of excessively large aliquot injections of fat is critical because these grafts may progress to areas of fat necrosis or liquefaction that can create a large cystic cavity of saponified sterile fat cells (**Fig. 3**). A 3.7-mm cannula is used to inject the fat in an antegrade and retrograde fashion. The passes should be rapid, in a fanning motion, and avoidance of staying in one location is essential for graft survival and prevention of contour irregularities. With each pass, no more than 5 to 10 cc of fat is injected. The plane of injection is constantly changed and tactile feedback of tissue resistance is assessed throughout lipoinjection. As with liposuction, it is critical to perform multiple passes in multiple directions to ensure an even and homogenous

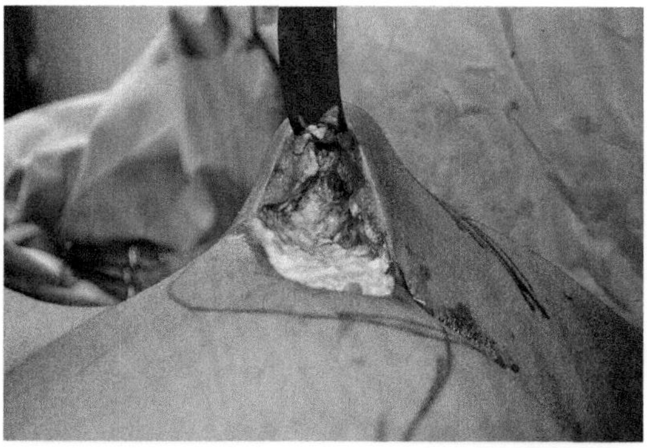

Fig. 3. Sterile fat necrosis caused by excessively large aliquots of fat graft.

distribution of fat. The planes of injection are into the superficial muscular/muscle fascial layer, deep subcutaneous, and lastly, superficial subcutaneous tissue layer in that order. Therefore, the injections begin deep and move more superficial and are repeated in multiple planes as needed for shape, contour, and size. During injection, avoidance of the deeper muscular layers is critical to avoid intravascular injection or injury to the sciatic nerve.[28] The safety of this procedure depends on injecting the fat into the appropriate planes, which requires understanding the gluteal anatomy as well as angling the cannula superficially from the superior and inferior access incisions (**Fig. 4**, Video 1).

An understanding of the anatomy is critical to avoiding incorrect injection planes and avoiding neurovascular structures. In addition, it is important to understand how the ligamentous and fascial anatomy can affect the injection cannulas. For example, the sacrocutaneous and ischiocutaneous ligaments are encountered by the injection cannula during this procedure. As the cannula passes through these structures, they have a tendency to torque the cannula, causing the tip of the cannula to dive deep into or below to the muscle. This can lead to large-vessel injury and potentially to fat embolization.[29,30] In order to avoid misdirection of the cannula, the surgeon should hold the cannula at an angle that avoids inadvertent misguidance from rigid tissue densities (ligaments and fascial condensations). Prerelease and intermittent rerelease of ligamentous structures as needed will aid cannula excursion through these structures while counteracting the torque the ligaments may place.

The fat placed in the injection syringes should not be excessively aqueous nor contain ligamentous and fibrous tissue. The presence of these additional tissues alters the necessary tension feedback required to optimally judge injection volume required per area. Ideally, during injection some tissue resistance should be encountered with every pass. Once a point of minimal resistance is felt, further injection should stop to avoid inadvertent pooling of fat lobules. This third spacing can cause future cyst formation and potential saponification of sterile fat as previously mentioned.

Overcorrection during gluteal fat transfer is not recommended, because excessive injection may result in greater pressure placed on the transplanted fat leading to a potentially cytotoxic event.[25–27] Excessively aqueous fat grafts will overestimate actual volume of viable fat cells injected. This may mislead patients because many seek a certain volume and determine success on this number. However, this leads to unrealistic expectations, and as the edema resolves, may lead to less than satisfactory patient outcomes. A viable fat ratio is approximately 30% to 50% of aspirate volume. For example, if 3 L is aspirated, up to 1500 mL may be usable fat grafts. This amount is determined by the density of fat cells per area. It is important to recognize that although the volume is not important to an excellent outcome, the volumes required are typically less in secondary cases, whereas weight loss patients typically require more. Many secondary patients have a fat transfer foundation and sufficient volume requiring only small volume additions to certain areas and contouring of the remainder of the buttock. Conversely, massive weight loss patients have more skin laxity and buttock ptosis, which requires more volume to correct. However, these patients can be challenging because they have a paucity of donor sites because of global fat loss. Areas of gluteal dimpling may be released with percutaneous aponeurotomy using a pickle fork device or flared Mercedes tip cannula on high oscillating vibration. The senior author (A.G.) prefers the flared cannula tip to release lower central fascial bands of the buttock and uses a pickle fork for very superficial irregularities. However, care must be taken to not overrelease too large of an area because this may lead to contour irregularities and a bubbling or fat compartment "blow-out" from rupture of fat compartment boundaries. Massaging is performed throughout the fat injection to avoid coalescence of fat lobules into clumps.

Access incisions are closed using a layered technique for sterility and viability of fat-grafted sites. The buttock and lumbar regions require watertight closure of incisions. Open drainage should not be used. Compression of the areas of liposuction is important to prevent seromas and ensure good adherence of the skin and superficial fat layers to the musculoskeletal framework. One or 2 layered Topifoam pads (Mentor, Irvine, CA, USA) are placed over the area of the lower back central (sacral/suprasacral) fat pad to help enhance the

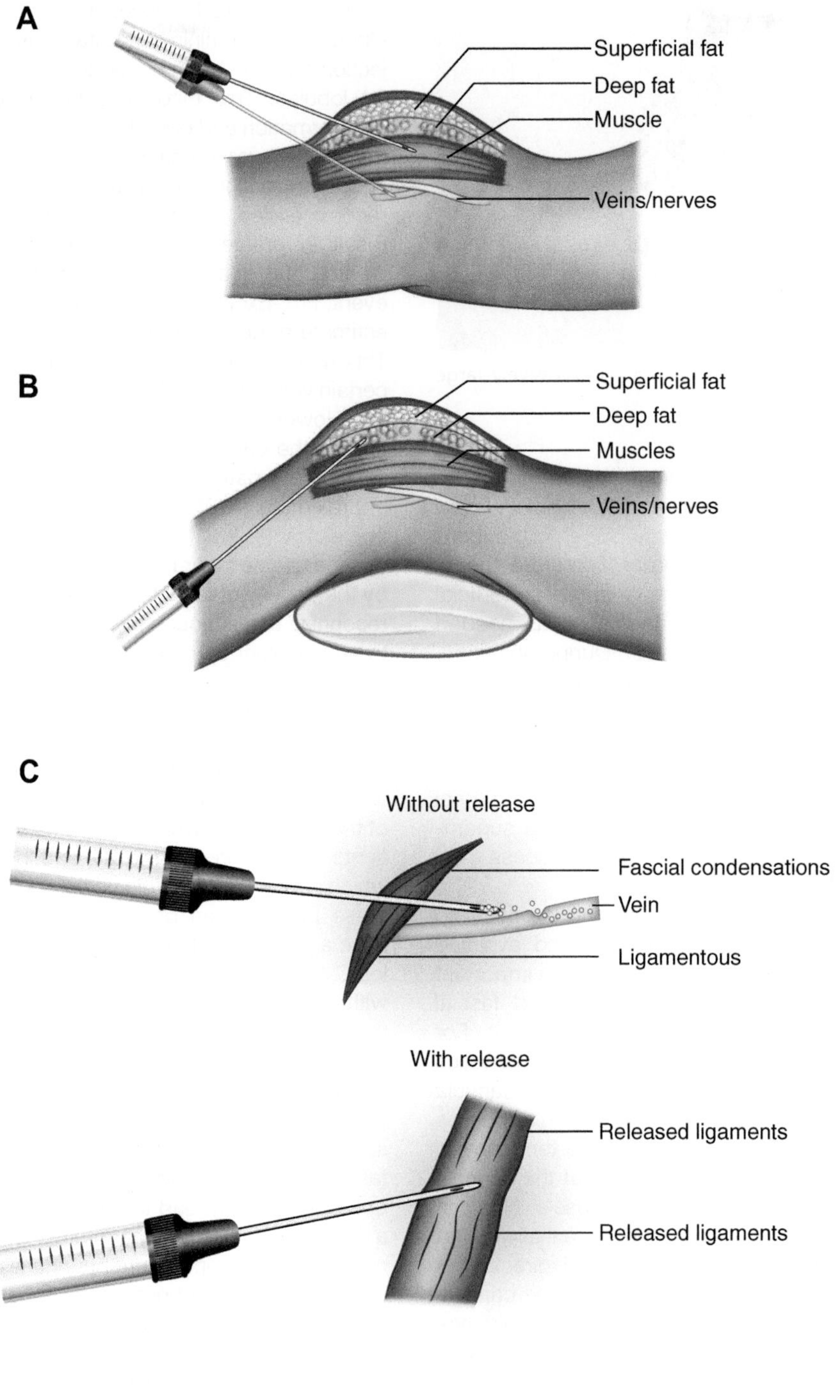

Fig. 4. (*A*) Improper hand position and cannula trajectory angle with misguidance facilitated by surrounding ligamentous structures. Ligaments require release before and throughout injection and change in injection angle to avoid deep veins and nerves. (*B*) Patient positioned with a bump under the groin along with operating room table flexed in a kidney position. This along with dropping the injection hand toward the floor and angling cannula superficially helps avoid deeper structures and inadvertent intravenous fat graft siphoning/migration. (*C*) Ligamentous and fascial condensations must be released before and throughout fat injection, particularly when using the infragluteal crease access incision. Misguidance of cannula into an undesired deeper intramuscular and submuscular space.

desired lower back lordosis. TopiFoam is also placed over the areas that have undergone liposuction, and the patient is placed into a compression garment. The authors encourage the use of garments that are looser or open over the buttocks for approximately 6 to 8 weeks.

POTENTIAL COMPLICATIONS AND MANAGEMENT OF COMPLICATIONS

Asymmetry

Although asymmetry is not a common source of patient complaints, it is often subtle. Preoperatively, it is important to identify and discuss asymmetries with the patient. Patient photographs aid this discussion by clearly defining the asymmetries for the patient. Many asymmetries can be improved with the procedure and should be a "soft" objective. Differential fat viability is actually an uncommon cause of unplanned postoperative asymmetries. The best management for asymmetries is patient education and preoperative planning. Hip asymmetries and pelvic tilting should be pointed out to patients preoperatively. Often iliac bone size and shape varies between sides. Patients who favor one hip over another can cause discrepancy in initial buttock/hip volume and the gluteal footprint. Despite meticulous technique, if substantial asymmetries are noted postoperatively, it is important to wait 3 to 6 months to ensure complete evaluation of graft take. If the asymmetry is significant at this point, then reoperation with fat grafting can be performed. More commonly, patients may request larger buttocks or improved density as fat graft take is finalized. Regrafting (if fat donor is available) can be attempted after 9 to 12 months. Weight gain may be required to increase remaining fat lobule size.

Contour Abnormalities

Management of contour abnormalities is performed similar to the technique used for asymmetry. Patient education and prevention are the most effective approaches to avoid contour abnormalities. As with asymmetries, it is important to note any preexisting contour abnormalities before the operation and discuss them in detail with the patient. One of the most challenging aspects of buttock augmentation with fat transfer is to fully correct cellulite, wavy skin contour, a flat lower pole, and dimples. Superficial skin contours are very difficult to reverse or correct completely, as are adherent lower pole or lateral areas that lack a native fat scaffold to build upon. Meticulous surgical technique with an eye toward recognition and prevention of contour abnormalities is the best approach.

Iatrogenic contour abnormalities of the buttock may also be seen postoperatively. In most cases, it is important to wait at least 3 to 6 months after the operation to accurately evaluate the deformity. If the deformity has been caused by excessively superficial fat injection, the irregularity may be treated with steroid injection or localized superficial liposuction with small cannulas. Inadequate fat injection to a particular region may be treated with additional fat transfer. Skin irregularities due to tethering from scar may be treated with percutaneous aponeurotomy and additional fat transfer. Skin dimpling may also be treated in a similar manner with release and superficial injection of smaller fat aliquots.

Fat Necrosis and Cysts

Avoidance of fat necrosis and cyst can be accomplished with meticulous fat injection technique and accurate assessment of the regional ability of the buttocks to expand where desired. The fat transfer should be done in small aliquots with the goal to have the graft surrounded by healthy, well-vascularized tissue that allows diffusion of nutrients and oxygen to all of the transplanted fat cells. When injection of too much fat in one pass occurs, there is an increased risk that the fat will pool within the gluteal tissue and the central core of the aliquot will not receive adequate nutrition to survive the grafting procedure. This central fat necrosis results in oil cysts or firm areas of fat necrosis. Small areas typically do not pose a clinical problem needing correction, whereas large areas may lead to larger cyst formations or create regional soft tissue depressions, or ptosis from fat graft loss. Complete fat loss and full buttock ptosis are rare. If they occur, a direct superiorly based buttock lift will treat the ptosis, and subsequent secondary fat injection for volume can be later performed.

The management of oil cysts depends on the size of the cyst. Small oil cysts may be allowed to resorb, be drained with needle aspiration or wall suction and a small cannula, or with formal incision and drainage. Large oil cysts may need to be drained under direct palpation or with ultrasound guidance. The lead author have only seen one case of a large saponified fat cyst, which was associated with a mature capsular wall. Following drainage, packing may be required to help the dead space close. As with oil cysts, areas of fat necrosis are treated depending on size. Small areas of fat necrosis, less than approximately 2 cm in diameter, may resolve with time and should be observed. Large areas of fat necrosis may require surgical excision.

Infection

Perioperative intravenous antibiotics, postoperative oral antibiotics, and mixing the patient's fat with antibiotics before transfer minimize wound infections. Patients are instructed to perform a chlorhexidine rinse before surgery and are instructed to maintain good hygiene postoperatively with the use of antibiotic ointment on access incisions and regular showers. Even with the most careful approach, wound infections can occur.

If a patient develops localized erythema concerning for cellulitis in the postoperative period, a very low threshold to treat with antibiotics should be present. Treatment is typically initiated with a fluoroquinolone for 7 to 10 days. If an abscess develops, it is promptly drained and cultures are obtained to guide appropriate antibiotic coverage. The wound is typically packed until it heals. Ideally, access to the abscess is obtained through one of the fat-transfer or liposuction incisions. This may be performed by lengthening the incision. In some cases, the abscess must be accessed with a new incision on the buttock. It is recommended that mycobacterial cultures be obtained at the time of abscess drainage. Rarely, mycobacterial infections have been noted in patients undergoing gluteal fat transfer. Referral to infectious disease specialists for appropriate treatment and surveillance is important. In these cases, interrogation of the operating room

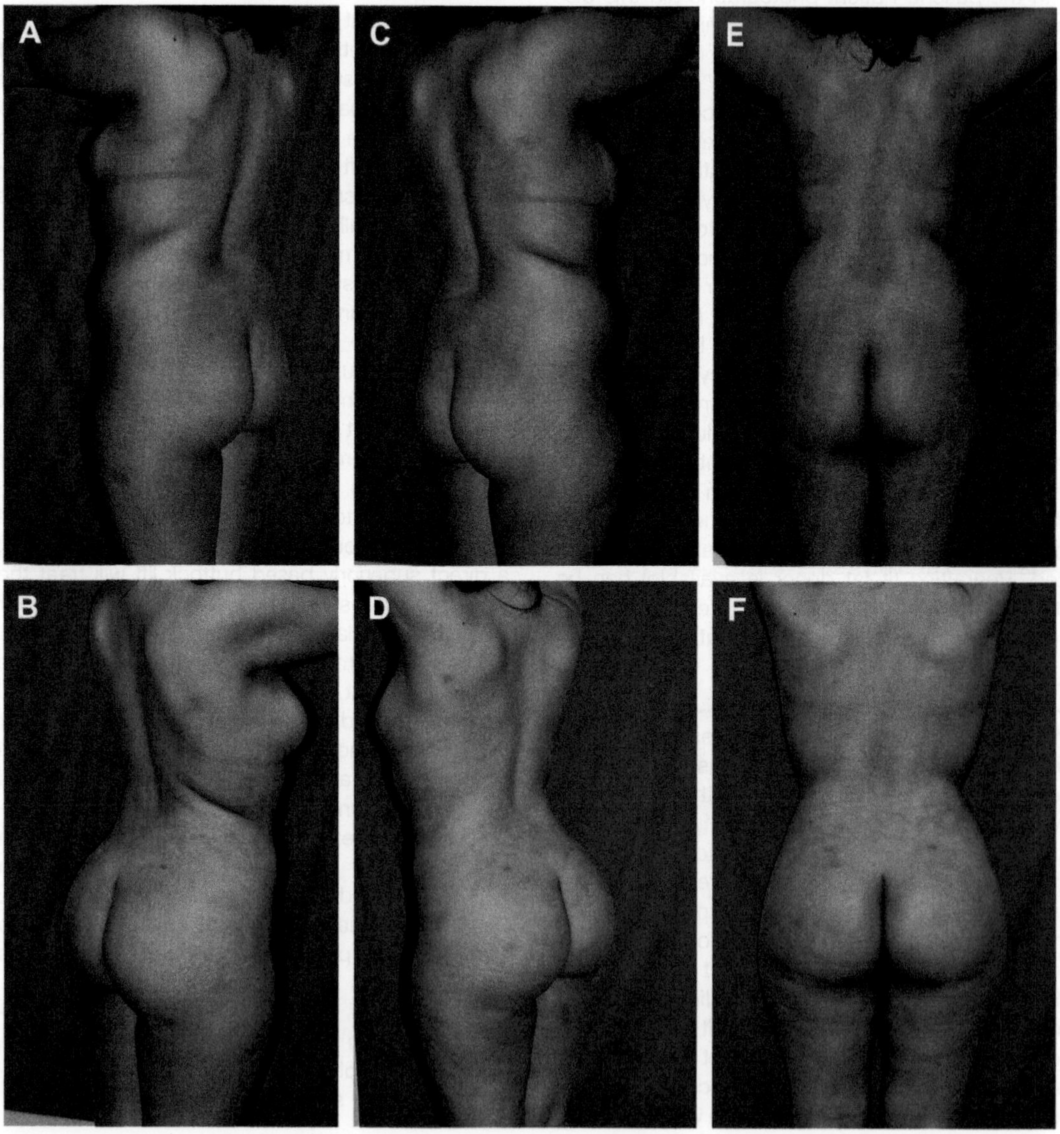

Fig. 5. (*A*) (*Left*) Before global liposuction and fat augmentation to the buttocks. (*B*) (*Right*) After fat transfer to bilateral buttocks and liposuction of arms, back, flanks, abdomen, and inner thighs. (*C, D*) Note the difference in left and right sides based on variations in pelvic bony tilt. (*E*) Distance and angle variation between right iliac bone and lowest rib versus left side. (*F*) Right has a deeper shorter distance between the iliac bone and rib cage.

for a source may be warranted. Fungal infections are very rare, but require antifungal antibiotics and direct excision of the spores may be necessary.

Seroma

Seroma can occur in the donor area and should be treated by needle aspiration and use of compression garments. Seromas that are clinically relevant in the recipient site or sites are rare and can be treated with simple aspiration as well. Repeated drainage may be necessary.

Fat Embolism

Microfat and macrofat embolization has been noted to occur with even low-volume gluteal augmentation procedures.[18,20] Macrofat embolization has been reported as a macroscopic, mechanical obstructive event in which large quantities of fat occlude the cardiovascular system. Fat embolism syndrome is a microscopic inflammatory event in which embolism of small quantities of fat results in a systemic inflammatory response.[17–20,28] In all cases, the greatest care should be placed on prevention of this complication. Fat should be injected in small aliquots only on advancement and withdrawal of the cannula with constant motion. Fat should be transferred into the subcutaneous and superficial muscular tissue only. Larger blood vessels have been noted deeper within the muscle and should be avoided. Theoretically, a partial laceration of these vessels may allow entry of fat grafts along a negative pressure gradient. In addition, avoidance of deep injection minimizes the risk of sciatic nerve injury. As noted above, proper injection angle and cannula guidance throughout injection are mandatory to avoid inadvertent ligamentous misguidance.

Fat embolism presents with acute or progressive cardiovascular compromise. In either setting, if there is suspicion of fat embolization, the patient should be supported with fluids and oxygen and promptly transferred to a hospital for evaluation and treatment.

POSTPROCEDURAL CARE

Postoperatively, the patients are placed on a 5-day course of antibiotics. The Topifoam pads are removed 7 to 10 days after the operation and are replaced as needed. The patient is instructed to use the surgical garment for up to 2 months after

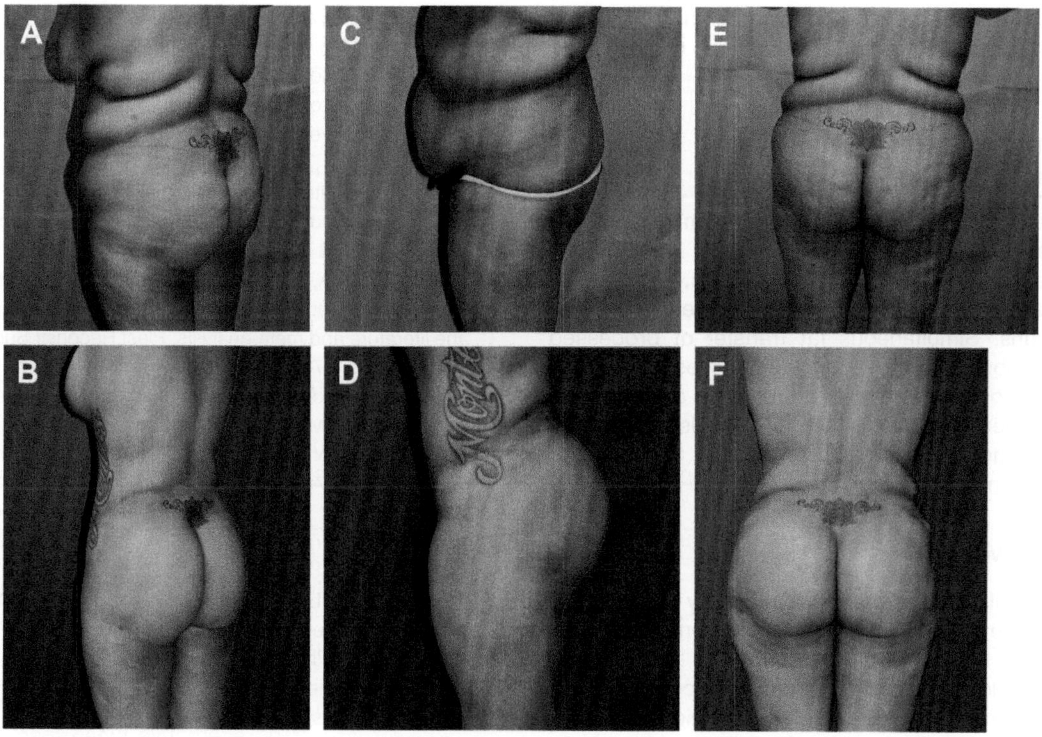

Fig. 6. (*A*) (*Left*) Before global liposuction, abdominoplasty, and fat augmentation to the buttocks. (*B*) (*Right*) After stages 1 and 2. (*C, D*) Abdominoplasty, fat transfer to bilateral buttocks and liposuction of arms, upper and lower back, flanks, lower abdomen, and inner thighs. (*E, F*) (Second stage) Six months later, liposuction mid back, abdomen, and arms with another session of fat transfer to bilateral buttocks.

the operation. After 7 to 10 days, patients are transitioned from the first-stage compression, which uses 2 zippers to second-stage compression, which only uses one zipper. Compression of the augmented buttocks can result in fat graft death; therefore, the patient is instructed to avoid sitting or lying on the buttocks for the first 2 weeks and up to 8 weeks as much as feasible, including prone positioning when sleeping and sitting with pillows under the thighs, keeping the gluteal region off the chair. These specialized pillows are now widely available commercially. Another approach some patients use is to sit on an inflatable exercise ball or sit on the thighs with the buttocks off the edge of a sitting stool or chair with no back.

Patients should be educated on meticulous hygiene. Patients are instructed to ambulate immediately after surgery.

REHABILITATION AND RECOVERY

Postoperatively, patients are instructed to have a relatively high caloric intake for the first 1 to 3 months after surgery to ensure better fat nutrition and retention. Patients are allowed to engage in light exercise 4 weeks after the operation. The authors recommend that patients focus on exercises that will build and tone muscle (yoga, Pilates, weight training, and so forth) rather than strenuous fat-burning exercises and excessive cardiocentric programs in the first 6 months.

OUTCOMES

Case Examples

Case examples in **Figs. 5** and **6** demonstrate the patient before global liposuction. Liposuction (reduction) was performed on arms, entire back, flanks, abdomen, as well as inner and outer thighs. Simultaneous fat transfer of processed fat lobules to the buttocks provides a powerful transformation of the entire body contour in a 360 degree fashion. Case in **Fig. 6** also underwent a staged abdominoplasty and fat transfer was performed in 2 stages.

SUMMARY

Gluteal fat transfer is an increasingly popular procedure that has the ability to transform a patient's entire body silhouette and gluteal appearance. With close attention to following proper perioperative protocols and meticulous technique, the procedure can be performed safely with powerful and consistent results. When performed carefully, gluteal fat transfer has an extremely low complication profile.

SUPPLEMENTARY DATA

Supplementary data related to this article can be found online at https://doi.org/10.1016/j.cps.2017.12.009.

REFERENCES

1. Surgeons, A.S.o.P. 2016 National Clearinghouse of Plastic Surgery Statistic Report. 2017. Available at: https://www.plasticsurgery.org/news/plastic-surgery-statistics. Accessed February 17, 2017.
2. Lewis CM. Correction of deep gluteal depression by autologous fat grafting. Aesthetic Plast Surg 1992; 16(3):247–50.
3. Pereira LH, Radwanski HN. Fat grafting of the buttocks and lower limbs. Aesthetic Plast Surg 1996; 20(5):409–16.
4. Cardenas Restrepo JC, Munoz Ahmed JA. Large-volume lipoinjection for gluteal augmentation. Aesthet Surg J 2002;22(1):33–8.
5. Mendieta CG. Gluteal reshaping. Aesthet Surg J 2007;27(6):641–55.
6. Cardenas-Camarena L, Silva-Gavarrete JF, Arenas-Quintana R. Gluteal contour improvement: different surgical alternatives. Aesthetic Plast Surg 2011; 35(6):1117–25.
7. Nicareta B, Pereira LH, Sterodimas A, et al. Autologous gluteal lipograft. Aesthetic Plast Surg 2011; 35(2):216–24.
8. Rosique RG, Rosique MJ, De Moraes CG. Gluteoplasty with autologous fat tissue: experience with 106 consecutive cases. Plast Reconstr Surg 2015; 135(5):1381–9.
9. Toledo LS. Gluteal augmentation with fat grafting: the Brazilian buttock technique: 30 years' experience. Clin Plast Surg 2015;42(2):253–61.
10. Condé-Green A, Kotamarti V, Nini KT, et al. Fat grafting for gluteal augmentation: a systematic review of the literature and meta-analysis. Plast Reconstr Surg 2016;138(3):437e–46e.
11. Mofid MM, Mendieta CG, Senderoff DM, et al. Buttock augmentation with silicone implants: a multicenter survey review of 2226 patients. Plast Reconstr Surg 2013;131(4):897–901.
12. Senderoff DM. Buttock augmentation with solid silicone implants. Aesthet Surg J 2011;31(3): 320–7.
13. Hidalgo JE. Submuscular gluteal augmentation: 17 years of experience with gel and elastomer silicone implants. Clin Plast Surg 2006;33(3):435–47.
14. Vergara R, Amezcua H. Intramuscular gluteal implants: 15 years' experience. Aesthet Surg J 2003; 23(2):86–91.
15. Cardenas-Mejia A, Martínez JR, León D, et al. Bilateral sciatic nerve axonotmesis after gluteal lipoaugmentation. Ann Plast Surg 2009;63(4):366–8.

16. Astarita DC, Scheinin LA, Sathyavagiswaran L. Fat transfer and fatal macroembolization. J Forensic Sci 2015;60(2):509–10.
17. Cardenas-Camarena L, Bayter JE, Aguirre-Serrano H, et al. Deaths caused by gluteal lipoinjection: what are we doing wrong? Plast Reconstr Surg 2015;136(1):58–66.
18. Rosique RG, Rosique MJ. Deaths caused by gluteal lipoinjection: what are we doing wrong? Plast Reconstr Surg 2016;137(3):641e–2e.
19. Sinno S, Chang JB, Brownstone ND, et al. Determining the safety and efficacy of gluteal augmentation: a systematic review of outcomes and complications. Plast Reconstr Surg 2016;137(4):1151–6.
20. Mofid M, Teitelbaum S, Suissa D, et al. Report on mortality from gluteal fat grafting: recommendations from the ASERF task force. Aesthet Surg J 2017;37(7):796–806.
21. Gutowski KA, ASPS Fat Graft Task Force. Current applications and safety of autologous fat grafts: a report of the ASPS fat graft task force. Plast Reconstr Surg 2009;124(1):272–80.
22. Gould MK, Garcia DA, Wren SM, et al. Prevention of VTE in nonorthopedic surgical patients: antithrombotic therapy and prevention of thrombosis, 9th ed: American College of Chest physicians evidence-based clinical practice guidelines. Chest 2012;141(2):e227S–77S.
23. Mendieta CG. Classification system for gluteal evaluation. Clin Plast Surg 2006;33(3):333–46.
24. Stulberg JJ, Delaney CP, Neuhauser DV, et al. Adherence to surgical care improvement project measures and the association with postoperative infections. JAMA 2010;303(24):2479–85.
25. Sinno S, Wilson SC, Brownstone ND, et al. Techniques and outcomes in fat grafting: using evidence to determine fact or fiction. Plast Reconstr Surg 2015;136(4S):131–2.
26. Rohrich RJ, Sorokin ES, Brown SA. In search of improved fat transfer viability: a quantitative analysis of the role of centrifugation and harvest site. Plast Reconstr Surg 2004;113(1):391–5.
27. Gir P, Brown SA, Oni G, et al. Fat grafting: evidence-based review on autologous fat harvesting, processing, reinjection, and storage. Plast Reconstr Surg 2012;130(1):249–58.
28. Wall S Jr, Del Vecchio D. Commentary on: report on mortality from gluteal fat grafting: recommendations from the ASERF task force. Aesthet Surg J 2017;37(7):807–10.
29. Ghavami A, Villaneuva NL, Amirlak B. Gluteal ligamentous anatomy and its implication in safe buttock augmentation. Plast Reconstr Surg, in press.
30. Ghavami A. Commentary: gluteal augmentation with silicone implants: a new proposal for intramuscular dissection. Aesthetic Plast Surg 2017;41(5):1148–9.

Autologous Flap Gluteal Augmentation
Purse-String Technique

Joseph P. Hunstad, MD, Mark A. Daniels, MD,
John C. Crantford, MD*

KEYWORDS

• Gluteal augmentation • Purse-string gluteoplasty • Buttock ptosis • Massive weight loss

KEY POINTS

- The ideal patient for purse-string gluteoplasty has buttock deflation and ptosis, and wishes to improve projection.
- Key elements of the procedure are buttock lifting combined with auto-augmentation, no undermining of auto-augmentation tissue, complete vascular preservation and use of a purse-string suture to enhance projection of auto- augmentation tissue.
- Purse-string gluteoplasty is a safe and effective technique to correct buttock ptosis and atrophy.

INTRODUCTION

Buttock atrophy and ptosis after massive weight loss or secondary to aging is a common complaint of many patients. First described in 2009,[1] the purse-string gluteoplasty is an alternative to existing methods of autologous buttock augmentation. Autologous buttock augmentation has been described by several authors.[2–8] Previously described methods involve undermining, rotational flaps, or flaps with a narrow base that are based on named perforator vessels. These methods relied on rotation flaps, which theoretically were axial pattern flaps, but in reality had random vascularity that frequently was associated with vascular embarrassment and tip loss. The purse-string gluteoplasty method of autologous buttock augmentation uses the patient's own redundant soft tissues to augment the atrophic buttocks in conjunction with lifting of the buttocks. This procedure has been shown to dramatically improve the result compared with a buttocks lift with excision of the redundant tissues, which can lead to a very lifted, but deflated buttocks.

The purse-string gluteoplasty was developed owing to inconsistent results with rotation flaps as a safe and predictable method of autologous buttock augmentation. This procedure involves no undermining or rotation of the augmented tissue, thereby simplifying the procedure and increasing the reliability of the augmented tissue. As one of its hallmarks, this method involves complete vascular preservation. The purse-string suture also lends shape and additional projection to the buttocks. The procedure can be done as an isolated procedure or in conjunction with circumferential abdominoplasty or bodylift.

The increasing number of obese patients and success of weight loss surgery has led to more demand for body contouring procedures.[9] Significant psychological stress owing to the deformities of massive weight loss is seen in this patient population.[10] It has also been suggested that buttock auto-augmentation during buttock lifting leads to

Disclosure Statement: The authors have nothing to disclose.
Department of Plastic Surgery, Hunstad Kortesis Bharti Plastic Surgery & MedSpa, 11208 Statesville Road, Suite #300, Huntersville, NC 28078, USA
* Corresponding author.
E-mail address: Clayton.crantford@gmail.com

Clin Plastic Surg 45 (2018) 261–267
https://doi.org/10.1016/j.cps.2017.12.008

greater patient satisfaction than buttock lift without auto-augmentation.[11] The purse-string gluteoplasty provides these patients with high satisfaction and aesthetically pleasing body contouring results.

The ideal purse-string gluteoplasty candidate is a patient with redundant skin and soft tissues of the lower back and gluteal region with deflation of the buttocks. This habitus can be determined using bimanual pinch and palpation. This procedure is not exclusive to the massive weight loss population. Patients with buttock atrophy and ptosis can greatly benefit from this procedure.

Patients should be medically healthy enough to undergo body contouring surgery, and have adequate cardiopulmonary status to tolerate prone positioning during surgery. Smoking cessation is imperative for at least 6 weeks before surgery (our policy) and until complete healing has occurred. Caution should be used in patients with diabetes or vascular disease. Blood loss is typically minimal; however, the surgeon should be aware of the patient's preoperative hemoglobin and coagulation status.

In consultation, patients often demonstrate their desired result by pulling up on their buttocks and thigh tissue. Patients may also wish to discuss other options such as buttock fat grafting or buttock implants. The classic massive weight loss patient requires skin removal to achieve satisfactory lifting of the ptotic and deflated buttock. Patients with "complete weight loss" will not have adequate body fat to harvest via liposuction for buttock fat grafting.[12] Prosthetic buttock implants come in a limited size range and are not typically recommended for use in conjunction with buttock lifting. Autologous tissue is usually plentiful, natural feeling, and redundant in virtually all massive weight loss patients, making the purse-string gluteoplasty, for many patients, an ideal body contouring procedure.

PROCEDURAL DETAILS

The patient is marked while standing. The point of maximum buttocks projection is identified, as previously described by Centeno and Mendieta,[13] as a line from the trochanter across the buttocks to the coccyx. This line identifies the point of ideal buttocks maximum projection. This is the intended final incision line because it centers the autologous buttocks augmentation (purse-string gluteoplasty) at the point of maximum ideal projection (**Fig. 1**).

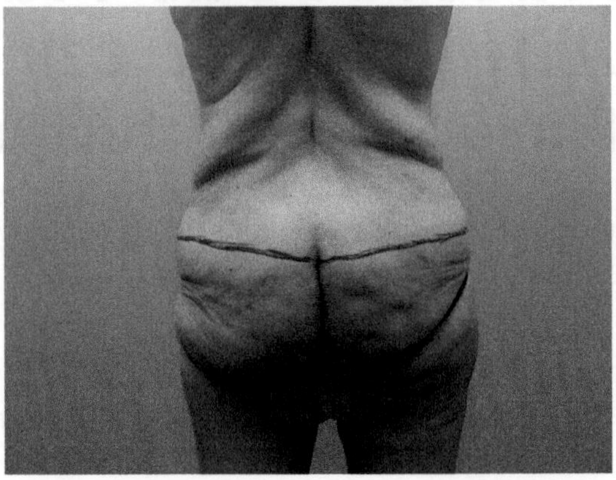

Fig. 1. The planned level of final scar. This overlies the point of maximal projection. The ideal incision is placed on a line drawn from the trochanter to the coccyx.

The first bimanual palpation markings are performed in the midaxillary line (**Fig. 2**). Because patients want to help us with the markings they tend to lean toward the surgeon when they are marked. This may lead to an excessive amount of skin being removed, so we ask the patient to lean slightly away from us when we mark the midaxillary line. If this is being performed with a body lift, the incision continues anteriorly into the lower body lift incision across the abdomen. The upper abdominal incision is an estimate that will definitively be determined intraoperatively with the use of a tissue demarcator.

Bimanual palpation then gathers up the excess tissue across the entire buttocks bilaterally (**Fig. 3**). There is always less tissue gathered up in the midline because of the strong midline zone of adherence. Realignment marks are then placed to facilitate reapproximation. The purse-string gluteoplasty is drawn from the medial aspect of the buttocks curvature to the lateral aspect of the buttocks curvature within the upper and lower lines of bimanual palpation. In the midline, a butterfly shape of tissue is identified, which will serve as

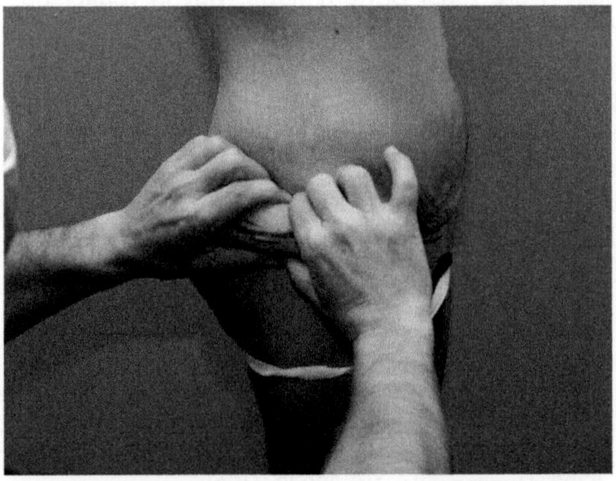

Fig. 2. The first bimanual pinch is performed at the anterior axillary line. Having the patient lean slightly away from the surgeon minimizes the risk of excessive tension.

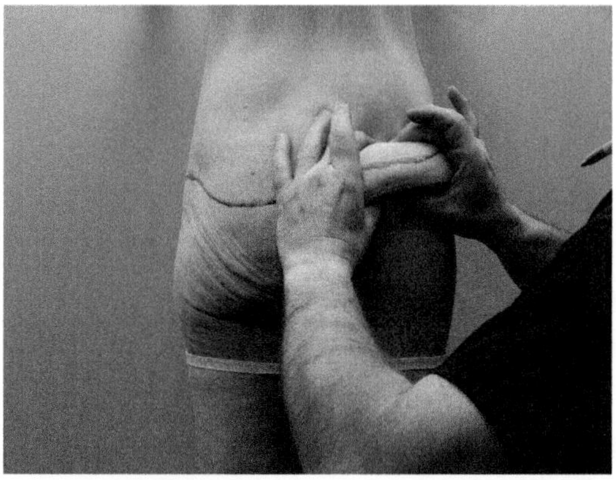

Fig. 3. Bimanual gathering is continued across the buttocks to mark the planned skin resection. Resection in the midline is less owing to the zone of adherence.

an anchoring point to the purse-string gluteoplasty autologous tissue to prevent lateral displacement (**Fig. 4**).

The lateral tissue excision pattern extends from the lateral edge of the purse-string gluteoplasty tissue to the anterior axillary line full thickness excision down to the muscular fascia.

Photographs are taken and the patient is placed in the prone position under anesthesia. The marks are rechecked with a penetrating towel clamps to ensure that excessive tissue is not being resected. Failure to close, or closure under very high tension, is problematic and can lead to the most dreaded complication of this procedure, namely, wound dehiscence. Wound dehiscence takes a significant amount of time to heal secondarily and is difficult for the patient and surgeon alike. Surgical scar revision is often indicated once the resulting scar has fully matured.

For those beginning the procedure, a good rule of thumb is to begin the actual skin incision 1 cm in from the originally planned superior and inferior markings. This will provide satisfactory tension when accommodating the purse-string gluteoplasty tissue. As experience is gained, slightly more aggressive skin excisions can be performed safely.

After careful confirmation of the markings, the incision lines are infiltrated with a dilute lidocaine-epinephrine solution. The area circled for the purse-string gluteoplasty flap is infiltrated superficially to facilitate deepithelization. Where the skin will be resected laterally, deeper infiltration is performed to minimize bleeding. A full prep and draping is performed in the usual fashion. The superior and inferior incision lines are then made with a #10 blade into the dermis and deeper dissection is performed with electrocautery to minimize bleeding. The central tissue over the purse-string gluteoplasty is deepithelialized sharply or with electrocautery. The dissection is then deepened to the muscle fascia all around the purse-string gluteoplasty tissue. The tissue anterior to this is resected full thickness to the muscle fascia. The central bowtie shaped tissue is reduced to the level of the superficial fascia and separated from the surrounding tissues. This is necessary because anchoring of the autologous buttocks tissue is necessary to the midline to prevent lateral displacement. Dissection of the incisions around the purse-string gluteoplasty are taken straight down to the muscle fascia creating a true island of skin and subcutaneous tissue without undermining and with complete preservation of all perforating vessels (**Fig. 5**).

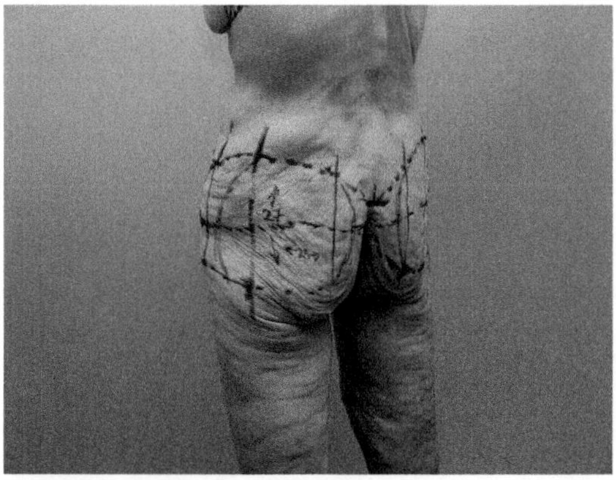

Fig. 4. Final skin markings. The area in purple marks the planned auto-augmentation. Realignment marks are essential because significant shifting can occur secondary to skin laxity.

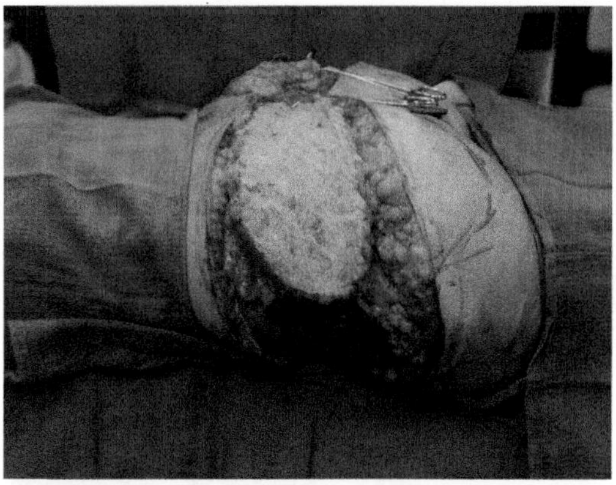

Fig. 5. Deepithelialized gluteal flaps. Dissection is carried straight down to the underlying deep fascia, maintaining the underlying vasculature. Skin is deepithelialized to preserve volume and provide a strong anchoring point to the midline.

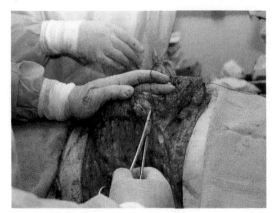

Fig. 6. Placement of the purse string suture at the level of the superficial fascial system; #1 Mersilene or equivalent is used for this process. The suture must glide easily through the tissues.

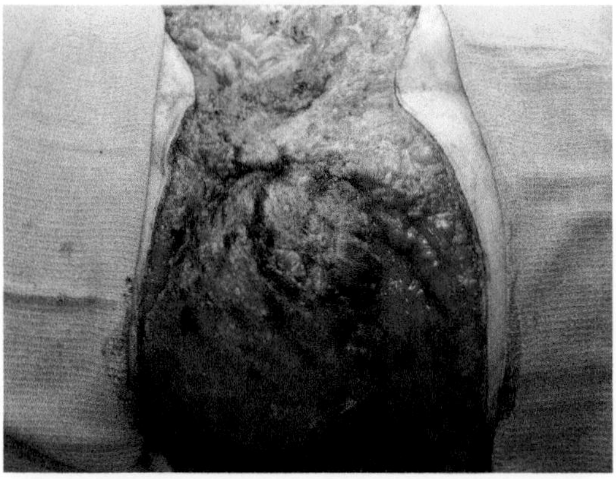

Fig. 8. The newly created mound is anchored to the central remnant previously preserved. The same suture as used for the purse string may be used here. This anchoring is critical to prevent lateral displacement of the autologous tissue. It is crucial to preserve the superficial fascia between the autologous flaps for a strong anchoring point.

The superficial fascial system can be marked for easier delineation and then a running, #1 Mersilene suture using a large taper needle is placed so that it glides through the tissue at the level of the superficial fascia (**Fig. 6**). The suture is then tied very tightly and secured with multiple knots. The purse-string tissue assumes an ideal configuration or shape similar to that of a high projecting full-size buttocks implant (**Fig. 7**). It is then anchored to the preserved residual superficial fascia medially. Usually, 3 Mersilene sutures are placed (**Fig. 8**). No venous congestion of this tissue has been observed to date.

A pocket is created inferiorly to the purse-string gluteoplasty based on the width of the formed autologous buttocks tissue. This pocket is elevated superficial to the gluteal fascia (**Fig. 9**). The pocket dissection is checked frequently to confirm adequacy to house the purse-string gluteoplasty. A closed suction drain is then placed and secured as with an isolated buttocks lift, or coiled beneath the skin and removed supine when a body lift is being performed.

Closure is performed by temporarily stapling the incision closed. Then, using 0 or #1 Vicryl sutures based on tension and body habitus, interrupted superficial fascia sutures are placed eliminating all tension on the skin closure. The skin closure is then performed with interrupted buried 2-0 Vicryl sutures in the deep dermis and then an intracuticular 4-0 Monocryl. Interrupted simple 3-0 Prolene sutures can be placed to act as security sutures, preventing skin separation during the early postoperative period of maximum swelling (**Fig. 10**).

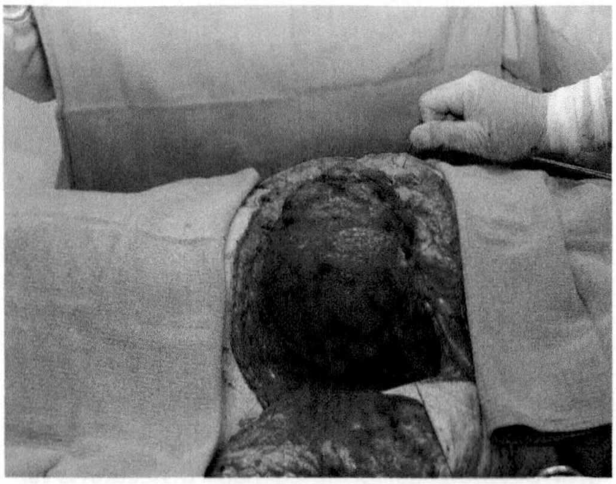

Fig. 7. The suture is secured as tightly as possible with approximately 6 knots. Once tightened, the suture leads to a narrowing of the gluteal mound and subsequent increased projection.

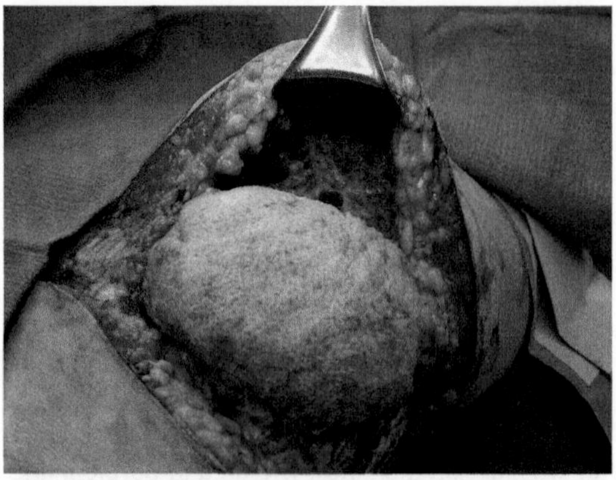

Fig. 9. A pocket is created to precisely fit the newly created mound by undermining the soft tissue directly below the flap, preserving the gluteal fascia.

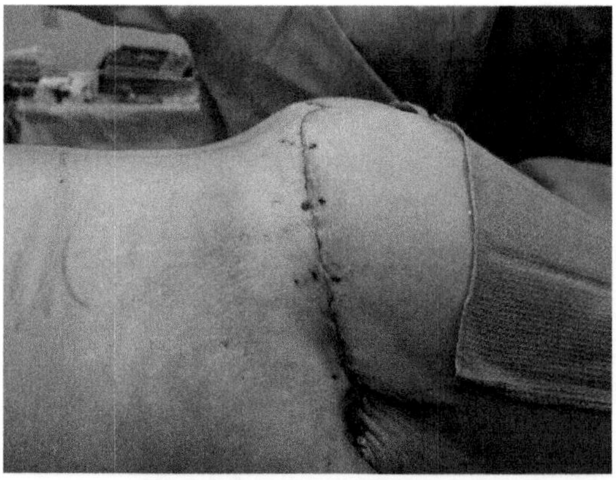

Fig. 10. Closure on the operating table (the dog ear seen was removed when the abdominoplasty was completed). Three-layer closure is performed with #1 Vicryl in the superficial fascia to minimize tension on final skin closure. Before final closure, a single drain is placed in the lower back to drain both pockets.

They can be usually removed without leaving behind suture marks in 4 or 5 days.

Dressings are minimal and include taping of the incision with 1-inch paper tape. This is split every 3 or 4 cm to allow for expansion and to minimize shearing forces that can cause blistering and subsequent hyperpigmentation. No compression dressings are applied for fear that they may pull across the incision line and cause separation.

Postoperatively, we allow the patient to sit gently on a pillow or soft padding as well as lay on their side. The tissues are examined frequently during the early postoperative recovery to ensure proper healing.

DISCUSSION

We have performed this technique in more than 40 patients to date. As can be expected with any body contouring procedure, skin laxity will ultimately recur to some degree. However, the newly created gluteal mounds maintain their projection over time. The most frequent complications are areas of wound dehiscence and widened scars. Undesirable scarring may be corrected with a simple scar revision or, if necessary, a revision lift. We have not encountered any episodes of fat necrosis or deep space infections. Advancement of this technique has included lowering the incision over the point of maximal projection, which has subsequently decreased elongation of the gluteal cleft. Patients report high levels of satisfaction with this procedure. The increase in gluteal volume and projection are unique advantages that this method offers over traditional gluteoplasty techniques (**Figs. 11–13**).

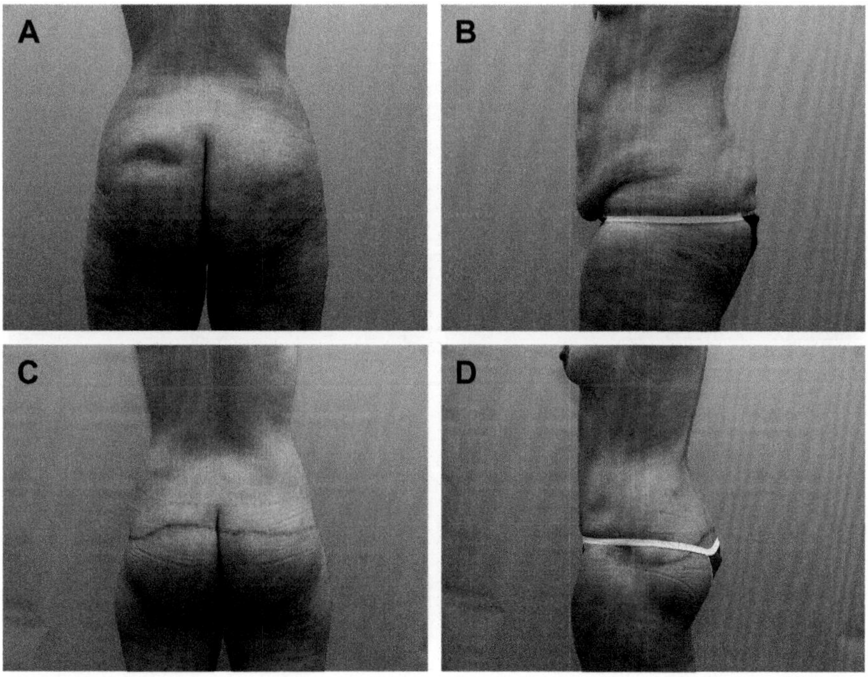

Fig. 11. (*A, B*) A 59-year-old woman with loose skin and buttock ptosis. (*C, D*) Two years after circumferential abdominoplasty with purse string gluteoplasty. She also underwent a scar revision after focal wound dehiscence.

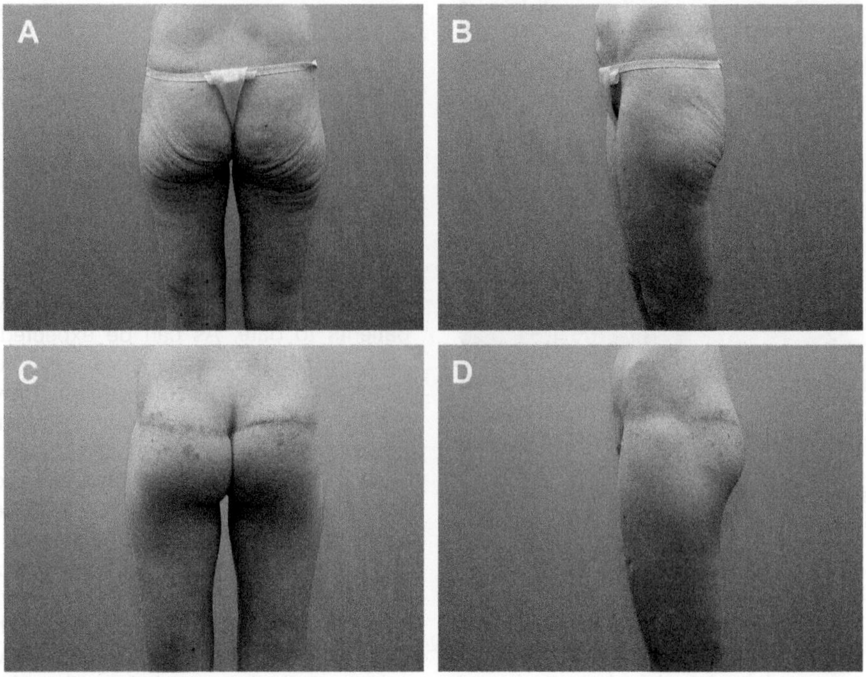

Fig. 12. (*A, B*) A 37-year-old woman with significant deflation and ptosis of her buttocks. (*C, D*) Eight months after circumferential abdominoplasty and purse string gluteoplasty.

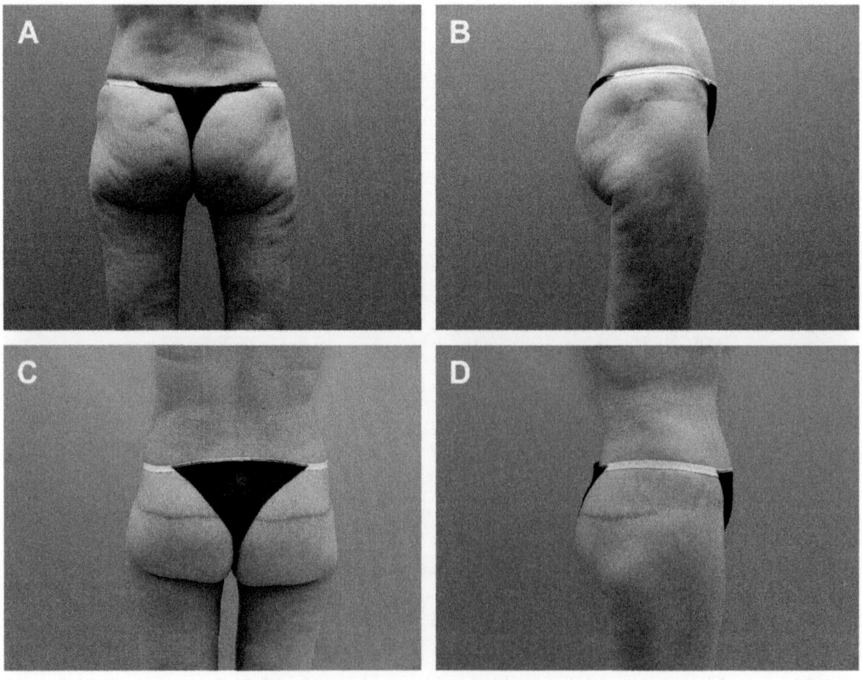

Fig. 13. (*A, B*) A 62-year-old woman with buttock ptosis and poor projection. (*C, D*) At 1 year and 4 months after purse string gluteoplasty (patient underwent prior abdominoplasty).

REFERENCES

1. Hunstad JP, Repta R. Purse string gluteoplasty. Plast Reconstr Surg 2009;123:123e–5e.
2. Centeno RF. Autologous gluteal augmentation. Clin Plast Surg 2006;33:479–96.
3. Balague N, Combescure C, Huber O. Plastic surgery improves long-term weight control after bariatric surgery. Plast Reconstr Surg 2013;132:826–33.
4. van der Beek ES, Geenen R, de Heer F. Quality of life long-term following bariatric surgery: sustained improvement after 7 years. Plast Reconstr Surg 2012;130:1133–9.
5. Rohde C, Gerut Z. Augmentation buttock-pexy using autologous tissue following massive weight loss. Aesthet Surg J 2005;25:576–81.
6. Raposo-Amaral CE, Cetrulo CL, de Campos Guidi M. Bilateral lumbar hip dermal fat rotation aps: a novel technique for autologous augmentation gluteoplasty. Plast Reconstr Surg 2006;117:1781–8.
7. Sozer SO, Francisco JA, Wolf C. Autoprosthesis buttock augmentation during lower body lift. Aesthetic Plast Surg 2006;29:133–7.
8. Oranges CM, Tremp M, di Summa PG, et al. Gluteal augmentation techniques: a comprehensive literature review. Aesthet Surg J 2017;37(5): 560–9.
9. Kitzinger HB, Aayev S, Pittermann A. The prevalence of body contouring surgery after gastric bypass surgery. Obes Surg 2012;22:8–12.
10. Azin A, Zhou C, Jackson T, et al. Body contouring surgery after bariatric surgery: a study of cost as a barrier and impact on psychological well-being. Plast Reconstr Surg 2014;133: 776e–82e.
11. Srivastava U, Rubin JP, Gusenoff JA. Lower body lift after massive weight loss: autoaugmentation versus no augmentation. Plast Reconstr Surg 2015;135: 762–72.
12. Hunstad JP, Aiken ME. Circumferential body contouring. In: Aly A, editor. Body contouring after massive weight loss. Boca Raton (FL): CRC Press; 2006. p. 183–212.
13. Centeno RF, Mendieta CG, Young VL. Gluteal contouring surgery in the massive weight loss patient. Clin Plast Surg 2008;35:73–91.

Autologous Flap Gluteal Augmentation
Split Gluteal Flap Technique

Sadri Ozan Sozer, MD[a,*], Osman Erhan Eryilmaz, MD[b]

KEYWORDS

- Split gluteal muscle flap • Autoprosthesis buttock augmentation • Lipografting • Adiopocutaneous

KEY POINTS

- The split gluteal muscle flap for autoprosthesis buttock augmentation is an autologous alternative to the other solutions such as lipografting, gluteal implants, and adipocutaneous flaps.
- Gluteal implants have been described with various rates of complications and difficulties.
- Lipografting is an effective means of moderately increasing buttock volume.
- Adipocutaneous flaps originate within the superior gluteal region and maintain volume in the top half of the buttocks, lacking the ability to reach the midportion of the buttocks.

Video content accompanies this article at http://www.plasticsurgery.theclinics.com/.

INTRODUCTION

Recently, there has been an increase in the number of patients seeking buttock augmentation and contour restoration.[1–4] Postbariatric surgery and cosmetic patients seeking circumferential body lifts also seek a way of avoiding a flattened buttock contour. Gluteal implants have been described with various rates of complications and difficulties. Lipografting is an effective means of moderately increasing buttock volume; neither of these procedures, however, directly addresses ptosis. Although the procedure described in this article readily addresses the volume deficit, it is especially indicated for those cases where ptosis and volume are the main concerns. Several adipocutaneous flaps to address gluteal augmentation in different settings have been described in this region. Most of these flaps originate within the superior gluteal region and maintain volume in the top half of the buttocks, lacking the ability to reach the midportion of the buttocks.

TREATMENT GOALS AND PLANNED OUTCOMES

The ideal flap should be versatile and not vascularly compromised, result in a superior gluteal concavity, and give the maximum projection at the midlevel of the buttocks.

Surgical scars should correspond to natural curves, and be hidden by a bikini or an underwear.

PREOPERATIVE PLANNING AND PREPARATION

The gluteal flap is based randomly on superior gluteal artery perforators. Perfusion to the skin overlying the gluteal region is supplied by 20 to 25 perforating branches of the superior and inferior gluteal arteries, both of which branch from the internal iliac artery.[5,6,7] The abundant vascular supply of the gluteal region provides robust perfusion to surrounding tissue flaps.

The estimated final scar is marked first. The intersection of the inguinal crease line with

The authors have nothing to disclose.
[a] El Paso Cosmetic Surgery, 651 S. Mesa Hills, El Paso, Texas 79912, USA; [b] Estetik Istanbul, Maçka cad No.24, Kat1 Daire2 Tesvikiye, İstanbul 34365, Turkey
* Corresponding author.
E-mail address: ozansozer@gmail.com

Clin Plastic Surg 45 (2018) 269–275
https://doi.org/10.1016/j.cps.2017.12.007

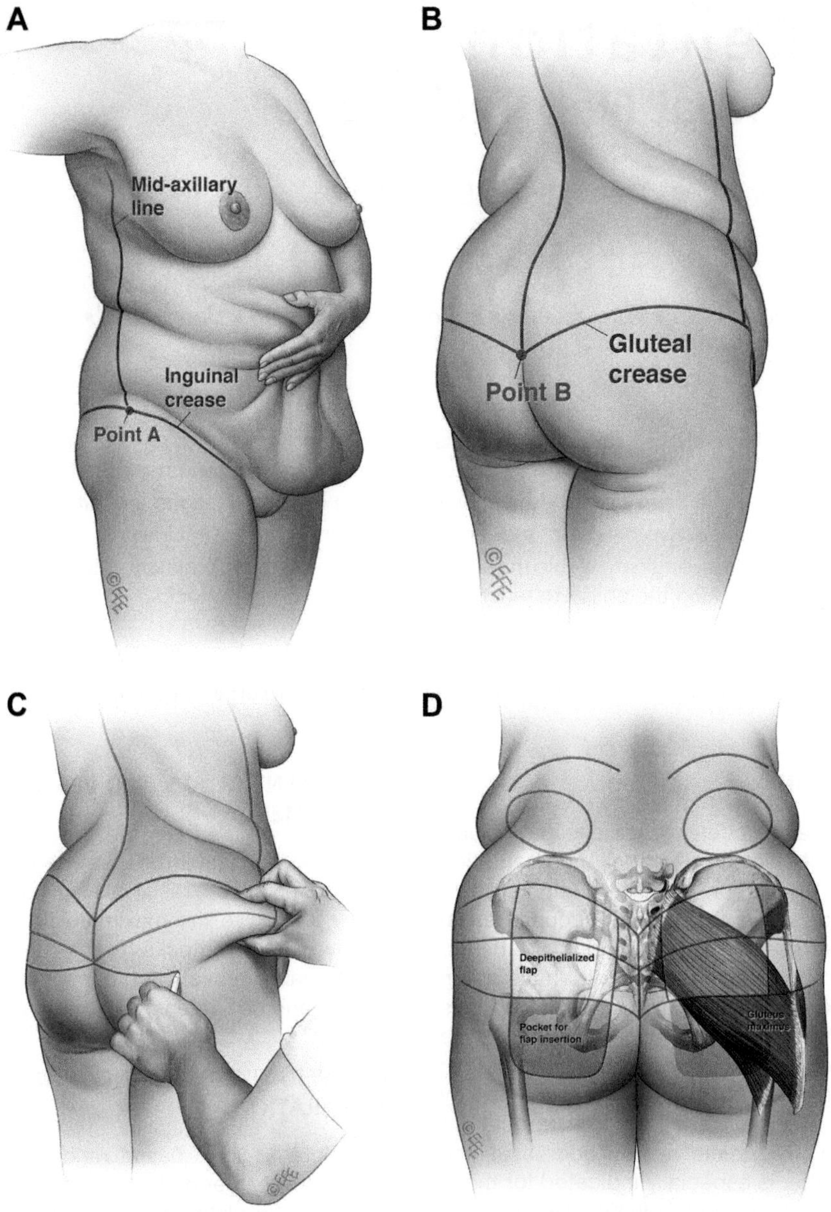

Fig. 1. Markings and anatomic landmarks.

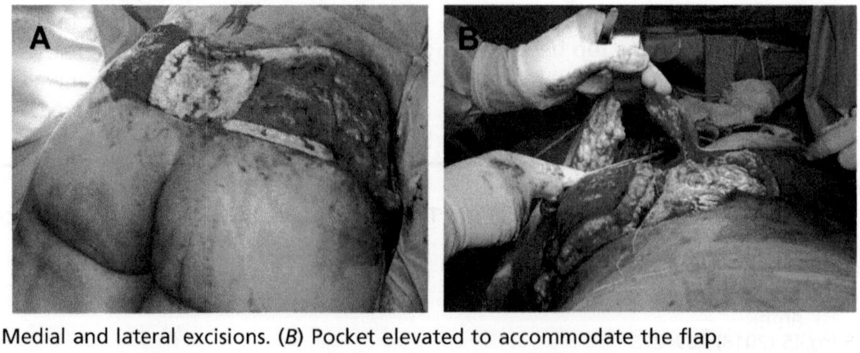

Fig. 2. (*A*) Medial and lateral excisions. (*B*) Pocket elevated to accommodate the flap.

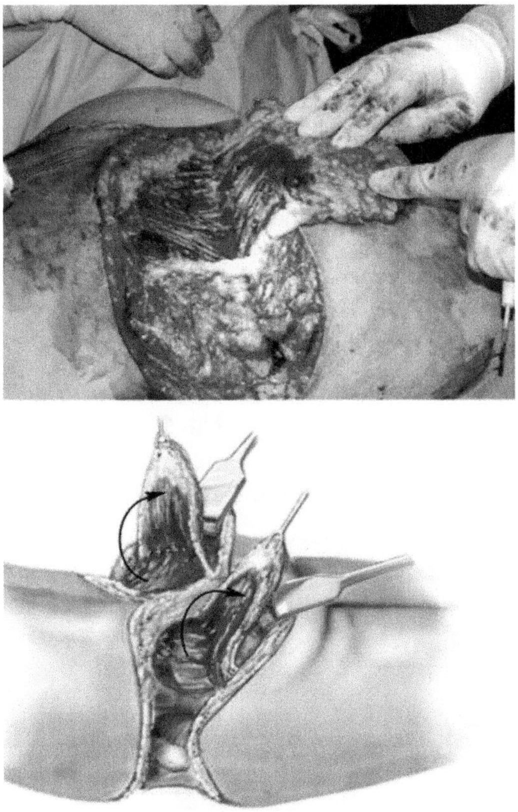

Fig. 3. Flap is rotated 180° after splitting the muscle.

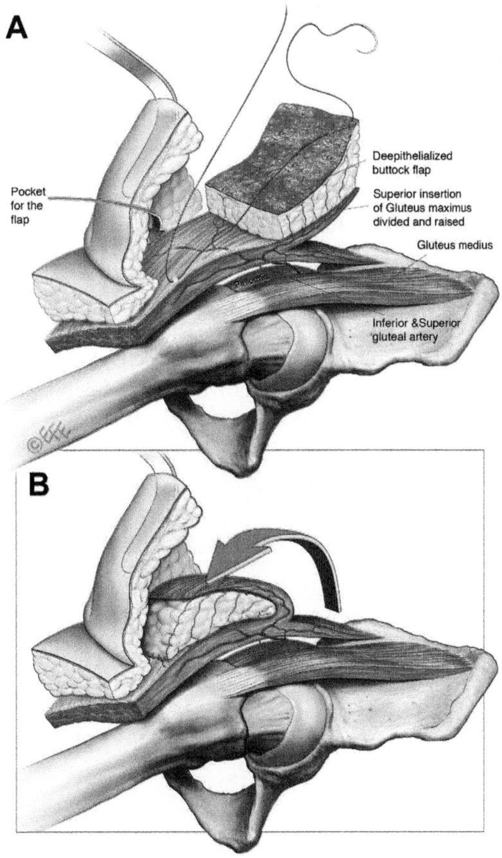

Fig. 4. Vascular distribution and 180° rotation.

midaxillary line is point A (**Fig. 1**A). The cephalad endpoint of intergluteal crease is point B (**Fig. 1**B). A line is drawn starting above the point B extending in a curvilinear fashion to point A. At the sacrum, the line from the contralateral side is joined, forming a V and creating an aesthetically pleasing V-shaped crease. This will form a scar that is slightly arched, follows the skin's tension lines, and is easily concealed by underwear. The pinch method is then used to estimate the amount of possible skin resection (**Fig. 1**C). The flap is drawn within this resection zone, with 80% of the flap centered over the gluteus maximus muscle.

The direction of elevation of the ptotic buttocks is cephalad and slightly medial. These lines can be continued anteriorly with abdominoplasty or spiral lift markings given the appropriate indications. They may also meet anteriorly at the flanks in an isolated buttock lift. A flap originating between the superior and inferior lines is marked within the medial two-thirds of the supragluteal tissue marked for excision. The flap is demarcated medially 2 to 3 cm lateral from the midline. The lateral demarcation of the flap is approximately three-fourths of the distance from the midline to the posterior axillary line and may range between 5 and 15 cm in width, depending on the patient's body habitus, buttock contour, and desired result (**Fig. 1**D).

Depending on the patient's contour deformities, liposuction is routinely performed in the flanks, sacrum, and posterior thigh, following the aesthetic units of the buttocks and accentuating their final contour.

Table 1
Potential complications of autologous flap gluteal augmentation

Potential Complications	Incidence	Prevention
Skeletonized flap appearance	Rare	Fat injection around the pocket
Fat necrosis	Rare	Appropriate flap design
Seroma/ hematoma	Rare	Flap dermal side down fixation Hemostasis Drain
Muscle animation	Very rare	

PATIENT POSITIONING

In the prone position, a silicone gel pad should be placed under the bilateral iliac crest and shoulders, accentuating the natural lumbar lordosis to facilitate liposuction and flap elevation.

PROCEDURAL APPROACH

The marked wedge of supragluteal skin to be excised is resected, leaving the subscarpal fat to aidin lymphatic drainage (Video 1). The marked gluteal flap is then de-epithelialized (see **Fig. 1**D; **Fig. 2**A).

The flap is dissected down to the fascia at a perpendicular angle superiorly, medially, and laterally. The inferior border of the flap is dissected inferiorly in an oblique angle to the level of the fascia. A pocket is created for insertion of the flap by undermining the buttock in the plane above the gluteus maximus fascia (**Fig. 2**B). The fascia in the superior, medial, and lateral borders of the dermal fat flap is divided. The flap is then raised by partially dividing the superior insertion of the gluteus maximus muscle to the posterior iliac spine and sacrum (see **Fig. 2**). The gluteus maximus is then split (5–6 cm) to allow the flap to rotate caudally 180° (**Fig. 3**).

The flap is rotated caudally into the pocket, and the free dermal edges are anchored with 3-0 Quill sutures to the gluteal fascia (**Fig. 4**).

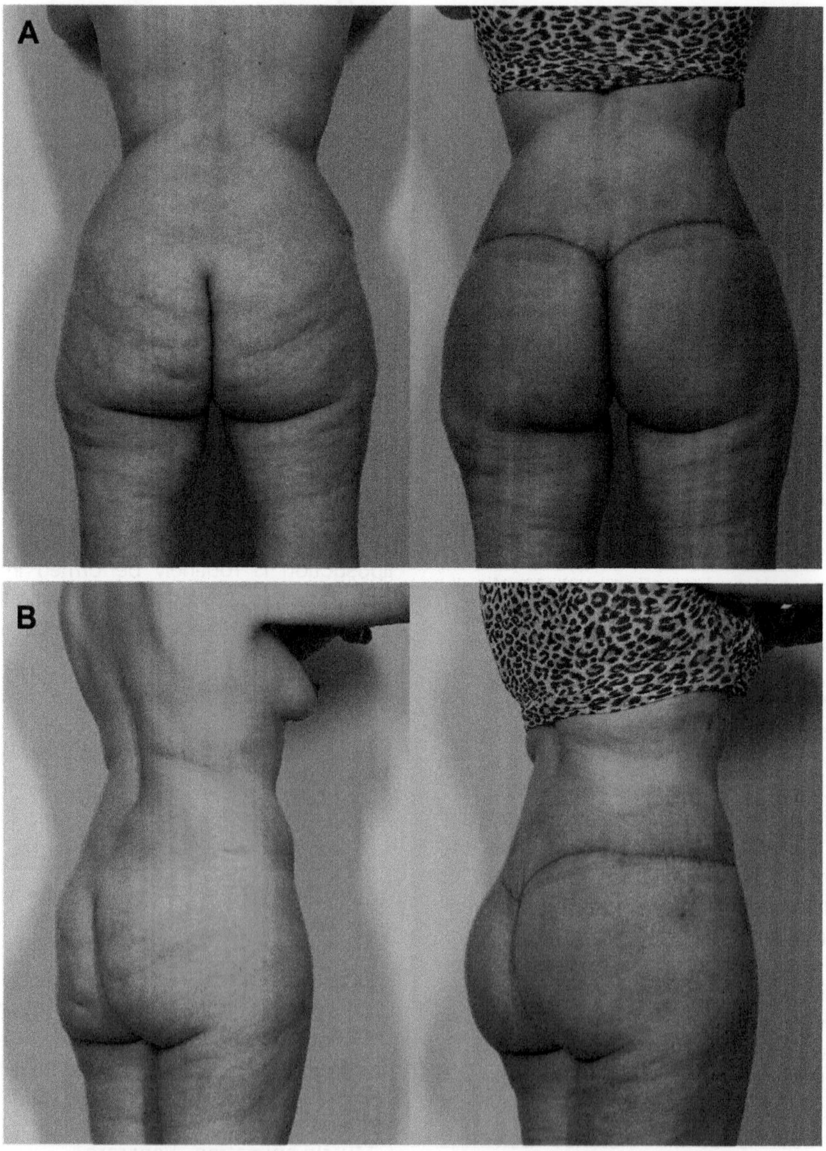

Fig. 5. Before and after, demonstrating improvement in shape and elimination of cellulite.

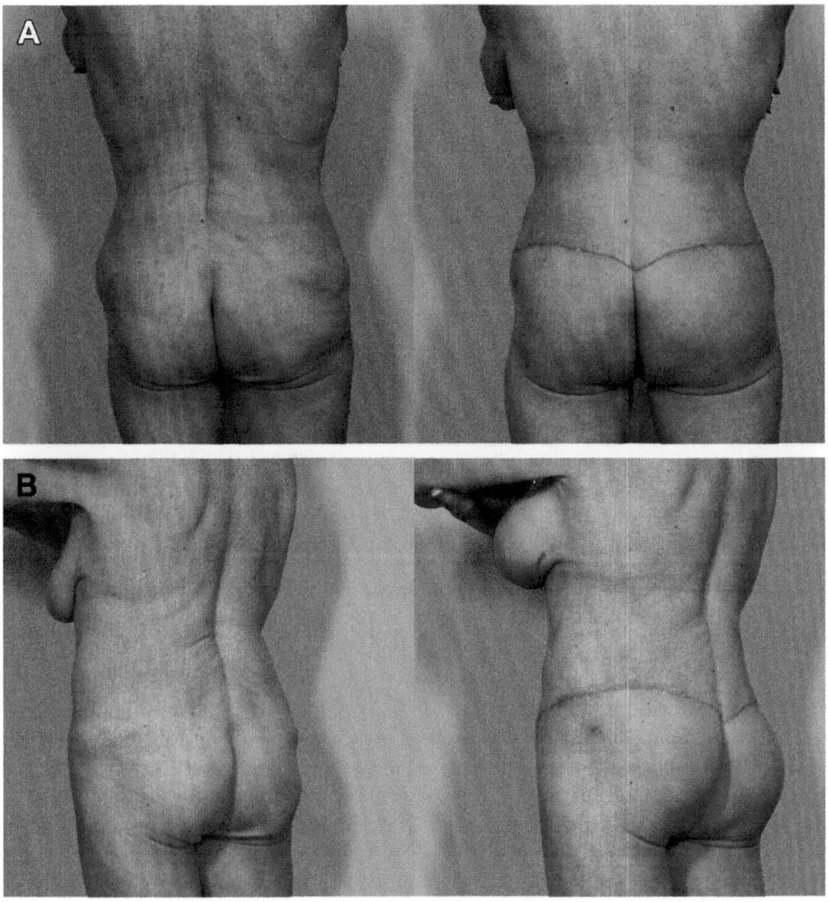

Fig. 6. Before and after, demonstrating shape improvement on patient with limited amount of tissue available.

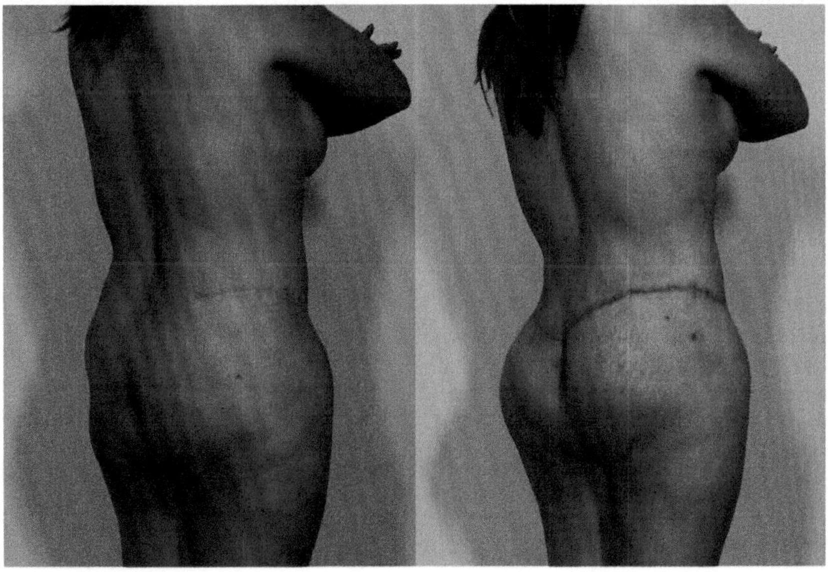

Fig. 7. Before and after of a patient who had pervious abdominoplasty, demonstrating the versatility of the techniques in terms of customization of scar location.

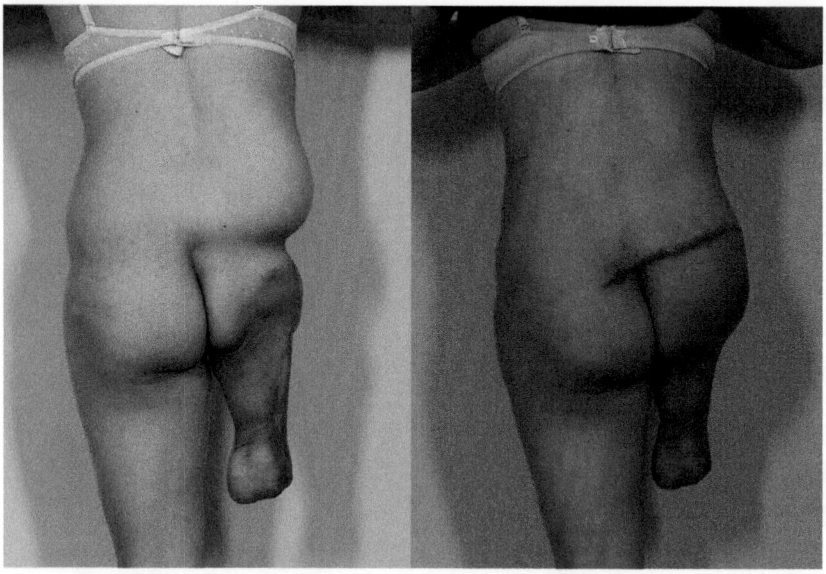

Fig. 8. Before and after, demonstrating correction achieved on a patient with almost complete absence of buttock.

Lipografting should be added to the procedure to camouflage the possibility of visibility along the lateral, medial, and inferior borders of the flap and to obtain a softer transition contour.

Securing the de-epithelialized surface upside down gives the flap a more rounded and implant-like shape. The remaining buttock skin is pulled cranially to cover the flap. The patient is then placed in the supine position and other concurrent procedures may be performed.

POTENTIAL COMPLICATIONS AND MANAGEMENT OF COMPLICATIONS

Incorporation of the split gluteus maximus muscle facilitates the mobilization of the flap caudally to reach the gluteal crease and increase the vascular supply to the flap when compared with the dermal fat flap (**Table 1**). There have been no cases of total flap loss or necrosis and no cases of any degree of fatty necrosis. The authors have not had any cases of hematomas or seromas in their series. This observation maybe attributed to several factors, including preservation of lymphatic drainage, minimizing dead space, postoperative compression of the area, and the use of drains. Only 1 revisionary procedure has been performed on these patients to date. Scar revision was performed in a delayed fashion after partial dehiscence caused by a seroma.

POSTPROCEDURAL CARE

Early mobilization in the recovery room and at home is encouraged.

Antiembolic stockings and compression garments are also utilized routinely. Closed suction drains are removed when output is less than 50 mL per 24 hours.

The authors do not restrict normal patient positioning postoperatively. Patients may sleep in any position and sit immediately. Patients may return to work in 10 to 15 days.

PUBLISHED CLINICAL RESULTS

In the authors' published series, 800 flaps have been performed in 400 patients. Seventy percent of those were postbariatric patients and the remainder cosmetic patients. Patients have uniformly expressed satisfaction with their outcomes.

SUMMARY

Clinical endpoints considered aesthetically pleasing in gluteal augmentation include a point of maximum projection at the midlevel of the buttocks This is verified by a horizontal line from the point of maximal projection of the mons pubis. Additionally, the correction of gluteal ptosi is verified by elevation of the gluteal mass and shortening of the infragluteal fold and improvement of the natural downward slope. The oblique dissection of the flap superiorly increases the length and reach of the flap. The flap can be custom-shaped to meet each individual patient's needs.

Other advantages of this flap compared with others is the caudal reach once it is mobilized, allowing for maximal projection at the midportion of the buttocks. At the same time, moving the tissue from the area above the buttocks inferiorly automatically creates a pleasing concavity or lumbar hyperlordosis. It also delivers significant improvement in the waist contour by removing the excess skin from the flanks. The tradeoff is a longer scar, which in the authors' experience is well accepted, adds minimal morbidity, and is well concealed when properly planned (**Figs. 5–8**).

SUPPLEMENTARY DATA

Supplementary data related to this article can be found online at https://doi.org/10.1016/j.cps.2017.12.007.

REFERENCES

1. Sozer SO, Agullo FJ, Palladino H. Split gluteal muscle flap for autoprosthesis buttock augmentation. Plast Reconstr Surg 2012;129:766–76.
2. Sozer SO, Agullo FJ, Wolf C. Autoprosthesis buttock augmentation during lower body lift. Aesthetic Plast Surg 2005;29:133–7 [discussion: 138–40].
3. Sozer SO, Agullo FJ, Palladino H. Autologous augmentation gluteoplasty with a dermal fat flap. Aesthet Surg J 2008;28:70–6.
4. Sozer SO, Agullo FJ, Palladino H. Spiral lift: medial and lateral thigh lift with buttock lift and augmentation. Aesthetic Plast Surg 2008;31:120–5.
5. Sozer SO, Erhan Eryilmaz O. Split gluteal muscle flap for autoprosthesis buttock augmentation. In: Strauch Berish, Vasconez LO, Herman CK, et al, editors. Grabb's encyclopedia of flaps. 4th edition. Wolters and Kluvert; 2016. p. 1533–6.

Autologous Gluteal Augmentation with the Moustache Transposition Flap Technique

Robert F. Centeno, MD, MBA[a,b,*]

KEYWORDS

• Gluteal augmentation • Circumferential body lift • Belt lipectomy • Buttock augmentation
• Autologous gluteal autoaugmentation • Gluteal flaps • Moustache flap • Massive weight loss

KEY POINTS

- Massive weight loss patients experience significant gluteal deformities that are often not amenable to correction with fat transfer or implants alone.
- The circumferential body lift or excisional buttock lift are inherently flattening procedure in the gluteal region and can permanently exacerbate preexisting deformities.
- Autologous gluteal autoaugmentation with circumferential body lift or excisional buttock lift can be used to address gluteal deformities by correcting buttock ptosis, restoring contour, and increasing projection.
- Autologous gluteal autoaugmentation with circumferential body lift or excisional buttock lift can combine with liposuction or surrounding gluteal aesthetic units, fat transfer, and adjunctive excisional techniques to refine results.
- Autologous gluteal autoaugmentation with the moustache flap transposition technique allows for significant gluteal contour correction, lowers the point of maximum projection, and fills the lower pole of the ptotic buttock.

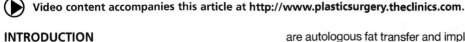

Video content accompanies this article at http://www.plasticsurgery.theclinics.com.

INTRODUCTION

The ongoing demand for bariatric surgery procedures its effect on massive weight loss (MWL) patients presenting with severe body contour deformities has unexpectedly driven demand for gluteal contouring procedures. Changing sociocultural gluteal aesthetic norms and exposure in popular culture media channels has also increased demand for aesthetic gluteal contouring procedures across the nation.[1] Although most procedures performed today are autologous fat transfer and implant procedures, the MWL patient can present with unique gluteal deformities, demanding alternative body contouring solutions. The dramatic increase in the popularity of aesthetic gluteal contouring has also increased the demand for circumferential body lifts (CBLs) and excisional buttock lifts (EBLs) with autoaugmentation in weight loss patients and non–weight loss patients with significant skin laxity or hypoplasia. Several techniques for autologous gluteal autoaugmentation (AGA) with CBL and EBL have been

Disclosure Statement: The author has nothing to disclose.

[a] Department of Plastic Surgery, The Ohio State University, 915 Olentangy River Road, Suite 2100, Columbus, OH 43212, USA; [b] Private Practice, Columbus Institute of Plastic Surgery, 6499 East Broad Street, Suite 130, Columbus, OH 43213, USA
* Private Practice, Columbus Institute of Plastic Surgery, 6499 East Broad Street, Suite 130, Columbus, OH 43213.
E-mail address: drcenteno@instituteplasticsurgery.com

Clin Plastic Surg 45 (2018) 277–293
https://doi.org/10.1016/j.cps.2017.12.011

posited as a solution to this problem. Although 3 general categories of autologous flaps are described in this article, the main focus is on the transpositional, "moustache" flap technique. Experience and knowledge of the variety of techniques allow an expanded application to the aesthetic patient presenting with gluteal hypoplasia in addition to the MWL population. Indications, technical variations, surgical planning, results, complications, and postoperative management are discussed.

MASSIVE WEIGHT LOSS AND AESTHETIC GLUTEAL DEFORMITIES

As one ages, anatomic changes that occur in the torso and gluteal region contribute to decreased gluteal projection and aesthetics. Accumulation of subcutaneous fat in areas surrounding the gluteal region detracts from the aesthetic appearance of the buttock. The accumulation of intraabdominal fat in women that accompanies perimenopausal changes coupled with rectus diastasis negatively affects the contour of the torso. Age-related skin laxity and ptosis of the subcutaneous fat also decreases projection of the gluteal region. Dramatic loss of adipose volume in the buttock of weight loss patients uniquely contributes to decreased projection and ptosis. The average female patient gets wider at the hips and the infragluteal crease lengthens with age.[2–5] Many of these findings prompt aesthetic patients to seek consultation for body contouring procedures. The CBL has proven to be a very effective procedure in addressing many of these concerns and is often recommended. Unfortunately, significant flattening of the buttock can occur with aggressive lifting posteriorly (**Fig. 1**, Video 1). Preexisting platypygia is also worsened by the procedure and is of concern to many aesthetic patients.

The MWL patient represents another end of the spectrum. Weight loss secondary to exercise or bariatric procedures often occurs in a variable

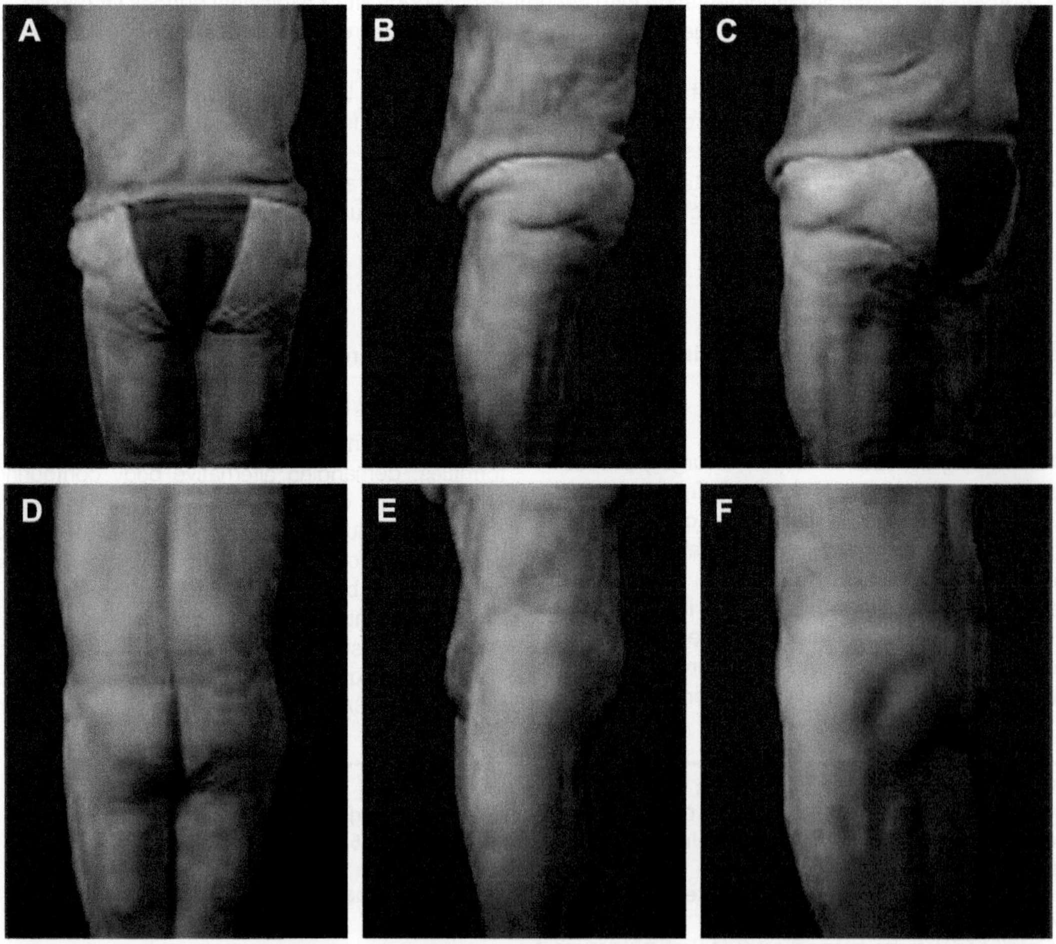

Fig. 1. Circumferential body lift/excisional buttock lift and buttock flattening. (*A–C*) Preoperative PA, Lateral, Oblique Views. (*D–F*) Postoperative PA, Lateral, Oblique Views.

manner. There are data to suggest that certain areas of adipose tissue on the body are more resistant to weight loss than others. The genetic programming of the resistant adipocytes differ from more responsive areas, suggesting a genetic role of different somatotypes. Some somatotypes such as "apples" seem to have less adipose tissue in the gluteal region. "Pears" tend to retain more tissue in the gluteal region. These somatotypes can also affect the shape of the pelvis and buttock shape. Finally, post weight loss body mass index (BMI) has a significant impact on these findings, irrespective of body shape. Many MWL patients tend to lose some volume in the gluteal region.[5]

The MWL patient also develops skeletal changes that may contribute to platypygia (**Fig. 2**). Morbid obesity is a restrictive lung disease with an obstructive component that is more pronounced in the supine position. Expiratory flow limitation in the supine position may lead to pulmonary hyperinflation and intrinsic positive end-expiratory pressure. This phenomenon is thought to play a role in positional orthopnea reported by obese patients.[6,7] Over time, obese patients are hypothesized to develop thoracic skeletal expansion to accommodate this increased need for functional reserve capacity and to accommodate hyperinflation. Thoracic kyphosis or scoliosis secondary to thoracic spine compression and anterior inclination of the pelvis also occurs.[8] Inadequately treated postbypass hypocalcemia, vitamin D malabsorption, secondary hypoparathyroidism, and independent negative bone remodeling modulated by either sex hormones or serum telopeptides may also worsen these weight-related skeletal changes.[9] These skeletal changes are permanent and worsen preexisting primary or secondary platypygia caused by loss of adipose tissue in the gluteal region. These skeletal findings also contribute significantly to asymmetry that is resistant to body contouring. It is imperative that these asymmetries and skeletal limitations are discussed with patients to manage their expectations.

EVOLUTION OF AUTOLOGOUS GLUTEAL AUTOAUGMENTATION TECHNIQUES

As demand for gluteal enhancement and the collective experience with the various forms of alloplastic and AGA has expanded, a consensus has emerged that limitations in gluteal implant design have limited the success and widespread acceptance of alloplastic gluteal augmentation in the United States. Nonetheless, these techniques are still applicable in certain subsets of well-informed patients. Alloplastic techniques are very successful in enhancing the gluteal aesthetic, but have limited applicability because of their significant long-term complication rates. The aesthetic success of these alloplastic procedures has inspired the authors and others to continue refinement of several autologous flap techniques for gluteal

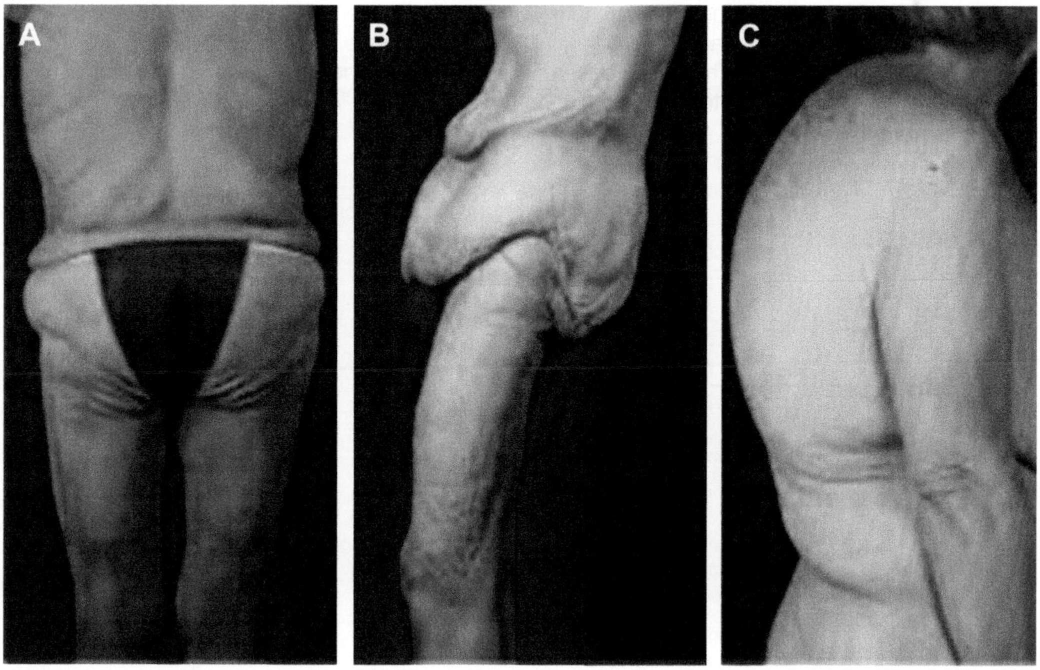

Fig. 2. Skeletal changes with massive weight loss. (*A*) Scoliosis & Chest Expansion. (*B*) Pelvic Rotation & Tilt. (*C*) Kyphosis & Chest Expansion.

augmentation.[10–13] Furthermore, the impact of implant position on buttock projection and aesthetics has significantly influenced autologous augmentation techniques.

Submuscular implants have the highest point of maximum projection in comparison with the ideal at the level at the mons pubis. Intramuscular implants lower the point of maximum projection, but they are still higher than ideal. Subfascial implants lower the point of maximum projection closest to the ideal at the level of the mons pubis (**Fig. 3**).

The MWL patient, with significant skin excess and buttock ptosis, is not the ideal candidate for either alloplastic augmentation in any of the 3 accepted planes: subfascial, intramuscular, submuscular, or autologous fat transfer. The combination of an excisional procedure (CBL/EBL) characterized by a higher than average minor complication rate, with alloplastic augmentation procedures where infection would be catastrophic, seems imprudent.[14,15] Deepithelialized flaps have been used in gluteal contouring for some time.[16–18] Published references to the use of autologous tissue in preventing gluteal deformities with CBL were also reported, but lacked significant detail and did not substantiate their potential for augmentation.[19,20] The description of the superior gluteal artery, inferior gluteal artery, and transverse lumbosacral back flaps and their vascular supplies also bolstered the clinical viability of this approach.[21] More recent anatomic studies have further refined our knowledge of the vascular anatomy of the gluteal region.[22,23]

The island AGA flap, one of the earliest techniques, simulated the round, nonanatomic design of submuscular gluteal implants. This flap is based on perforators from the superior gluteal artery, which are preserved by restricting undermining of the flaps. Hunstad has reported a variation of the island flap, an imbrication flap, that uses a purse string suture to enhance the projection of the flap. Colwell described a variation of the island flap based on a superior gluteal artery perforator flap design (**Fig. 4**) Pascal, Raposa-Amaral, and Kohler all proposed variations of the superior gluteal artery perforator flap island flap with incremental recruitment of additional surrounding tissue to enhance outcomes (**Fig. 5**). Although projection is enhanced significantly with these incremental flaps, the point of maximum projection remains high compared with alternative flap designs. Flap dissection that limits undermining and mobilization of the flap from the original donor site to preserve vascularity is the main limiting factor. Long-term augmentation results with these approaches have been disappointing in the author's experience. Higher than ideal gluteal projection and lack of inferior pole projection continue to plague the aesthetic outcomes of these techniques. These shortcomings led to the development of the author's preferred technique, the moustache AGA flap (**Fig. 6**A), which is one variation of a transpositional flap. The moustache AGA flap uses the back and lateral flank tissue as a partial island and partial transposition flap based on perforators from the superior gluteal artery and lumbar perforators.[24,25] Inferomedial transposition of the "handle bar" part of the moustache AGA flap allows for the recruitment of additional tissue for augmentation purposes, as well as lowering the point of maximum projection to the level of the mons pubis, which is more aesthetically harmonious. Loose imbrication of the flap with sutures allows for the formation of an "anatomically" shaped autologous

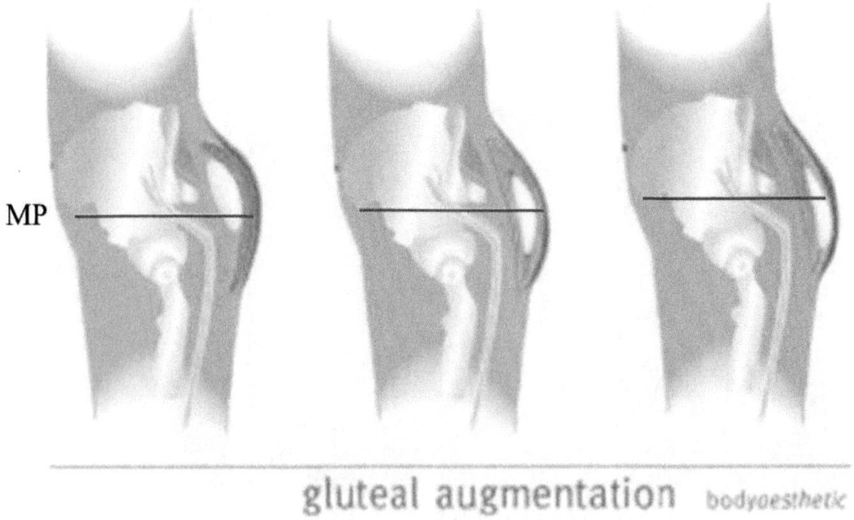

Fig. 3. Implant position and gluteal point of maximal projection. MP, mons pubis.

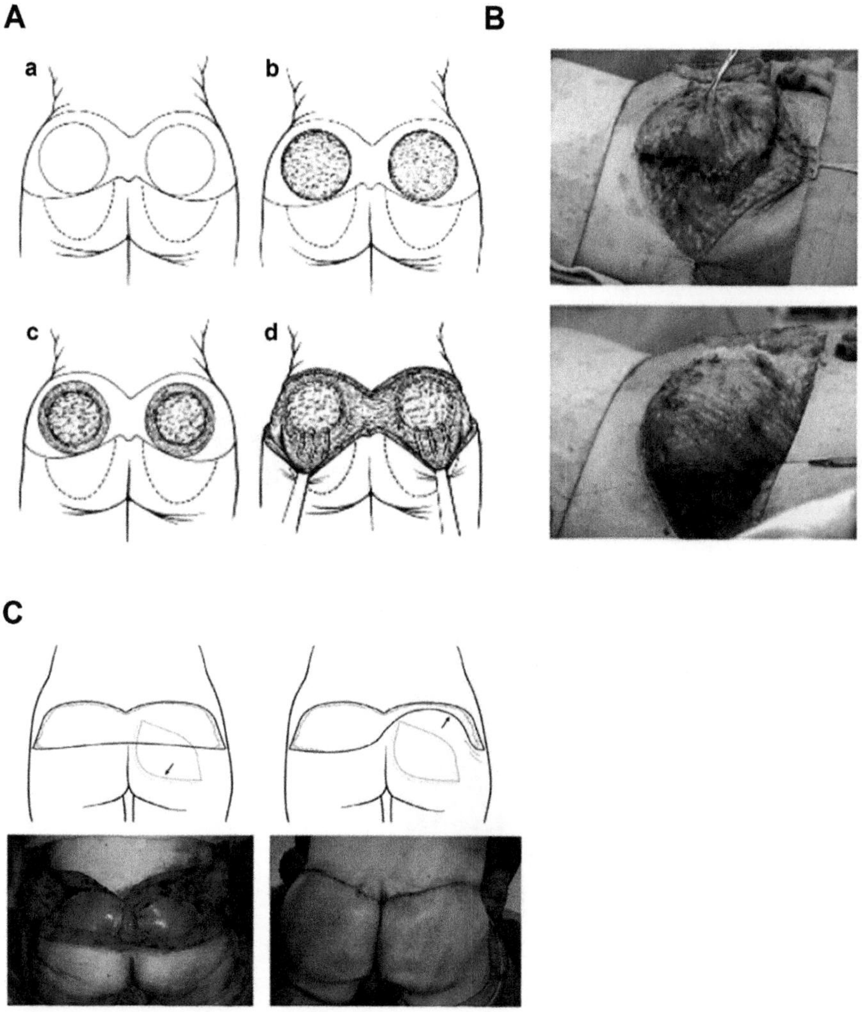

Fig. 4. Island gluteal flaps. (*A*) Centeno island. (*B*) Hunstad purse string. (*C*) Colwell, Borud superior gluteal artery perforator flap. (*a*) Markings. (*b*) Depithelialized Flaps. (*c*) Dissected Flaps. (*d*) Anchoring & Shaping Sutures.

implant reminiscent of the alloplastic procedures. The central area of the flap tissue is typically divided to allow for easier closer and turned inferolaterally to be incorporated into the flap. Rhode also proposed a partial transposition flap to lower the point of maximum projection of the autologous flaps to enhance outcomes.[26] Sozer and colleagues[27–30] proposed a gluteus maximus muscle turnover flap based on partial dissection of the gluteus maximus muscle to enhance projection and reach of the flap to the mid to lower pole of the buttock with pleasing results. Based on the published results and a critical assessment of aesthetic outcomes, the Centeno-moustache transposition flap or one of the other iterations, as described by Rohde or Sozer and colleagues, likely represent the procedures of choice where significant, long-lasting aesthetic augmentation is desired and a lower point of maximum projection is critical for a harmonious outcome (**Fig. 6**).

GLUTEAL AESTHETIC ANALYSIS

Selection of a technique for gluteal contouring in the MWL or aesthetic patient begins with a careful aesthetic analysis of the nature and causes of the gluteal deformity. The status of the subcutaneous adipose tissue in the gluteal region as well as the surrounding gluteal aesthetic units of the torso and lower extremities is the first step of the analysis (**Fig. 7**).[31] Volume excess or paucity is precise enough for technique selection purposes. The buttock shape as described by Mendieta[32] is then determined (**Fig. 8**). V-Shaped buttocks are the most difficult to correct and require the greatest volume of tissue in the lower pole and lateral aspect of the buttocks. Muscle and bony skeletal height and width are then identified to determine if the buttock needs apparent shortening or lengthening, and to

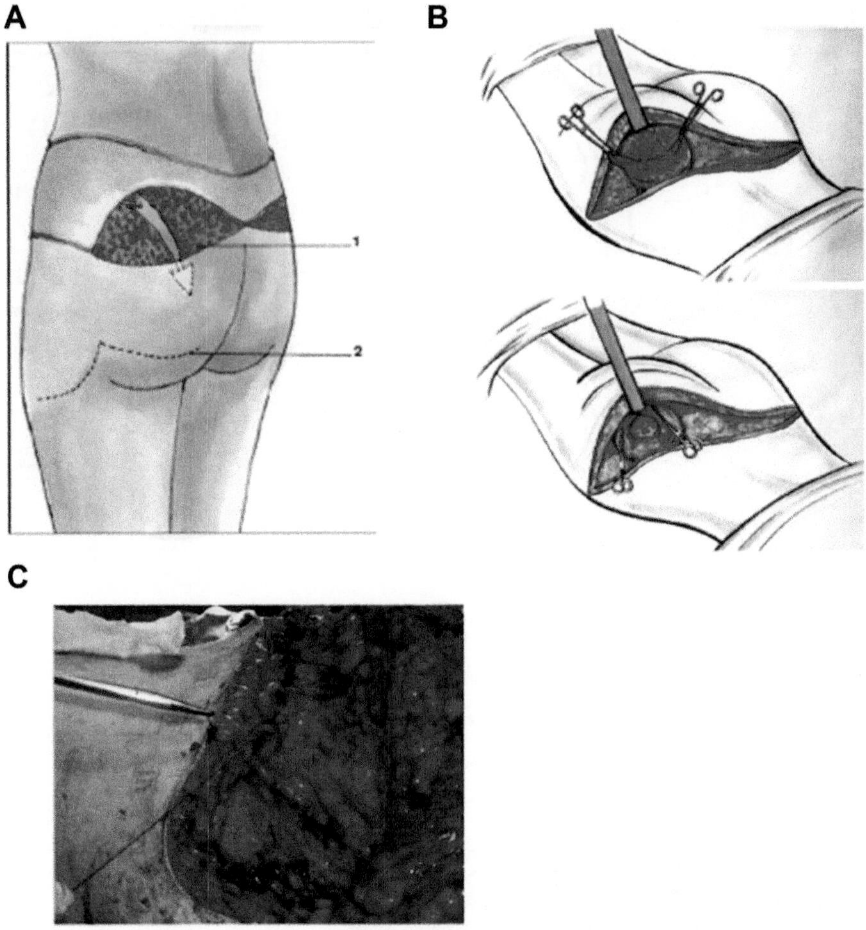

Fig. 5. Incremental gluteal flaps. (*A*) Pascal. (*B*) Raposa-Amaral. (*C*) Koller.

determine the final location of the point of maximum projection (**Fig. 9**).[32] This analysis is important to incision height placement as it relates to flap selection and final incision location. High-riding CBL/EBL incisions can enhance waist definition while lengthening the buttocks favorably in patients with shorter buttocks and unfavorably in patients with longer buttocks (**Fig. 10**). Shorter buttocks characterized by a short gluteus maximus muscle and pelvic height can be favorably treated more efficiently with shorter flaps such as the island or incremental flaps. Buttocks characterized by longer muscle, bony, and visual length as well as V-shaped buttocks are more appropriately treated with a transposition flap. The transposition flaps recruit additional tissue to fill the lower one-third of the buttock and the lower lateral aspect of V-shaped buttock; the lower the point of maximum projection closer to the ideal. Finally, the quality and laxity of the skin of the abdomen, flanks, hip, back, buttock, anterior thigh, lateral thigh, and posterior thigh are noted. The results of this analysis are then used to guide you through a gluteal contouring algorithm for body contouring (**Fig. 11**). Once the decision is made that gluteal augmentation is desirable and that an excisional procedure is indicated owing to posterior skin laxity, then a CBL or EBL is considered. If CBL or EBL are indicated, then autologous augmentation with a vascularized gluteal flap becomes the procedure of choice in patients with a BMI of less than 30 kg/m^2. The gluteal augmentation algorithm in indicates preferred choices for gluteal augmentation under various conditions. Over time, the use of autologous tissues either as a flap or in fat transfer have become the procedures of choice in the author's practice. If significant lateral deficiency is present, as in a V-shaped buttocks, autologous fat transfer can be combined with a moustache flap for further refinement. The moustache flap and other transpositional flaps have made supplemental procedures such as adjuvant or staged fat transfer

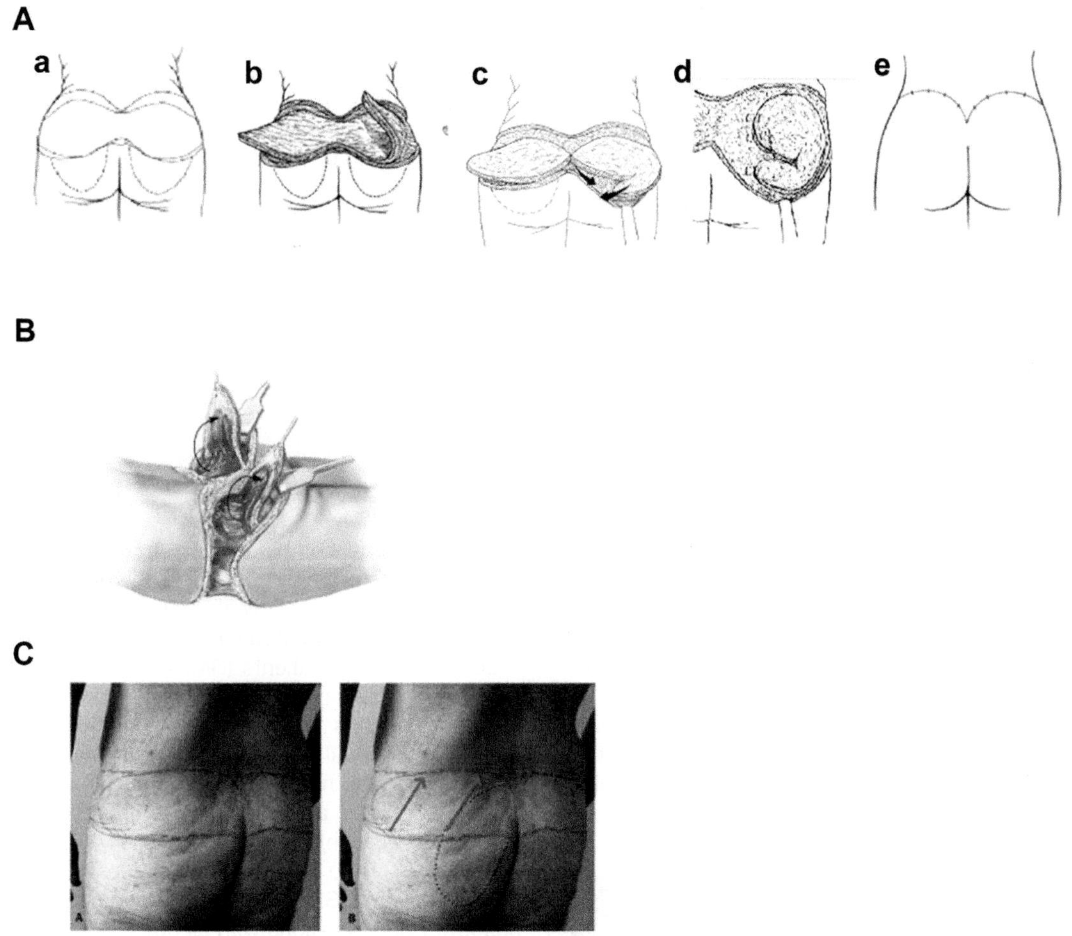

Fig. 6. Transpositional gluteal flaps. (*A*) Centeno moustache flap. (*B*) Sozer-split gluteal turnover flap. (*C*) Rhode. (*a*) Markings. (*b*) Moustache Flap De-epithelialized and Dissected. (*c*) Flap Rotation. (*d*) Flap Inset. (*e*) Inverted V Closure.

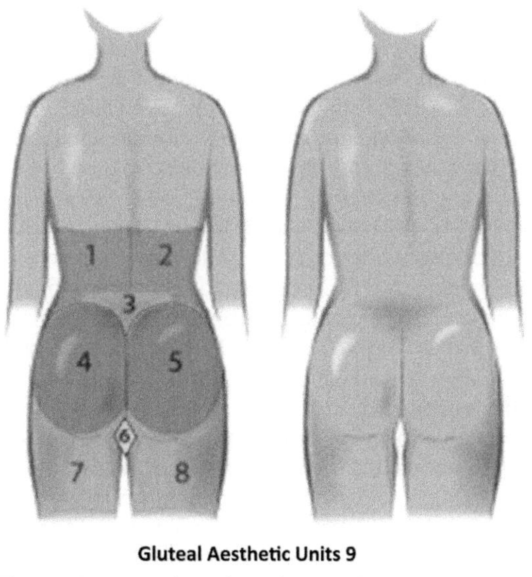

Fig. 7. Centeno-gluteal aesthetic units.

or alloplastic implants less necessary owing to the significant augmentation achieved. The high complication rates experienced with the various forms of implant augmentation has also relegated these procedures to last resort procedures in only the most well-informed and compliant patients.

BODY MASS INDEX AND PROCEDURAL INDICATIONS

Obese patients with a BMI of greater than 30 kg/m^2 have been shown to be at higher risk for perioperative complications in aesthetic and MWL body contouring. Wound healing dehiscence, delayed healing, seromas, infection, and deep venous thrombosis are some of the common complications observed in obese patients. These patients are far from the generally agreed upon ideal aesthetic goals and should be managed more conservatively. Less risky approaches such as staged liposuction and excisional procedures,

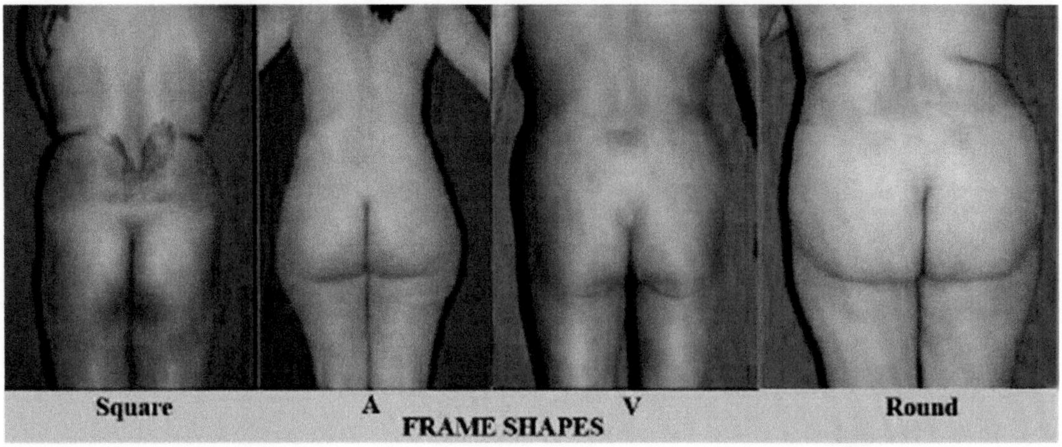

Fig. 8. Mendieta buttock shapes.

and limited dissection can reduce morbidity in this group. AGA with CBL/EBL is not recommended in this group.

Midrange BMI patients (BMI 25–30 kg/m^2) also benefit from excisional procedures, adjunctive liposuction, and the addition of autologous fat transfer for further shaping. Younger patients without comorbidities in the lower part of this range can benefit from AGA with CBL/EBL. Which procedures are combined and how they are staged is determined by combining aesthetic judgment, preoperative medical status, age, BMI, physical findings, and patient desires.

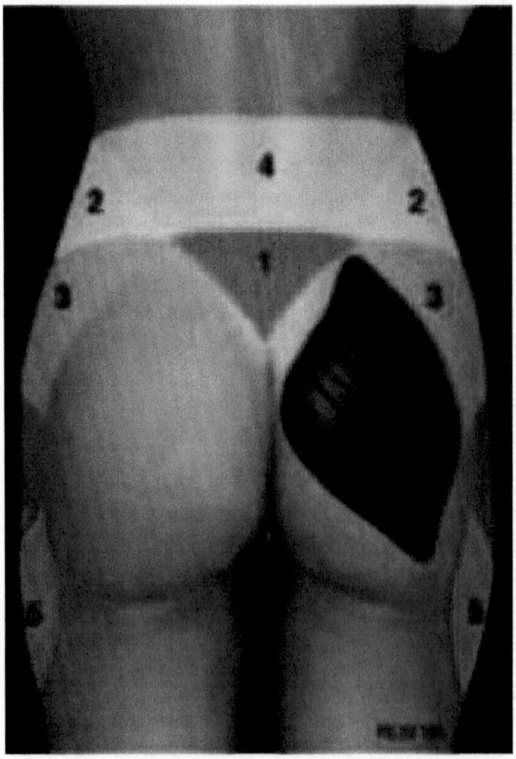

Fig. 9. Mendieta gluteus maximus and pelvic height.

Low-range BMI patients (BMI <25 kg/m^2) with skin laxity, gluteal hypoplasia, and no other viable long-term options for gluteal augmentation likely represent the ideal group for AGA with CBL/EBL. They typically do not have enough fat for autologous fat transfer and prosthetic implants alone would pose any unjustifiable risk in the MWL population. This group benefits the most aesthetically from AGA with CBL/EBL procedure and typically has fewer complications with all other factors being equal (**Table 1**).

AUTOLOGOUS GLUTEAL AUTOAUGMENTATION FLAP INDICATIONS

Once the patient has been determined to be a good candidate for AGA with CBL/EBL, the selection of the appropriate flap design to meet the aesthetic goals is paramount (see **Fig. 11**). The island AGA flap with our without imbrication and its variations are the procedures with the smallest volume of tissue and consequently the least augmentation. The position of these flaps usually sits on the upper one-third or mid two-thirds of the gluteus maximus muscle, making them appropriate for shorter buttocks. They are only indicated for prevention of the flattening effect of the CBL/EBL. Preoperative buttock projection should either be "normal" or as close to what is desired by the patient. The island AGA flaps' point of maximum projection usually lies at, or slightly above, the transposed level of the mons pubis. As such, they may be more aesthetically applicable in African American or Asian women, as well as in male patients. A desire for a higher point of maximum projection or a shorter vertical height of

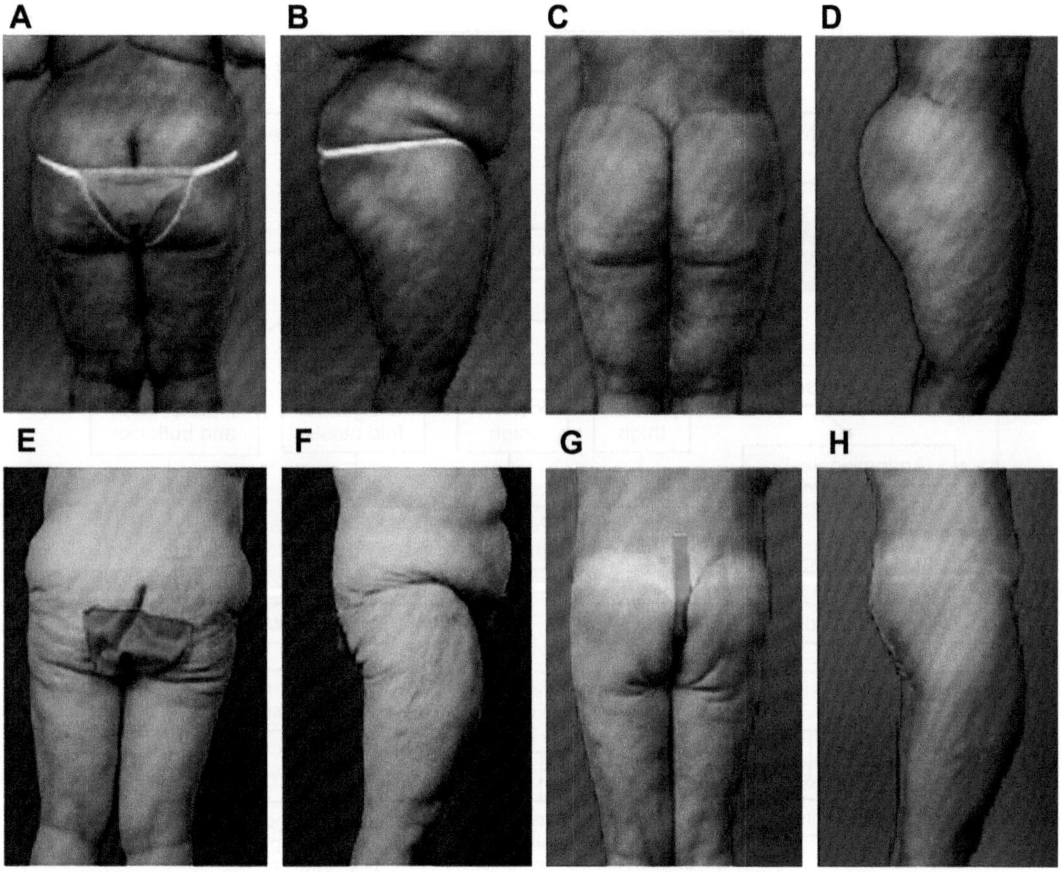

Fig. 10. Incision placement and buttock lengthening, shortening. (*A*) Preoperative PA View. (*B*) Preoperative Lateral View. (*C*) Postoperative PA View High Incision. (*D*) Postoperative Lateral View High Incision. (*E*) Preoperative PA View. (*F*) Preoperative Lateral View. (*G*) Postoperative PA View Low Incision. (*H*) Postoperative Lateral View Low Incision.

the pelvis may contribute to these aesthetic preferences. These aesthetic findings are thought to be more desirable in these subsets of patients.[33] Finally, use of the island flap design is discouraged in the V-shaped buttock because inferomedial and lateral volume restoration is critical to a good aesthetic outcome. They may be effective in the appropriate A-shaped, square, and round buttocks.

Incremental AGA flap designs that incorporate additional nonundermined tissue inferior or lateral to an island flap design are thought to represent the next level of AGA. They are indicated in patients who have mild preoperative platypygia and desire modest augmentation. This outcome was accomplished by designing a larger flap with significantly more volume inferiorly and laterally. These flap designs are effective in padding the gluteal region slightly more effectively than the island flaps. Because the point of maximum projection remains significantly higher than the transposed level of the mons pubis, the inferior pole of the buttock is not addressed. This approach can work in a patient with significant buttock ptosis and an A-shaped, round, or square buttocks. The incremental flaps can be particularly helpful in improving lateral buttock deficiency in patients with these buttock shapes.

Transpositional AGA flap designs are the flap designs of choice when definitive augmentation is desired. These flaps have the greatest volume and the versatility to restore volume in all regions of the buttock, including the upper, middle, and lower thirds of the buttock. The final desired volume can be easily adjusted to suit the patient's aesthetic wishes by varying both the height and width of the flap. By recruiting lateral trunk tissue inferomedially or superior gluteal tissue inferiorly, their final point of transposed maximum projection is at the level of the mons pubis and characterizes the most generally accepted gluteal aesthetic. The inferior pole and lateral aspect of the buttock and lateral hip can be augmented significantly to enhance the gluteal aesthetic in a square or V-shaped buttock, making it the flap design of choice. The transpositional AGA flaps such as the moustache flap are the procedures of choice because of their wide applicability, good long-term aesthetic outcome, and ease of downstaging as the clinical situation demands.

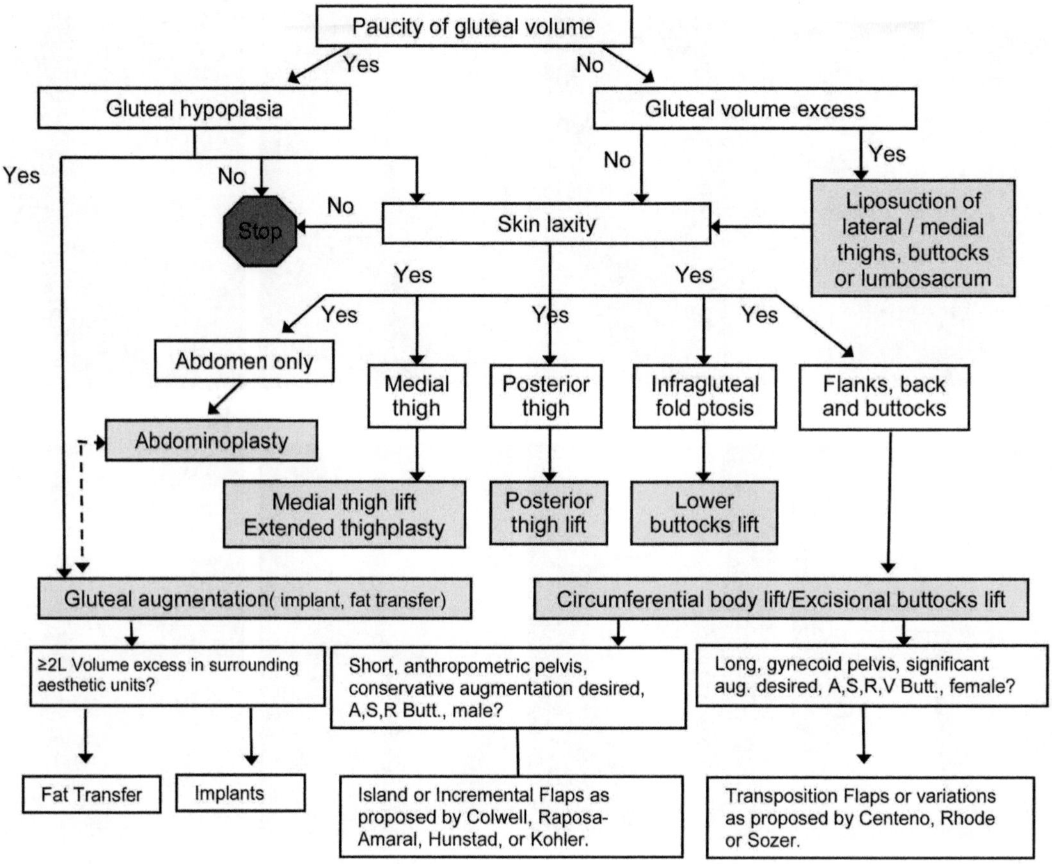

Fig. 11. Gluteal contouring algorithm.

Irrespective of the final flap design chosen, the volume of the flap can be adjusted as required by the clinical situation and patient wishes. The primary limitation to greater flap volume is the upper limit of the skin marking pattern used for the CBL/EBL. Smaller flaps can also be used for an increased safety margin in terms of tissue perfusion, or to avoid excessive tension on the posterior CBL/EBL flaps. All flaps can be downstaged or completely resected for patient safety if there is any concern about tissue perfusion, excessive tension on the CBL closure, or an inability to close the flaps over the autologous implant.

Table 1
BMI and procedure selection

BMI (kg/m^2)	Gluteal Contouring Procedures
<25	CBL/EBL with AGA, with or without fat transfer, with or without adjunctive excisional procedures
25–30	Fat transfer, with or without adjunctive excisional procedures, with or without CBL with AGA
>30	CBL/EBL, liposuction, with or without fat transfer, with or without adjunctive excisional procedure

Abbreviations: AGA, autologous gluteal autoaugmentation; BMI, body mass index; CBL, circumferential body lift; EBL, excisional buttock lift.

CLINICAL ANATOMY

The integrity of the superficial anatomic structures of the lateral trunk, posterior trunk, and gluteal region are most at risk of injury during the posterior portion of a CBL/EBL. The iliohypogastic and ilioinguinal nerves are both branches of the L1 nerve root and originate in the sacral plexus. These nerves travel inferomedially between the transversus abdominis and internal oblique muscles. The iliohypogastric nerve divides into lateral and anterior cutaneous branches to supply skin overlying the lateral gluteal region and above the pubis. CBL incisions made at or below the inguinal crease can put these nerves at risk. The lateral cutaneous branch of the iliohypogastic and the intercostal nerves also can be entrapped laterally during surgery. This entrapment can occur if aggressive lateral plication of the external oblique muscle is performed to enhance waist definition or if 3-point sutures or quilting sutures are used laterally to close the dead space. Sensation to the gluteal region and lateral trunk has several sources: the dorsal rami of sacral nerve roots 3 and 4, the cutaneous branches of the iliohypogastric nerve arising from the L1 root, and the superior cluneal nerves originating from the L1, L2, and L3 roots and then passing over the iliac crest. The protective cutaneous sensation transmitted by these nerves is temporarily disrupted during the CBL and AGA with CBL. Patients should be counseled about frequent positional changes and avoidance of heating pads and blankets to avoid pressure necrosis or burns.

Perfusion to the skin overlying the gluteal region is supplied by perforating branches of the superior and inferior gluteal arteries, both of which branch from the internal iliac artery. The lumbosacral region is also supplied by lumbar perforators. Some of these perforators must be sacrificed during the posterior portion of the CBL/EBL, or AGA with CBL/EBL, but the abundant supply provides robust perfusion to surrounding tissue flaps.

The fascial anatomy of the gluteal region has significant clinical implications for the aesthetic of the aging buttock. Relaxation of the fascial "apron" is implicated in gluteal ptosis in conjunction with volume loss and skin laxity. Resection and tightening of this superficial fascial apron can not only improve gluteal ptosis, but plays a significant role in the CBL/EBL procedure and AGA with CBL/EBL. This fascial apron is analogous to the superficial fascial system. The deep gluteal fascia plays a significant role in AGA with CBL as a fixation point, but also as a strong retaining fascia in the subfascial approach to alloplastic gluteal augmentation. The superficial apron and the deep gluteal fascia fuse and become tightly adherent to form the infragluteal fold, a structure that should not be violated because it is exceedingly difficult to recreate.[34]

OPERATIVE MARKINGS

Marking a patient for AGA with CBL/EBL begins with marking the patient for a modified version of the traditional CBL/EBL. The posterior CBL/EBL markings are placed lower than usual to allow for augmentation of the mid or lower pole of the buttock and to conform to gluteal aesthetic units. The lowering of the posterior markings also serves to visually shorten the gluteal region to enhance aesthetics. The point of maximum gluteal projection is first projected from the level of the mons pubis to the back and marked. This projected point is used to help determine the level of maximum projection for the augmentation component. The position of the superior markings of the CBL/EBL is then chosen based on a number of factors. These factors include the transposed point of maximum projection, the desire to visually shorten or lengthen the buttock, and how much lower pole augmentation is needed. A useful anatomic landmark described by Mendieta[32] is the sacral promontory that corresponds to the origination site of the gluteal maximus muscle or the "buttock proper." A gull-wing–shaped superior incision is used to 2 purposes: (1) to place the incision between the sacral and gluteal aesthetic units thereby enhancing aesthetics, and (2) to prevent or improve unfavorable intergluteal fold lengthening associated with buttock lifting. The iliac crest is too high of an anatomic landmark for the superior markings and will excessively lengthen the buttock, limit inferior augmentation of the gluteal region, and unfavorably lengthen the intergluteal sulcus. Then, inferior markings of the CBL/EBL are marked by pulling and pinching the ptotic, lax gluteal skin up to meet the superior markings. This amount of skin resection is sufficient to correct gluteal laxity while safely accommodating the newly placed AGA flaps without undue tension. Two symmetric gluteal pockets are then measured and marked below the inferior CBL/EBL markings starting 2 to 3 cm above the infragluteal fold.

The desired flap design is then marked beginning at the most inferior resection mark in the gluteal region. The size of the flap is determined by the preexisting gluteal dimension, the amount of augmentation desired, and the upper limits of the CBL or buttock–flank lift markings. The flaps are centered from medial to lateral over each gluteal region. When using a transpositional or moustache flap, the lateral handle bar tissues of the desired width and length are then drawn. A towel or tape measure is used to determine adequate inferior rotation of the turnover flap or inferomedial transposition of the handle bars of the moustache transpositional flap. The limiting point to the arc of rotation is 12 cm from the midline for the moustache traspositional flap and the inferior border of the gluteus maximus muscle for the turnover flap. Once in the prone position on the operating table, the central (sacral) superior and inferior markings for the posterior portion of the CBL/EBL can then be adjusted inferiorly 1 to 3 cm to accommodate the superior displacement of lax tissues, to ensure the safety of the central resection, to preserve the gluteal aesthetics, and to shorten a long intergluteal sulcus. Traditional descriptions of the posterior CBL/EBL markings result in a final incision that is either aesthetically too high, violates the gluteal aesthetic units, or gives the buttock an elongated or square appearance.[35–37] The final placement of the posterior CBL/EBL with AGA markings represents somewhat of a compromise. To develop a flap that allows for augmentation of the middle and lower poles of the buttock and is between gluteal aesthetic units, the markings have to be lower than traditional descriptions. The permanent placement of the incision at the junction between the gluteal aesthetic units improves the appearance of the buttock in the posteroanterior view at the potential cost of harming waist definition by widening it. This problem can be overcome by performing adjunctive liposuction in patients with excess flank fat. In contrast, a traditionally high posterior CBL/EBL incision improves lumbar lordosis and apparent gluteal projection in the lateral view and waist definition in the posteroanterior view, but at the expense of a permanently elongated buttock on the posteroanterior view. The traditional high incision may also be visible above normal underwear or clothing.

OPERATIVE TECHNIQUE

The procedures all begin with deepithelialization of the AGA flap design of choice. The island and incremental flaps are both dissected in a beveled fashion with electrocautery down through the superficial fascial system, gluteal fascia, and lumbosacral fascia. The sacral fascia is left intact. The surrounding tissue is resected as planned to complete the CBL/EBL, leaving a layer of fat above the muscular fascia. The gluteal pockets centered over the gluteal region are symmetrically dissected below the superficial fascial system but above the gluteal fascia down to, but not beyond, the infragluteal crease. A lateral tissue bridge is left in place as a border to the pocket to prevent lateral malposition of the AGA flap. When using a transpositional flap or moustache flap, the handle bar extensions of the flap are then dissected from the posterior thoracic fascia up until 12 cm from the midline to preserve the superior gluteal artery perforators. In contrast, the extend of the gluteus maximus muscle limits the inferior dissection of the split gluteal turnover flap. The dermis of the distal handle bar or of the split turnover flap is anchored to the gluteal fascia in the most inferomedial aspect of the gluteal pocket. The medial portion of the moustache flap is divided centrally and rotated inferolaterally and sutured to the dermis of the flap. The moustache transpositional AGA flap is loosely imbricated with sutures to refine projection, shape and symmetry (see **Fig. 6**A, B). The flaps are further anchored to the medial aspect of the gluteal pocket with absorbable sutures to enhance the final shape and prevent lateral displacement. Drains are placed bilaterally in the inferior most aspect of the dissection pocket. The CBL incision is closed temporarily with towel clips. Once symmetry is confirmed, the superficial fascial system is closed with the preferred suture. The deep and superficial dermis are closed in the usual fashion. The incision is dressed with the preferred dressing, but care is taken to avoid shearing forces caused by restrictive dressings.

COMPLICATIONS

Complications directly related to the AGA do not seem to be increased significantly when compared with historical standards for CBL/EBL. The reported rates of delayed wound healing, epidermolysis, or skin necrosis is in the range of 0% to 77%, and the overall complication rates in the range of 10% to 80%.[35–39] The robust vascularization of the flaps seen in MWL patients and limitation of flap dissection to no more than 2 contiguous angiosomes seems to provide good flap perfusion and viability. Only 1 series of AGA with CBL reported a significantly higher wound healing complication rate when compared with the CBL only cohort of MWL patients.[40] Despite these complications, surgeons and patients alike expressed greater satisfaction with the aesthetic outcomes of the AGA group. By the authors' own admission, patients in the AGA cohort were heavier on average even though BMIs were comparable and the markings for the AGA with CBL procedure were quite aggressive. These findings suggest potential confounding variables such as flap design, obesity-associated risk, and patient selection issues that could affect the conclusions. A recently published metaanalysis found no difference in the complication rates between MWL patients who underwent body lift alone in comparison with those who underwent body lift with an autologous flap gluteal augmentation.[41] In the author's series, 1 case of minor flap necrosis was likely a result of an excessively long handle bar lateral extension of the moustache flap into the posterior–intercostal angiosome as described by Taylor's unit.[22,23] Because this lateral extension is undermined to allow inferomedial transposition in the moustache variation of the transpositional AGA flap, the 2 adjacent angiosomes limitation of perforator flap perfusion may have been exceeded.

An aggregate, retrospective comparison of delayed wound healing rates and complications for CBL patients and for AGA with CBL does not suggest a significantly increased complication rate (**Figs. 12** and **13**, **Table 2**). The delayed wound

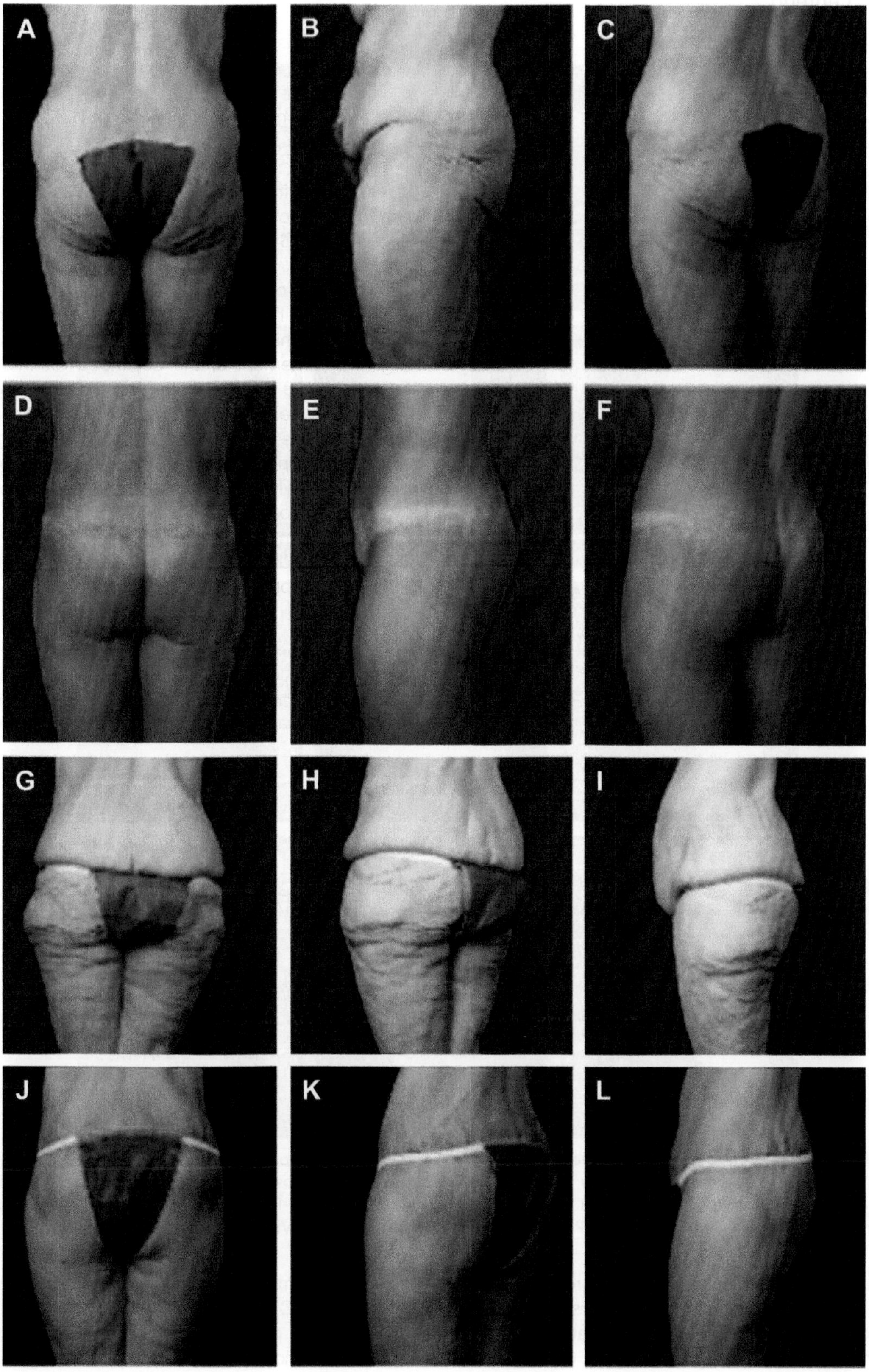

Fig. 12. Circumferential body lift/autologous gluteal autoaugmentation island flap results. (*A*) Preoperative PA View. (*B*) Preoperative Lateral View. (*C*) Preoperative Oblique View. (*D*) Postoperative PA View. (*E*) Postoperative Lateral View. (*F*) Postoperative Oblique View. (*G*) Preoperative PA View. (*H*) Preoperative Oblique View. (*I*) Preoperative Lateral View. (*J*) Postoperative PA View. (*K*) Postoperative Oblique View. (*L*) Postoperative Lateral View.

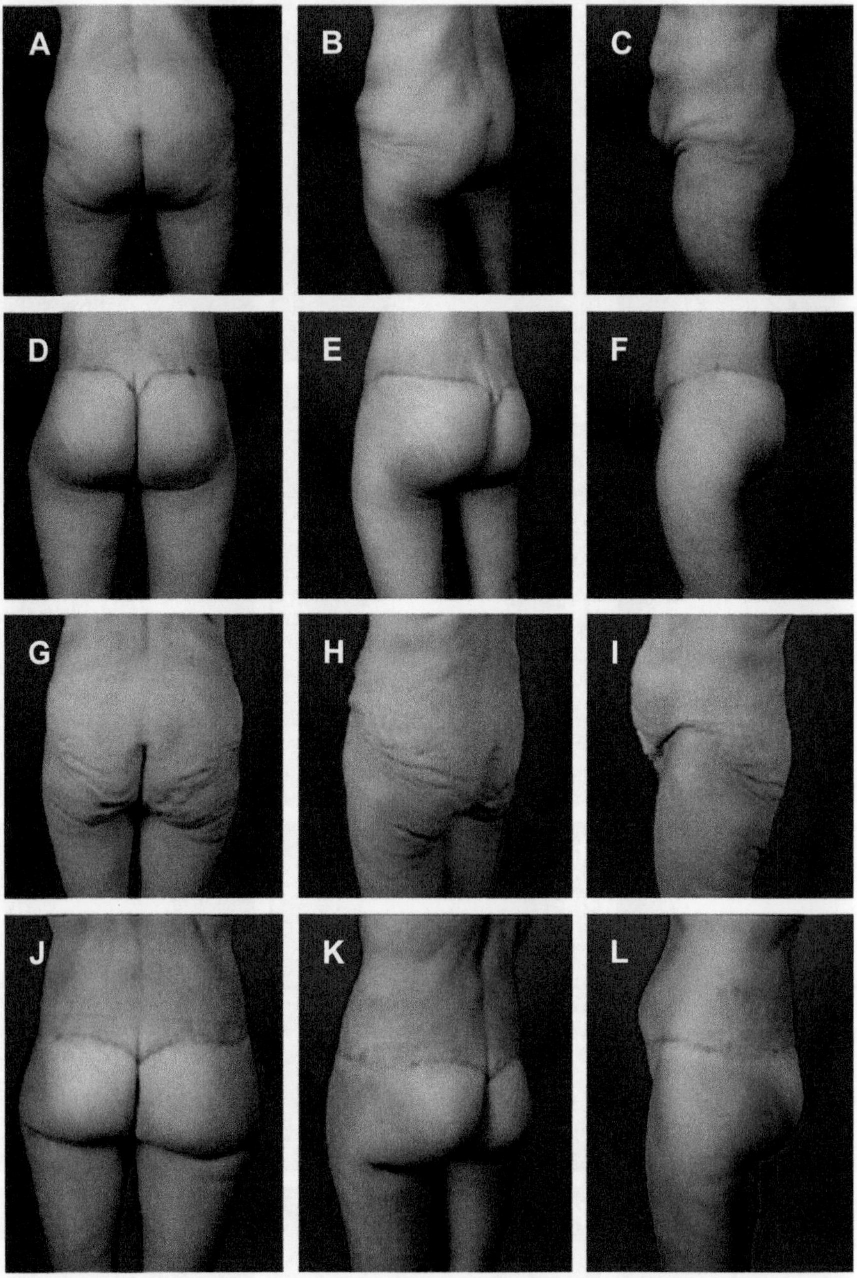

Fig. 13. Circumferential body lift/autologous gluteal autoaugmentation moustache flap results. (*A*) Preoperative PA View. (*B*) Preoperative Oblique View. (*C*) Preoperative Lateral View. (*D*) Postoperative PA View. (*E*) Postoperative Oblique View. (*F*) Postoperative Lateral View. (*G*) Preoperative PA View. (*H*) Preoperative Oblique View. (*I*) Preoperative Lateral View. (*J*) Postoperative PA View. (*K*) Postoperative Oblique View. (*L*) Postoperative Lateral View.

healing rates noted in these 2 series are comparable with the delayed wound healing rates for CBL and body contouring in MWL or obese patients in these published series. The MWL patient, who compromised the majority of the patients in the series, likely represents a more "at-risk" patient when compared with a normal, healthy aesthetic patient. Nonetheless, the undermining of the inferior flap and tension on the closure may be more significant when AGA is added to the CBL. This combination can lead to wound healing problems, especially in the central aspect of the incision in the "water-shed" region of tissue perfusion. To help ameliorate this problem, the patient is marked for the central resection in the bent over posture to simulate the tension placed on the incision when in the postoperative semi-

Table 2
Centeno CBL/Moustache AGA complication rates (n = 52)

Complication	% (n)
Minor delayed wound healing	17 (9)
Superficial wound dehiscence	7 (4)
Major wound dehiscence	4 (2)
Infection	4 (2)
Temporary anal overexposure	4 (2)
Seroma requiring drainage	2 (1)
AGA flap malposition	2 (1)
Minor fat necrosis	2 (1)
Major fat necrosis	0
Skin necrosis	0
DVT/PE	0
Pressure sores	0
Long-term palpability	0

Abbreviations: AGA, autologous gluteal autoaugmentation; CBL, circumferential body lift; DVT, deep venous thrombosis; PE, pulmonary embolism.

Fowler's position and the extent of central resection is limited. Careful preoperative planning to avoid posterior overresection and conservative flap size initially is helpful in avoiding serious wound healing problems, skin necrosis, and dehiscence. Proper selection of lower BMI patients who are at a lesser risk of wound healing problems is also helpful. Although these restrictions may limit the quality of your initial results, significantly better results can be achieved once more experience is gained.

Large, clinically significant seromas owing to dead space can be reduced by putting drains in the most dependent portion of the gluteal pocket. Doxycycline sclerosis is used in postoperative seroma or excessive drain output management in CBL patients in the author's practice. Tissue sealants are not currently used owing to cost considerations and the absence of convincing data in this application. Quilting sutures are not routinely used owing to the inefficiency and tethering effect that these sutures may cause.

In addition to these precautions, the importance of proper patient selection cannot be overstated when contemplating AGA with CBL/EBL. Using the appropriate procedure for the proper BMI group and matching physical characteristics will significantly reduce the complication rates. Patients with a BMI of greater than 30 kg/m^2 are at risk for wound healing complications from virtually all body contouring procedures and do not represent ideal candidates for these procedures. Less risky approaches are recommended.

PERIOPERATIVE SAFETY

On average, AGA with CBL patients prefer 1 to 2 days of hospitalization, but it can be safely performed as an outpatient procedure. AGA with EBL patients typically tolerate the procedure well as an outpatient. Multiprocedure MWL cases are physically demanding on the patient and require attentive postoperative management. Blood loss, temperature, electrolyte, fluid, and deep venous thrombosis/pulmonary embolism prophylaxis issues are routinely monitored. The patient is placed in the prone position on an operative bed covered with a full-length gel mattress and gel rolls under the torso. Adequate padding of the face, eyes, axilla, breasts, genitals, elbows, knees, and feet are confirmed to prevent injury.[42,43] Hemodynamic and ventilatory stability are confirmed once the patient is in the final operative position.[44,45] Intraoperative FiO_2 is increased to 80% and a "nonrebreather" mask may be used in the postanesthesia care unit for 2 hours postoperatively because of the evidence that this intervention reduces the incidence of postoperative infection and nausea.[46,47] Routine postoperative laboratory studies include a complete blood count and basic metabolic panel, and serum calcium, magnesium, and phosphate measurement when combined cases are performed. Other studies such as glucose monitoring, total protein, albumin, and coagulation studies are performed as indicated.[48] Protein supplementation and nutritional optimization plays a key role in recovery in the MWL and aesthetic patients.[49,50] Foley catheter placement for monitoring urine output is also routine. Prophylactic antibiotics are used for 24 hours. Sequential compression devices and early ambulation are routinely used for deep venous thrombosis prophylaxis. Postoperative injectable or oral anticoagulants are used synergistically with compression devices if the patient is at moderate to high risk for deep venous thrombosis or pulmonary embolism or has a history of previous deep venous thrombosis or pulmonary embolism.[51–53] The dosing of these medications are based on lean body weight and should be adjusted in the obese patient. Postoperative hematomas, although possible, are not common if a delayed anticoagulant start protocol is used. A low index of suspicion should be maintained and appropriate diagnostic studies ordered when postoperative anticoagulation is used.

Compression garments are not routinely used postoperatively. Concerns about skin perfusion and pressure necrosis over drains relegates their use to the late postoperative period. Traditional dressings have been replaced by tissue glues to allow monitoring of skin perfusion and to reduce blistering caused by shear forces and postoperative edema. Drains are removed once the output is below 30 mL in 24 hours. If drainage is excessive or prolonged, sclerosis can be performed with a high concentration doxycycline solution (500 mg in 10 mL 0.9% normal saline solution) by infusing it through the drain, clamping for 15 to 30 minutes, and then returning to suction. Before performing sclerosis, local anesthesia can be achieved by infusing a weight appropriate dose of 0.5% bupivacaine (Marcaine) into the seroma cavity. Postprocedure pain can be experienced for 8 to 24 hours after sclerosis and oral narcotics are recommended. This procedure may need to be repeated several times before a significant reduction in drainage output is observed. This doxycycline concentration is higher than the recommended intravenous dosage because of its inflammatory properties. It is an off-label use of the medication and patients should be informed of this status. Alternatively, if a seroma occurs after drain removal, the seroma cavity may be injected with the solution followed by aspiration. Special precautions should be taken to ensure that the solution is not injected into the subcutaneous tissue because fat and skin necrosis may ensue. Office-based ultrasound guidance during aspiration or injection has been a useful tool in the author's practice. Pain is usually indicative of subcutaneous infusion and the procedure should immediately be aborted. In uncommon situations, seroma cavity excision or imbrication can be performed.[54]

SUMMARY

AGA with CBL/EBL in the MWL or aesthetic patient is a useful adjunct in body contouring surgery. The moustache flap technique represents an alternative to alloplastic augmentation and other less applicable autologous techniques for improving gluteal contour in both the MWL and aesthetic patient for whom an excisional procedure is indicated. AGA with CBL/EBL using the mustache flap technique seems to achieve long-lasting correction of platypygia with an acceptable safety profile. Further refinement of these techniques and improved patient selection have led to fewer complications and improved aesthetic outcomes.

SUPPLEMENTARY DATA

Supplementary data related to this article can be found online at **https://doi:10.1016/j.cps.2017.12.011**.

REFERENCES

1. American Society for Aesthetic Plastic Surgery 2016. Cosmetic Surgery National Data Bank Statistics.
2. Bauccu O, Gozil R, Ozmen S, et al. Gluteal region morphology: the effect of the weight gain and aging. Aesthetic Plast Surg 2002;26:130–3.
3. Da Rocha RP. Surgical anatomy of the gluteal region's subcutaneous screen and its use in plastic surgery. Aesthetic Plast Surg 2001;25:140–4.
4. Toth MJ, Tchernof A, Sites CK, et al. Menopause-related changes in body fat distribution. Ann N Y Acad Sci 2000;904:502–6.
5. Kopelman PG. The effects of weight loss treatments on upper and lower body fat. Int J Obes 1997;21:619–25.
6. Ferretti A, Giampiccolo P, Cavalli A, et al. Expiratory flow limitation and orthopnea in massively obese subjects. Chest 2001;119:1401–8.
7. Watson RA, Pride NB. Postural changes in lung volumes and respiratory resistance in subjects with obesity. J Appl Physiol (1985) 2005;98:512–7.
8. De Souza SAF, Faintuch J, Valezi AC, et al. Postural changes in morbidly obese patients. Obes Surg 2005;15:1013–6.
9. Giusti V, Gasteyger C, Suter M, et al. Gastric banding induces negative remodeling in the absence of secondary hyperparathyroidism: potential role of serum c telopeptides for follow-up. Int J Obes 2005;29(12):1429–35.
10. Vergara R. Intramuscular gluteal implants: fifteen years' experience. Aesthet Surg J 2003;23(2):86–91.
11. De la Pena JA. Subfascial technique for gluteal augmentation. Aesthet Surg J 2004;24:265–73.
12. Gonzalez-Ulloa M. Gluteoplasty: a ten-year report. Aesthetic Plast Surg 1991;15:85–91.
13. Mendieta CG. Gluteoplasty. Aesthet Surg J 2003; 23(6):441–55.
14. Sinno S, Chang JB, Brownstone ND, et al. Determining the Safety and Efficacy of Gluteal Augmentation: A Systematic Review of Outcomes and Complications. Plast Reconstr Surg 2016;137(4):1151–6.
15. Mofid MM, Gonzalez R, de la Peña JA, et al. Buttock augmentation with silicone implants: a multicenter survey review of 2226 patients. Plast Reconstr Surg 2013;131(4):897–901.
16. Gonzalez M, Guerrerosantos J. Deep planed torso-abdominoplasty combined with buttocks pexy. Aesthetic Plast Surg 1997;21:245–53.
17. Guerrero-Santos J. Secondary hip-buttock-thigh plasty. Clin Plast Surg 1984;11:491–503.
18. Pitanguy I. Surgical reduction of the abdomen, thighs and buttocks. Surg Clin North Am 1971;51:479–89.
19. Pascal JF, Le Louarn C. Remodeling body lift with high lateral tension. Aesthetic Plast Surg 2002;26:223–30.
20. Regnault P, Daniel R. Secondary thigh-buttock deformities after classical techniques. Prevention and treatment. Clin Plast Surg 1984;11(3):505–16.

21. Strauch B, Vasconez LO, Hall-Findlay EJ. Grabb's encyclopedia of flaps. 2nd edition. Philadelphia: Lippincott-Raven; 1988.
22. Taylor GI, Corlett RJ, Dhar SC, et al. The anatomical (angiosome) and clinical territories of cutaneous perforating arteries: development of the concept and designing safe flaps. Plast Reconstr Surg 2011;127(4):1447–59.
23. Pan WR, Taylor GI. The angiosomes of the thigh and buttock. Plast Reconstr Surg 2009;123(1):236–49.
24. Centeno RF. Autologous gluteal augmentation with circumferential body lift in the massive weight loss and aesthetic patient. Clin Plast Surg 2006;33:479–96.
25. Young VL, Centeno RF. The role of large-volume liposuction and other adjunctive procedures. In: Rubin JP, Matarasso A, editors. Aesthetic surgery after massive weight loss. Philadelphia: Elsevier Saunders; 2007. p. 167–87.
26. Rohde C, Gerut ZE. Augmentation buttock pexy using autologous tissue following massive weight loss. Aesthet Surg J 2005;25(6):576–81.
27. Sozer SO, Agullo FJ, Wolf C. Autoprosthesis buttock augmentation during lower body lift. Aesthetic Plast Surg 2005;29:133.
28. Sozer SO, Agullo FJ, Palladino H. Bilateral lumbar hip dermal fat rotation flaps: a novel technique for autologous augmentation gluteoplasty. Plast Reconstr Surg 2007;119(3):1126–7.
29. Sozer SO, Agullo FJ, Palladino H. Autologous augmentation gluteoplasty with a dermal fat flap. Aesthet Surg J 2008;28(1):70–6.
30. Sozer SO, Agullo FJ, Palladino H. Split gluteal muscle flap for autoprosthesis buttock augmentation. Plast Reconstr Surg 2012;129(3):766–76.
31. Centeno RF. Gluteal aesthetic unit classification: a tool to improve outcomes in body contouring. Aesthet Surg J 2006;26(2):200–8.
32. Mendieta CG. The art of gluteal sculpting. St Louis (MO): Quality Medical Publishing; 2011.
33. Lee EI, Roberts TL III, Bruner TW. Ethnic considerations in buttock aesthetics. Semin Plast Surg 2009;23(3):232–43.
34. Centeno RF, Young VL. Clinical anatomy in aesthetic gluteal contouring surgery. Clin Plast Surg 2006;33: 347–58.
35. Gonzalez-Ulloa M. Belt lipectomy. Br J Plast Surg 1960;13:179–86.
36. Lockwood TE. Lower-body lift. Aesthet Surg J 2001; 21:355–70.
37. Lockwood TE. Maximizing aesthetics in lateral-tension abdominoplasty and body lifts. Clin Plast Surg 2004;31:523–37.
38. Aly AS, Cram AE, Chao M, et al. Belt lipectomy for circumferential truncal excess: the University of Iowa experience. Plast Reconstr Surg 2003;111(1):398–413.
39. Nemerofsky RB, Oliak DA, Capella JF. Body lift: an account of 200 consecutive cases in the massive weight loss patient. Plast Reconstr Surg 2006; 117(2):414–30.
40. Srivastava U, Rubin J, Gusenoff JA. Lower body lift after massive weight loss: auto-augmentation versus no augmentation. Plast Reconstr Surg 2015;135(3): 762–72.
41. Carlone R, Naudet F, Chaput B, et al. Are there factors predictive of postoperative complications in circumferential contouring of the lower trunk? A meta-analysis. Aesthet Surg J 2016;36(10): 1143–54.
42. Cheney FW, Domino KB, Caplan RA, et al. Nerve injury associated with anesthesia: a closed claims analysis. Anesthesiology 1999;90:1062–9.
43. Kroll DA, Caplan RA, Posner K, et al. Nerve injury associated with anesthesia. Anesthesiology 1990; 73:202–7.
44. Brodsky J. Positioning the morbidly obese patient for anesthesia. Obes Surg 2002;12:751–8.
45. Lincoln JR, Sawyer HP. Complications related to body positions during surgical procedures. Anesthesiology 1961;22:800–9.
46. Greif R, Laciny S, Rapf B, et al. Supplemental oxygen reduces the incidence of postoperative nausea and vomiting. Anesthesiology 1999;91(5):1246–52.
47. Mangram AJ, Horan TC, Pearson ML, et al. Guideline for prevention of surgical site infection. Infect Control Hosp Epidemiol 1999;20:247–8.
48. Rubin JP, Nguyen V, Schwentker A. Perioperative management of the post-gastric-bypass patient presenting for body contour surgery. Clin Plast Surg 2004;31:601–10.
49. Agha-Mohammadi S, Hurwitz DJ. Nutritional deficiency of post-bariatric surgery body contouring patients: what every plastic surgeon should know. Plast Reconstr Surg 2008;122(2):604–13.
50. Austin RE, Lista F, Khan A, et al. The Impact of protein nutritional supplementation for massive weight loss patients undergoing abdominoplasty. Aesthet Surg J 2016;36(2):204–10.
51. Young VL, Watson ME. The need for venous thromboembolism (VTE) prophylaxis in plastic surgery. Aesthet Surg J 2006;26(2):157–75.
52. Venturi ML, Davison SP, Caprini JA. Prevention of Venous thromboembolism in the plastic surgery patient: current guidelines and recommendations. Aesthet Surg J 2009;29(5):421–8.
53. Jeong HS, Miller TJ, Davis K, et al. Application of the Caprini risk assessment model in evaluation of non–venous thromboembolism complications in plastic and reconstructive surgery patients. Aesthet Surg J 2014;34(1):87–95.
54. Shermak MA, Rotellini-Coltvet LA, Chang D. Seroma development following body contouring surgery for massive weight loss: patient risk factors and treatment strategies. Plast Reconstr Surg 2008;122(1): 280–8.

Printed and bound by CPI Group (UK) Ltd, Croydon, CR0 4YY
08/05/2025
01864711-0009